Hospital Billing

Completing UB-04 Claims

second edition

Susan Magovern
Jean Jurek, MS, RHIA, CPC

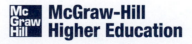 **McGraw-Hill Higher Education**

Boston   Burr Ridge, IL   Dubuque, IA   New York   San Francisco   St. Louis
Bangkok   Bogotá   Caracas   Kuala Lumpur   Lisbon   London   Madrid   Mexico City
Milan   Montreal   New Delhi   Santiago   Seoul   Singapore   Sydney   Taipei   Toronto

HOSPITAL BILLING: COMPLETING UB-04 CLAIMS

Published by McGraw-Hill, a business unit of The McGraw-Hill Companies, Inc., 1221 Avenue of the Americas, New York, NY, 10020. Copyright © 2009 by The McGraw-Hill Companies, Inc. All rights reserved. Previous edition © 2004. No part of this publication may be reproduced or distributed in any form or by any means, or stored in a database or retrieval system, without the prior written consent of The McGraw-Hill Companies, Inc., including, but not limited to, in any network or other electronic storage or transmission, or broadcast for distance learning.

Some ancillaries, including electronic and print components, may not be available to customers outside the United States.

This book is printed on acid-free paper.

Printed in the United States of America.

11 12 13 14 QTN/QTN 19 18 17 16

ISBN   978-0-07-352089-6
MHID   0-07-352089-6

Vice President/Editor in Chief: *Elizabeth Haefele*
Vice President/Director of Marketing: *John E. Biernat*
Senior sponsoring editor: *Debbie Fitzgerald*
Managing developmental editor: *Patricia Hesse*
Developmental editor: *Connie Kuhl*
Executive marketing manager: *Roxan Kinsey*
Lead media producer: *Damian Moshak*
Media producer: *Marc Mattson*
Director, Editing/Design/Production: *Jess Ann Kosic*
Project manager: *Marlena Pechan*
Senior production supervisor: *Janean A. Utley*
Designer: *Marianna Kinigakis*
Media project manager: *Mark A. S. Dierker*
Outside development house: *Wendy Langerud, S4Carlisle Publishing Services*
Typeface: *10.5/13 Times*
Compositor: *Aptara, Inc.*
Printer: *Quad/Graphics*

All brand or product names are trademarks or registered trademarks of their respective companies.

CPT codes are based on CPT 2008
HCPCS codes are based on HCPCS 2008
ICD-9-CM codes are based on ICD-9-CM 2008

CPT five-digit codes, nomenclature, and other data are copyright 2007 American Medical Association. All rights reserved. No fee schedules, basic unit, relative values, or related listings are included in the CPT. The AMA assumes no liability for the data contained herein.

All names, situations, and anecdotes are fictitious. They do not represent any person, event, or medical record.

Library of Congress Cataloging-in-Publication Data
Magovern, Susan.
    Hospital billing : completing UB-04 claims / Susan Magovern, Jean H. Jurek.
      p. cm.
    Includes index.
    ISBN-13: 978-0-07-352089-6 (alk. paper)
    ISBN-10: 0-07-352089-6 (alk. paper)
    1. Hospitals—Accounting. 2. Medical fees. 3. Health insurance claims. I. Jurek, Jean H. II. Title.
RA971.3.M237 2009
362.11068'1—dc22

                2007050417

The Internet addresses listed in the text were accurate at the time of publication. The inclusion of a Web site does not indicate an endorsement by the authors or McGraw-Hill, and McGraw-Hill does not guarantee the accuracy of the information presented at these sites.

www.mhhe.com

BRIEF CONTENTS

CONTENTS

Chapter 3   Hospital Insurance 57

Chapter 4   Medical Coding Basics 79

PREFACE

Welcome to *Hospital Billing*. This text/workbook introduces you to the basic concepts, knowledge, and skills you will need for a successful career in hospital billing. Health care continues to be one of the fastest growing industries in the United States. This growth is the result of the increased medical needs of an aging population, advances in technology, and the growing number of health practitioners. There is increasing need for health care administrative staff to support medical professionals in many capacities. One critical function in all health care settings is medical billing. Individuals who have an understanding of the revenue cycle and billing requirements in facilities are well prepared to handle these positions.

A POTENTIAL CAREER IN HOSPITAL BILLING

Patient account specialists in billing departments play important roles in the financial well-being of all health care facilities. Billing for services in health care is more complicated than in other industries. Government and private payers vary in payment for the same services, and health care providers deliver services to beneficiaries of several insurance companies at any one time. Patient account specialists in the hospital setting must be familiar with the rules and guidelines of Medicare in particular, as well as other health care plans, in order to submit correct claims for proper reimbursement. With an effective administrative staff, a hospital billing department receives maximum appropriate reimbursement for services provided.

Hospital billing is a challenging, interesting career, where you are compensated according to your level of skills and how effectively you put them to use. Those with the right combination of skills and abilities may have the opportunity to advance to management positions such as patient account managers or to positions such as outpatient or inpatient billing consultants. The more education the individual has, the more employment options and advancement opportunities are available. Individuals who have a firm understanding of the hospital billing process will find themselves well prepared to enter this ever-changing field.

OVERVIEW OF THIS PROGRAM

Whether your course of study is medical assisting, medical insurance and billing, or health information technology, this text/workbook gives you the background, knowledge, and skills needed to successfully carry out billing-related duties in a facility setting.

Entry-level hospital billers must have a basic grasp of the following:

- The hospital billing flow
- Basic coding and payment systems
- The data elements required to complete the newly mandated hospital billing form (UB-04)
- The relationship of the paper UB-04 billing form to its electronic equivalent
- The way in which form-completion requirements vary depending on the type of facility, the medical insurance plan, and the inpatient/outpatient status
- Job performance in compliance with HIPAA privacy and best practices regulations

Hospital Billing 2e presents clear, straightforward coverage of these topics reinforced by extensive application material.

TO THE STUDENT

The three instructional parts of the text/workbook follow this sequence:

- The five chapters in Part 1, *The Hospital Billing Environment,* provide essential background about the health care environment, the hospital revenue cycle, medical insurance, and coding and payment systems.

- The ten chapters in Part 2, *The UB-04 Claim Form,* cover each major section of this complex claim form, explaining the important terms, the purpose, and the correct completion of the section.

- The two chapters in Part 3, *Simulation,* provide an opportunity for you to apply what you have learned as you complete inpatient and outpatient UB-04 claim forms, either by hand or by using the simulated UB-04 form available at the book's Online Learning Center.

WHAT EVERY INSTRUCTOR NEEDS TO KNOW

WHAT'S NEW IN THE SECOND EDITION?

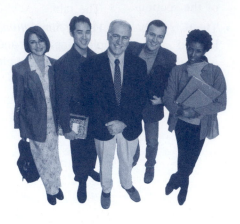

- **NEW section on HIPAA in Chapter 1:** Of special importance is the expanded coverage of HIPAA in Chapter 1. Professionals in the health care industry must understand current regulations. The most important is compliance with HIPAA rules concerning medical insurance and billing, because the law now provides for civil and criminal penalties when fraud or abuse is found, and billers are potentially liable along with their employers. In today's health care environment, claims cannot be simply correct. Claims, as well as the process used to create them, must also comply with the rules imposed by federal and state law and by government and private payer health care program requirements. HIPAA Tip feature boxes are included in each chapter, in addition to the necessary chapter content.

- **NEW approach to the hospital billing process in Chapter 2:** The established ten-step medical billing process that is used in other McGraw-Hill textbooks, such as Valerius et al: *Medical Insurance 3e,* Newby: *From Patient to Payment 5/e,* and Sanderson: *Computers in the Medical Office 5/e,* has been followed by defining it for the hospital environment. An illustration of this process is printed on the inside front cover of the text/workbook for easy reference. The illustration captures the ten-step billing cycle that is used to organize the text presentation in Chapter 2.

- **NEW chapters for hospital coding and payment methods:** The previous Chapter 4 on coding and payment has been replaced with two separate chapters—Chapter 4, "Medical Coding Basics," and Chapter 5, "Payment Methods and Billing Compliance." Patient account specialists must understand basic medical coding guidelines and principles in order to verify diagnosis and procedure codes that are used on charge slips and health care claims. For this reason, Chapter 4 in the new edition expands coverage of the fundamental principles of diagnostic and procedural coding in the hospital setting. Chapter 5 presents more detailed coverage of the inpatient and outpatient payment systems used by Medicare, together with the latest updates to each. A new section on billing compliance defines fraud and abuse and discusses the importance of compliance plans in today's regulatory environment.

- **NEW form-completion information for the newly mandated UB-04 claim:** The UB-92 claim form used in hospital billing was replaced by its successor, the UB-04, on March 1, 2007. The second edition of *Hospital Billing* has been fully revised to provide accurate and up-to-date information on UB-04 claim completion. Information on the UB-04's new format, fields, data elements, and billing requirements is provided in ten chapters that cover every section of the form. The information applies to claim preparation whether it is reported in electronic format or as a paper claim. The UB-04, like its predecessor the UB-92, represents a complex set of decisions. The text/workbook is designed to provide students with background information on the form so that they will understand the context in which it is prepared and have the knowledge to comprehend the decisions needed to complete it.

- **NEW UB-04 form-completion method for the computer-based exercises and application materials:** The second edition comes with a simulated UB-04 form that was created by McGraw-Hill for use with the text/workbook. The simulated form, which is designed to view, create, edit, and print UB-04 claims, is a pdf file that works with Adobe Reader. In Part 2 of the text/workbook, students analyze sample claims created with the form that apply information about each section of the form. In Part 3, students have the option to use the simulated form to complete the required inpatient and outpatient claims presented in the case studies.
- **UPDATED Appendix A:** The tables in Appendix A have been updated to reflect the new UB-04 claim form. The tables include listings of the following UB-04 codes: type of bill codes, occurrence codes, value codes, and revenue codes.
- **NEW Appendix B:** Appendix B, available at the text's Online Learning Center, contains two new tables. Table B-1: The Eighty-One UB-04 Form Locators, lists each field contained on the UB-04 form with a description of what the field contains and whether it is required by Medicare. Table B-2: A Comparison of the UB-92 and UB-04 Claim Forms, compares the old and new claims in terms of new data, deleted data, data with an expanded field size, and so on. Anyone already familiar with the UB-92 form can study Appendix B for a quick and concise introduction to the new form.

TEACHING SUPPLEMENTS

Teaching supplements for *Hospital Billing 2/e* are located at the text/workbook's Online Learning Center (OLC), www.mhhe.com/MagovernHospitalBilling2. The OLC contains an information center with general information about the text/workbook, as well as an instructor center and a student center with corresponding instructor and student resources.

For the Instructor

Instructor resources on the OLC include:

- Instructor's Manual: The Instructor's Manual is available in both Word and PDF format. A print on demand option is available if a printed copy is required. The Instructor's Manual includes:
  - Course overview
  - Correlation tables: AHIMA CCA, CCS-P, and CCS; SCANS; National Health Care Skill Standards; AAMA Role Delineation Chart Areas of Competence (2003); and AMT Registered Medical Assistant (RMA) Exam Topics.
  - Chapter-by-chapter lesson plans
  - End-of-chapter solutions
  - Part 3 Case Studies solutions

- PowerPoint® files for each chapter

- Electronic testing program featuring McGraw-Hill's EZ Test. This flexible and easy-to-use program allows instructors to create tests from book specific items. It accommodates a wide range of question types and instructors may add their own questions. Multiple versions of the test can be created and any test can be exported for use with course management systems such as WebCT, Blackboard, or PageOut.
- Sample claims for the Part 2 Computer Exploration activities
- Simulated claim form (UB04.pdf) for the Part 3 Case Studies

- Blank hospital billing claim form (BlankForm.pdf)
- Appendix B, containing Table B-1: The Eighty-One UB-04 Form Locators, and Table B-2: A Comparison of the UB-92 and UB-04 Claim Forms
- Links to professional websites
- PageOut link

For the Student

Student resources on the OLC include:

- Additional quizzes and other review activities
- Sample claims for the Part 2 Computer Exploration activities
- Simulated claim form (UB04.pdf) for the Part 3 Case Studies
- Blank hospital billing claim form (BlankForm.pdf)
- Appendix B, containing Table B-1: The Eighty-One UB-04 Form Locators, and Table B-2: A Comparison of the UB-92 and UB-04 Claim Forms
- Links to professional websites
- PageOut Link

WHAT EVERY STUDENT NEEDS TO KNOW

Many tools to help you learn have been integrated into the text.

CHAPTER FEATURES

Learning Outcomes

Present a list of the most important points you should focus on in the chapter.

LEARNING OUTCOMES

After completing this chapter, you will be able to define the key terms and:

1. Discuss the reasons for the increase in employment opportunities for patient account specialists.
2. Identify important duties performed by patient account specialists.
3. Describe the main types of patient-care facilities, and distinguish between inpatient and outpatient hospital services.
4. Describe the basic types of medical insurance plans.
5. List the major types of private-sector payers and government-sponsored health care programs.
6. Define the three main methods of payment for hospital services.
7. Discuss some ways in which hospitals are regulated.
8. Discuss the federal health care legislation known as the Health Insurance Portability and Accountability Act (HIPAA) of 1996.
9. Explain four rules connected with HIPAA: the Privacy Rule, the Security Rule, the Electronic Health Care Transactions and Code Sets Rule, and the HIPAA Final Enforcement Rule.

Key Terms

List the important vocabulary words alphabetically to build your hospital billing terminology. Key terms are highlighted when introduced in the text.

KEY TERMS

- accounts receivable (AR)
- adjustments
- admission
- aging
- ancillary charges
- appeal
- attending physician
- charge description master (CDM)
- charge explode
- charge slip
- compliance
- discharge
- DNFB (discharged/not final bill) list
- electronic health record (EHR) system
- encounter form
- explanation of benefits (EOB)
- guarantor
- inpatient-only procedures
- medical necessity
- precertification
- professional services
- Quality Improvement Organization (QIO)
- referring physician
- remittance advice (RA)
- routine charges
- uncollectible account
- utilization review (UR)

Opening Chapter Text

Explains how the information in the chapter relates to the hospital billing process.

Chapter 2 introduces the hospital billing process. When patients visit a hospital, the facility's business staff works together with the clinical staff of physicians and nurses and with the support staff, such as housekeeping and food service, to make the encounters as satisfactory as possible. Clinicians plan and perform medical treatments and procedures. The business staff follows a process that helps ensure that all services are documented and reimbursed.

After patients are registered, the medical care provided to them is documented in their medical records. Also recorded is the cost of each service or supply that is billable to a patient's account. At the end of the inpatient hospitalization or outpatient visit, the charges are collected and entered in the patient accounting system. Patient account specialists use this system to prepare insurance claims and patients' bills. This work is done carefully to avoid billing errors that might lead to incorrect charges, unpaid bills, or late payments. The process continues with sending insurance claims to third-party payers and bills to patients, processing payments, and collecting overdue accounts.

Margin Features

HIPAA Tips, Billing Tips, and Compliance Guides—connect you to the real world of hospital billing. These tips on HIPAA rules, billing points, and ensuring compliance with correct billing and coding practices are located near the related chapter topics.

HIPAA TIP

HIPAA Rules Apply

The Military Health System and the TRICARE health plan are required to comply with the HIPAA Privacy Rule. The Electronic Health Care Transactions and Code Sets and Security Rules also apply.

$$ Billing Tip $$

TRICARE Fiscal Year Different

Check the date when collecting TRICARE deductibles; TRICARE's fiscal year is from October 1 through September 30, so annual deductibles renew based on this cycle.

COMPLIANCE GUIDE
Medicare Coverage of Preventive Services

By law, Medicare does not cover general preventive services, such as routine annual examinations and tests, or most screening tests, such as a blood test to rule out the presence of cancer. However, each year Congress passes exceptions to these general rules to cover screening examinations that have proven to be very important. Some examples include screening mammography for breast cancer and a prostate specific antigen (PSA) test for prostate cancer. More recent screening procedures that are covered include a one-time physical exam for new Medicare enrollees, screening blood tests for cardiovascular disease, screening colonoscopies, and tests for people at risk for diabetes.

Figures, Flow Charts, and Tables

Illustrate the key concepts in the chapter visually.

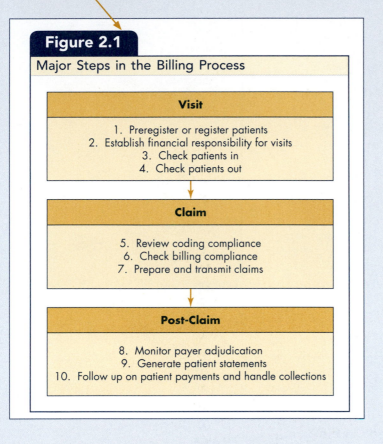

Figure 2.1

Major Steps in the Billing Process

Visit
1. Preregister or register patients
2. Establish financial responsibility for visits
3. Check patients in
4. Check patients out

Claim
5. Review coding compliance
6. Check billing compliance
7. Prepare and transmit claims

Post-Claim
8. Monitor payer adjudication
9. Generate patient statements
10. Follow up on patient payments and handle collections

837I Alert and "No Map" Fields—alert you to important differences in the paper UB-04 claim and its electronic equivalent, the 837I.

837I aler✚

Type of Bill

On the electronic 837I claim, the leading zero in the TOB code is not reported. The leading zero is a new element in TOB reporting beginning with the UB-04.

837I No Map Field

FL 66—ICD Version Indicator

Qualifier codes 9 and 0 are not used on the electronic HIPAA claim. Although the HIPAA claim is designed to accept the expanded size of future ICD-10-CM codes (ICD-9-CM codes are three to five digits long, and ICD-10-CM codes will be up to seven digits long), currently it does not contain a field for reporting the ICD version being used. In the future, it is likely that the electronic claim will add qualifier codes for this purpose.

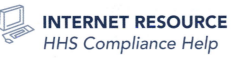 **INTERNET RESOURCE**
HHS Compliance Help

www.hhs.gov/ocr/hipaa/assist.html

FYI

No CMPs Imposed

In the first four years of implementation, over 24,000 privacy complaints were lodged with the OCR, but no CMPs were issued.

Internet Resources—provide website names and addresses of resources that reinforce concepts in nearby chapter text.

FYI—supply explanations of key terminology and concepts at critical points in the chapter.

CHAPTER REVIEW

REVIEW AND APPLICATIONS — CHAPTER 3

CHAPTER SUMMARY

1. Primary insurance is the first payer of a claim. Secondary insurance covers the balance due after the first-payer payment, based on the insurer's guidelines. Supplemental insurance is purchased to cover costs that primary and secondary insurance do not cover, such as deductible and coinsurance amounts.

2. When a beneficiary has more than one insurance plan, the coordination of benefits clause prohibits collecting more than 100 percent of the charges.

3. Medicare Part A covers inpatient hospital care, skilled nursing facility care, and home health, respite, and hospice care. Services covered under Medicare Part A are measured in benefit periods. A benefit period begins when a patient first receives Medicare-covered inpatient hospital care and ends when that patient has been discharged from the hospital or SNF for sixty consecutive days. Beneficiaries have unlimited benefit periods but are responsible for certain deductibles.

    Medicare Part B covers physicians' visits and procedures as well as supplies. For Original Medicare Plan (OMP) beneficiaries, Medicare pays 80 percent of approved charges after the deductible is met, and the patient or a secondary payer pays the remaining 20 percent. For people who enroll in one of the other Medicare plans, such as the Medicare managed care plans, other payment rules apply. Medicare managed care plans, called Medicare Advantage plans, make up Medicare Part C. Medicare Part D provides voluntary Medicare prescription drug plans that are open to people who are eligible for Medicare.

4. The Medicare Secondary Payer program controls Medicare benefits when Medicare beneficiaries are covered by other plans. A claim is sent first to the primary payer and then to Medicare with the remittance advice.

5. Medicaid is an entitlement program that pays for the health care needs of individuals and families with low incomes and few resources. The program is jointly funded by the federal government and state governments. Individuals who apply for Medicaid benefits must meet minimum federal requirements and any additional requirements of the state in which they live. To receive federal matching funds, states must cover certain services, including inpatient and outpatient hospital services and

Summary

Provides helpful review of the chapter's key concepts.

Check Your Understanding

Reinforces the important facts and points made in the chapter. Question formats include true-false, multiple choice, short answer, claim analysis, and partial claim fill-in.

✔ **CHECK YOUR UNDERSTANDING**

Write *T* or *F* to indicate whether you think the statement is true or false.

_____ 1. Patients usually buy secondary insurance and have supplemental insurance through their spouses.

_____ 2. The primary insurance carrier is sent the first claim.

_____ 3. Participating facilities can charge Medicare patients whatever the costs for their services are.

_____ 4. Medicare is primarily a medical insurance plan for people over age sixty-five.

_____ 5. Medicare Part A covers the work of physicians, such as surgeons or dermatologists.

_____ 6. The Medicare Part A cash deductible is due once a year.

_____ 7. The Medicare Modernization Act mandated that CMS replace the numerous LCDs and NCDs with Medicare administrative contractors (MACs).

_____ 8. HINN, also known as a hospital ABN, stands for Hospital-Issued Notice of Noncoverage.

_____ 9. The Medicare Secondary Payer program establishes the primary payer when the patient has another insurance plan.

_____ 10. Medicaid coverage is provided to people with low income and few resources.

Internet Applications

Describe relevant websites and direct you to use the Internet to research and report your findings. The goal of these activities is to extend your knowledge of the selected topics and to learn to use the Internet as a research tool.

Internet Applications

1. Locate the Medicare fiscal intermediary (FI) or Medicare administrative contractor (MAC) for your state. Also locate the Part B carrier or Part B MAC.

2. On the website for your FI or MAC, locate a local medical review policy (LCD). What service or procedure does it describe? What diagnoses does it list that support the medical necessity for the service or procedure?

3. The deductible amounts required for Medicare Part A and Part B change annually. Visit the CMS website, and find this year's (a) Part A cash deductible and (b) coinsurance rate. How do these rates compare with last year's rates?

4. The MSP questionnaire may be downloaded from the CMS website at the following address: www.cms.hhs.gov/ProviderServices/Downloads/pro_othertool.pdf. Read through the form. How many pages does the form contain? What is the primary purpose of the form and how does the format of the questionnaire accomplish this purpose.

5. Locate the address and telephone number of the TRICARE regional contractor for your state.

UB-04 Activity: Claim Analysis

Viewing FLs 1-7: Provider Information

Open the file **Sample01.pdf** in Adobe Reader, and answer the following questions:

1. Two important billing fields in the Provider section are FL 4 (TOB) and FL 6 (billing period). Based on the TOB in FL 4, is this claim for inpatient or outpatient services?

2. At what type of facility did the patient receive the services?

3. Can you determine if the patient completed the treatment, or is the treatment ongoing?

4. How do the service dates in FL 45 correlate with the dates reported in FL 6? Were all of the services received on the same day?

5. Are the dates in FL 6 the same as the Admission date in FL 12? Can you think of a circumstance when these would be different?

6. On what date was the bill prepared? How many days did it take for the hospital to prepare the bill after the services were received?

7. FL 43 lists "OR SERVICES," meaning operating room services. Refer to Table 7.1 on page 148. If this patient received the same surgery at an ambulatory surgery center, what TOB would you expect to see?

8. Does the billing provider have a separate billing address?

9. If the patient returns to this facility again for a different condition, will the information in FLs 3a and 3b change?

10. Does the information in FL 5 (Federal Tax Number) remain the same for all bills the facility prepares, or does it vary depending on the patient?

When finished viewing the claim, click Exit on the File menu.

UB-04 Claim Analysis Activities

Provide sample hospital claims with guided questions directed at helping you understand the complex way in which data elements interact on the hospital billing form.

CASE STUDY 1

PATIENT INFORMATION

Patient Name: Merez, Joseph F.	Medical Record Number: 1639870
Patient Address: 10 State St.	Date of Birth: 10-11-1960
City/State/Zip: Hartford, CT 06120	Occupation: Sales–Full-time employee
Telephone Number: 203-555-1867	Sex: M
Social Security Number: 231-87-9855	Marital Status: Married
Patient Control Number: 76341980	Employer: Handelsman Insurance

INSURANCE INFORMATION

Primary Insurance

Insured's Name: Merez, Joseph F.	Secondary Provider No.: R10
Patient's Relationship to Insured: self	Release of Information on File Y/N: Y
Insured's ID Number: 46-22	Accepts Assignment Y/N: Y

CHAPTER 17'S CASE STUDIES

The case studies in Chapter 17 give you practice in completing six outpatient and four inpatient hospital claims.

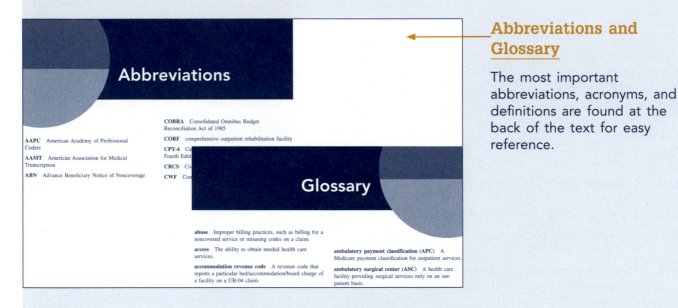

Abbreviations and Glossary

The most important abbreviations, acronyms, and definitions are found at the back of the text for easy reference.

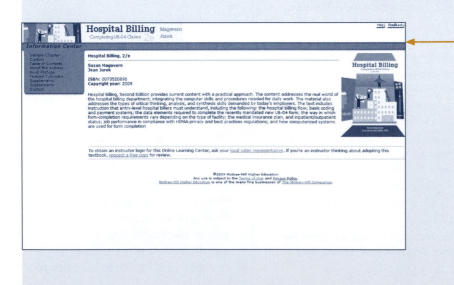

Online Learning Center (OLC)

www.mhhe.com/Magovern HospitalBilling2

The OLC offers additional learning and teaching tools.

ACKNOWLEDGMENTS

For insightful reviews, criticisms, helpful suggestions, and information, we would like to acknowledge the following individuals:

Cheryl Bauer, AS
High Tech Institute
Phoenix, AZ

Kathy Bode, MS, BS
Flint Hills Technical College
Emporia, KS

John W. Brandebura, BS, BA
Maric College
San Diego, CA

Gerry A. Brasin, CMA, AS, CPC
Premier Education Group
Springfield, MA

Janet L. Burr, RN, NCICS
Tri State Business Institute
Erie, PA

Candace M. Garland, AS
Sanford Brown Institute
Springfield, MA

Janet Hunter, BS, MBA, MS
Northland Pioneer College
Holbrook, AZ

Jane Kelly, PhD, CPC
Davenport University
Merrillville, IN

Philip A. Mayo, CPC
Seacoast Career Schools
Manchester, NH

Linda C. Napolitano, BS
F·E·G·S Trades & Business School
New York, NY

Joni Schlatz, MS, RHIT
Central Community College
Hastings, NE

Sandra Silvestro, MEd, CPC
Seacoast Career Schools
Manchester, NH

Cheryl Spears, RHIA
St. Philip's College
San Antonio, TX

Donna K. Thrasher, CPC
MedVance Institute
Cookeville, TN

Previous Edition Reviewers

Cathy Beaty, RHIA
Mountain View College
Dallas TX

Mona Burke, RHIA
Bowling Green State University-Firelands
Huron, OH

Ellen Callahan, CS, BS, MAT
Miller-Motte Technical College
Charleston, SC

Debra Cook, MAEd., RHIA
Catawba Valley Community College
Hickory, NC

Dianne Cunningham
Roane State Community College
Knoxville, TN

Dr. Barbara Fortuna
Miami-Dade Community College
Miami, FL

Debbie Gilbert, RHIA
Dalton State College
Dalton, GA

Jennifer Hornung-Garvin
Gwynedd-Mercy College
Gwynedd Valley, PA

Susan Gutjhar, RHIT, CCS, CPC
Southwestern Illinois College
Coulterville, IL

Loretta Horton, MEd., RHIA
Hutchinson Community College
Hutchinson, KS

Kathleen Kelly, RHIT
San Diego Mesa College
Ramona, CA

Karen D. Lockyer, RHIT, CPC
Montgomery College
Takoma Park, MD

Betty Mitchell, RHIA
Baltimore City Community College
Baltimore, MD

Dory Rincon, CMA, RHIT, CPC, CPC-H
City College of San Francisco
San Francisco, CA

Nanette Sayles
Macon State College
Lizella, GA

Rhonda Seibert, RHIA
Northeast Iowa Community College
Calmar, IA

Cheryl Spears, RHIA
St. Phillip's College
San Antonio, TX

Susan Wallace
Administrative Consultant Services, Inc.
Shawnee, OK

Previous Edition Technical Reviewers

Sheryl L. Fritz, RHIT, CCS-P
Amy L. Wood, CPC

The Hospital Billing Environment

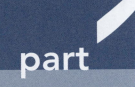

part 1

Introduction to Hospital Billing

LEARNING OUTCOMES

After completing this chapter, you will be able to define the key terms and:

1. Discuss the reasons for the increase in employment opportunities for patient account specialists.

2. Identify important duties performed by patient account specialists.

3. Describe the main types of patient-care facilities, and distinguish between inpatient and outpatient hospital services.

4. Describe the basic types of medical insurance plans.

5. List the major types of private-sector payers and government-sponsored health care programs.

6. Define the three main methods of payment for hospital services.

7. Discuss some ways in which hospitals are regulated.

8. Discuss the federal health care legislation known as the Health Insurance Portability and Accountability Act (HIPAA) of 1996.

9. Explain four rules connected with HIPAA: the Privacy Rule, the Security Rule, the Electronic Health Care Transactions and Code Sets Rule, and the HIPAA Final Enforcement Rule.

KEY TERMS

- acute care facility
- Administrative Simplification
- ambulatory surgical center (ASC)
- Centers for Medicare and Medicaid Services (CMS)
- coinsurance
- consumer-driven health plan (CDHP)
- copayment (copay)
- cost-based reimbursement
- covered entity
- deductible
- de-identified health information
- electronic data interchange (EDI)
- Health Insurance Portability and Accountability Act (HIPAA) of 1996
- health maintenance organization (HMO)
- HIPAA Electronic Health Care Transactions and Code Sets (TCS)
- HIPAA Privacy Rule
- HIPAA Security Rule

- home health agency (HHA)
- hospice
- indemnity plan
- inpatient
- intermediate care facility (ICF)
- managed care organization (MCO)
- minimum necessary standard
- outpatient
- per diem
- preferred provider organization (PPO)
- premium
- prospective payment
- protected health information (PHI)
- providers
- skilled nursing facility (SNF)
- treatment, payment, and health care operations (TPO)

Chapter 1 introduces the environment in which patient account specialists work. In the growing health care industry, patient account specialists help ensure the financial health of facilities by performing important tasks such as checking patients' medical insurance coverage and following up on delayed or unpaid bills. They are employed by a number of different types of facilities. This chapter covers the major inpatient care facilities and then describes the facilities that provide outpatient care.

Because the topic is critical to the billing function, Chapter 1 also discusses the sources of the payments hospitals receive for their services. Some patients pay for the services themselves. Many patients have medical insurance that covers a portion of the bill, but they are also responsible for some costs. Medical insurance companies use various methods of calculating the payments for facilities' services, which are explained in the chapter.

Patient account specialists work in a regulated environment. Federal and state laws govern physicians and clinical and administrative hospital staff members to ensure high-quality health care services for all patients. This chapter presents the major regulatory agencies, the groups that review facilities, and the standards for business conduct.

Federal health care regulation under the Health Insurance Portability and Accountability Act (HIPAA) requires hospitals to protect the confidentiality of patient information. This chapter provides background information on HIPAA and discusses four key areas of HIPAA legislation—the Privacy Rule, the Security Rule, the Electronic Health Care Transactions and Code Sets Rule, and HIPAA enforcement.

The Hospital Billing Environment

"This is patient Karl Castle calling. Can you explain all these charges on my bill for my recent hospital stay? Why didn't my insurance pay for these big items?"

"This is Gloria Rodgriquez, your representative from XYZ Insurance Company. We have one of your facility's claims here—number Y4646088—and there are questions about it."

"This is Bob over in the radiology department. We need help on the billing paperwork for a patient who was admitted for a workup. Do you know which tests are covered by the patient's insurance plan? Do we have to get the insurance company's OK before conducting the tests?"

Patient account specialists handle these kinds of questions every day. As important contributors to the hospital billing process, successful patient account specialists ensure that hospitals receive the maximum appropriate payment on time. Payments are essential in order to be able to pay for staff salaries and operating expenses while providing high-quality health care for all patients.

The Health Care Industry:
A Growing Opportunity

The health care industry offers many rewarding career paths. Hospitals must compete for patients and revenue in a complex environment of varying insurance coverage, managed care contracts, and federal and state regulations. Employment in positions that help handle these demands is growing, as are opportunities for career growth.

Higher Costs and an Aging Population

Health care spending in the United States, which the National Coalition on Health Care estimates reached $2 trillion in 2005, continues to climb. Health care costs have risen faster than the general economy for many years because of continued increases in the price of medical care and an aging American population that is living longer and requiring more health care services.

Many medical care costs have increased steadily. Hospital costs are rising more than 10 percent each year. Continual technological improvements—such as a new type of pacemaker that coordinates the action of both the sides of the heart—add costs in every area of medicine. A single piece of sophisticated diagnostic equipment, such as an advanced magnetic resonance imaging (MRI) machine, may cost over a million dollars. Health insurance premiums are higher as doctors build the increasing cost of malpractice insurance into their fees.

Also, the population of the United States is getting older. The baby boom generation (people born between 1946 and 1964) will reach retirement age during the coming decades. By 2030 the number of people over sixty-five will make up 20 percent of the population—65 million Americans. The elderly need more health care than do young people, so the aging population will require more health care services.

Pressure to Control Costs and Services

Higher health care costs and an aging population together create pressure on the health care industry to control costs and regulate services. Employers must offer medical benefits to employees to retain the best workers, so they want insurance companies to reduce or at least hold level the price of medical benefits that they buy for employees. In response, insurance companies adopt methods intended to manage medical care and costs. They continually scrutinize the need for—and at times deny payment for—various medical services. They negotiate lower prices for their contracts with health care **providers**—the facilities and physicians who provide medical or other health services and supplies. Insurance companies also closely examine each bill they pay to make sure it meets their guidelines and regulations.

Federal and state laws also aim to curtail fraudulent practices in the delivery of health care. Because fraud wastes taxpayers' resources and causes costs to rise, it is a serious crime that carries penalties and fines for the guilty. Complying with regulations to avoid accusations of improper or illegal actions, which can lead to fines and, in some cases, imprisonment, is essential.

Job Focus

Because of this competitive and complex situation, knowledgeable patient account specialists are in demand. Effective and efficient work is critical for the satisfaction of patients—the hospital's customers—and for the financial success of the facility. Employment may be in the department of a single facility or in a centralized business office that handles billing for a number of facilities. Figures 1.1 and 1.2 show two sample job descriptions, one for an entry-level position and the other for a position requiring work experience.

Figure 1.1

Patient Account Specialist, Facility-Based

Department: Accounting

Position Type: Full-Time/Regular

Reports to: Patient Accounts Supervisor

Position Summary: Completes billing process accurately and on time for a designated group of accounts, by payer classification or other assignment method; answers inquiries by mail, phone, or online as related to that designated account group.

Principal Duties and Responsibilities:

- Processes claim forms on time and accurately
- Makes inquiries, via telephone or online, according to policy, on delinquent accounts. Involves the patient as allowed under contract.
- Maintains excellent rapport with customers in this process.
- Continues to remain up to date concerning rules and regulations governing the billing process.
- Responds to all inquiries, billing denials, and other communications in an efficient and effective manner.
- Maintains all reports, files, and records as needed.

Qualifications:

High school diploma or equivalent education/experience. Post high school work in accounting and information technology preferred. Strong PC skills. Knowledge of medical terminology is a plus. Ability to communicate clearly and concisely. Strong analytical and organizational skills.

Figure 1.2

Outpatient Billing Consultant, Managed Care Organization

Department: Accounting

Position Type: Full-Time/Regular

Reports to: Outpatient Billing Manager

Position Summary: Develops, educates, and supports standards for efficient operations and compliance with federal, state, and local billing regulations.

Principal Duties and Responsibilities:

- Develops and maintains education materials for facilities that integrate operational processes, standards, system edits, and regulatory requirements.
- Develops and maintains computer-based training courses for billers.
- Assists with testing chargemaster-related products.
- Supports the Billing Helpline by performing research and/or reviewing responses for chargemaster-related questions submitted to the Billing Helpline.
- Stays abreast of new regulatory requirements and estimates future educational activities.

Qualifications:

High school graduate with 3–7 years experience in a health care business office, including management of personnel. Knowledge of operational, financial, and systems processes as well as Medicare regulatory requirements. Strong PC skills. Ability to communicate clearly and concisely. Strong analytical and organizational skills.

Duties that patient account specialists may perform include:

- Verifying patients' medical insurance coverage and other arrangements to pay for planned treatments and services
- Ensuring that insurance company rules are followed in all billing activities
- Reviewing and resolving problems so that claims can be sent to insurance companies for payment as soon as possible
- Completing insurance forms with technical accuracy so that insurance companies understand the health care services being reported for payment
- Following up on claims and bills that have not been paid
- Answering questions about charges and payments from patients and insurance companies
- Using interpersonal skills in dealing with insurance companies and patients to establish professional and courteous relationships that enhance the billing and reimbursement process

To perform these duties well, entry-level patient account specialists must have communication and computer skills, pay attention to detail, be flexible and honest, and be able to work as team members. For advancement, knowledge of medical terminology, medical coding systems, and types of payment systems is required.

Types of Facilities

Patient account specialists work in a variety of health care settings that offer a variety of services. Some facilities are tax-exempt and not-for-profit; others are owned by investors and operated to make a profit. There are religious and secular facilities, urban and rural settings, and general and specialty environments. Some hospital facilities offer short-term (acute) care, and others offer long-term care.

Facilities Providing Inpatient Care

Acute Care Facilities

INTERNET RESOURCE
Browse by Provider Type: Hospital Center

The website for the Centers for Medicare and Medicaid (CMS) provides a set of links under Browse by Provider Type on the Medicare home page. Each link displays up-to-date information regarding the Medicare program as it affects that particular provider type. The Hospital Center link provides the most up-to-date information on acute care facilities. www.cms.hhs.gov/center/hospital.asp

Hospital size is often measured in terms of the number of beds, which may range from under one hundred to over seven hundred. Hospitals may serve from five thousand to over fifty thousand patients every month. Hospitals must be licensed by state agencies in order to provide services.

Acute care facilities provide continuous professional medical care to patients who are in the acute stages of conditions or illnesses. These patients have severe symptoms, such as heart attacks, serious injuries from car accidents, and cancerous tumors that must be removed surgically. Patients who require acute care in hospitals are admitted as **inpatients.** They need continuous medical services from medical professionals. Unless they expire or are transferred to another facility on the first day, they usually require at least an overnight stay.

General hospitals accept all types of patients. Specialized health care hospitals offer services such as psychiatric care. Private hospitals are either for-profit, investor-owned institutions or nonprofit facilities. Public hospitals are owned by the federal government (such as veterans' and military hospitals), by states (such as long-term psychiatric facilities and teaching hospitals), or by local governments.

Skilled Nursing Facilities

Skilled nursing facilities (SNFs) provide daily care for inpatients who require medical or nursing care or rehabilitation services for injuries, disabilities, or sickness. Often the care provided in a SNF (pronounced "sniff") is for health maintenance since patients require services over a long period of time, sometimes for years. However, a SNF may also have a subacute rehabilitation unit. In this unit of a SNF, patients stay a much shorter period of time and treatment is directed at rehabilitation services such as physical or occupational therapy.

Skilled nursing care includes care given by licensed nurses under the direction of a physician, such as intravenous injections, tube feeding, and changing sterile dressings on a wound. Skilled nursing facilities must be licensed to provide this care. A SNF may be a part of a hospital or a separate facility, such as a nursing home. Often, patients are transferred from a hospital to a SNF in order to recuperate from surgery or other hospital treatment.

Intermediate Care Facilities

Some inpatients do not require either acute care or skilled nursing care. These patients are cared for in **intermediate care facilities (ICFs).** An example is a facility providing care for developmentally disabled people.

Hospice Care

A **hospice** is an organization that provides health care for people with terminal illnesses—meaning people who are not expected to live longer than six months—that emphasizes emotional needs and coping with pain and death, rather than cure. Hospice organizations provide support and counseling services for these people and their families, pain relief, and symptom management. Some hospice care is located in hospitals, and the patients being cared for are considered inpatients. Most hospice care is provided in patients' homes or in hospice centers.

Facilities Providing Outpatient Care

Outpatients receive care in a medical setting without inpatient hospitalization. Because of advances in medical technology and because the cost of an overnight stay is avoided, the use of outpatient care is increasing. This type of care may be provided in hospitals, where the length of stay is usually less than twenty-three hours, in outpatient physician clinics inside the hospital, in separate facilities, or in patients' homes. It includes services that help diagnose patients' conditions, treatments for these conditions and illnesses, surgery, and rehabilitation.

Hospital Departments

Hospitals often have outpatient departments in their facilities. Emergency departments—where care is required immediately—serve outpatients who can be treated and discharged without hospital admission as well as patients who need admission to the hospital. Emergency care involves a situation in which delay in treatment would lead to a significant increase in the threat to life or a body part. (Emergency care differs from urgently needed care, in which the condition must be treated right away but is not life-threatening.) Other hospital-based departments provide services for outpatients, such as a radiology department where a patient can have an X-ray or an MRI taken.

Ambulatory Surgical Centers or Units

Ambulatory surgical centers (ASCs), also called same-day surgery centers or units, provide surgical services only for ambulatory patients. Ambulatory patients' planned procedures do not usually require hospitalization, so ASCs do not have beds for patients to stay overnight. In case of emergency situations,

FYI

Common Outpatient Services

ASCs provide many common services, such as:

- Orthopedics and sports medicine, including arthroscopy of the knee, shoulder, ankle, and elbow; fracture and tendon repairs; and hand surgery including carpal tunnel release
- Gynecology and women's health, including breast biopsies and simple mastectomies
- General surgery, such as hernia repair and varicose vein ligation
- Ear, nose, and throat operations, including tonsillectomy and myringotomy (ear tube placement)
- Plastic surgery, including face and eyelid surgery and removal of skin lesions and skin grafts
- Urology, such as prostate biopsy
- Podiatry, including bunionectomy and hammer-toe repair
- Oral surgery, including extraction of impacted wisdom teeth and dental restorations
- Ophthalmology, such as cataract extraction with lens implant

ASCs are always staffed with medical personnel who are trained in cardiac life support. Patients who require hospitalization after their procedures are admitted to inpatient facilities. Those who need rehabilitation or extended recuperation are transferred to facilities such as a SNF.

Clinics

A *clinic* is an outpatient facility that provides scheduled medical services for patients. Examples include physical therapy after a joint replacement, such as rotator cuff surgery, and exercise programs.

Home Health Agencies

Home health agencies (HHA) are licensed to provide skilled nursing and other therapeutic services. These agencies include visiting nurse associations and hospital-based home care programs. Home health care services are usually furnished to patients in their homes and must be prescribed by a physician. Types of services include skilled nursing care, physical therapy, medical social services, medical supplies, and rehabilitation equipment.

Integrated Delivery Systems

Most hospitals are part of an organized health care approach usually called an integrated delivery system. In these systems, there is a network of acute care hospitals, ambulatory surgical centers, rehabilitation facilities, skilled nursing facilities, clinics, and home health agencies. There are also physicians who are employed by or affiliated with the network. At the center of the system is a single administration. Most integrated systems are locally organized, such as through the merger of local hospitals into large multifacility systems.

Integrated delivery systems are important because patients should receive care from facilities that best suit their illnesses and treatments. Just as there is no need to pay for hospitalization for a common cold, many conditions are best treated in skilled nursing facilities or at home. Integrated delivery systems help guarantee the best quality of health care possible while also controlling costs. A network helps deliver high-quality care because it connects health care services in an organized way. Patients' health information is provided to each facility as needed. Patients benefit from referrals to the right type of care and from well-organized follow-up. For example, when a patient has had a stroke, an acute care hospital, a rehabilitation hospital, a long-term care facility, and a home care program can coordinate services from the onset of the condition until the patient resumes normal activities. Patients' medical records can be quickly accessed in each facility as treatments and conditions require.

Paying for Hospital Services: Insurance Basics

Medical insurance, also known as health insurance, is bought by individuals to help pay for the costs of health care services.

The Medical Insurance Contract

Insurance is a written contract between a policyholder and an insurance company. Under this contract, the policyholder, also called the insured or the member, pays a periodic **premium.** The insurance company pays for medical services for a specified time period according to the schedule of benefits, which is a list of covered medical expenses.

Many insurance plans cover preventive medical services. These include annual physical examinations, routine cancer screening procedures such as mammograms, pediatric and adolescent immunizations, and prenatal care. A plan's schedule of benefits also lists treatments that are covered at different rates and services that are not covered. For example, a medical insurance plan often does not cover routine dental procedures.

Types of Plans

Insurance companies create a variety of plans (also called insurance products) that offer benefits for various prices. In each plan, they manage the risk that some individuals they insure will require extremely expensive medical services by spreading that risk among many policyholders. Either groups or individuals may be insured. In general, policies that are written for groups cost policyholders less than those written for individuals.

Group plans are usually offered to employers or other organizations (such as labor unions). The employer agrees to the contract, pays the premiums, and in turn offers the coverage to its group members (also called subscribers or enrollees) either at no cost as a job benefit or at a significantly reduced cost. People whose employers do not offer group insurance or who are not eligible for group insurance from employers—for example, independent contractors, temporary or part-time employees, or unemployed people—may purchase individual policies directly from insurance companies. In either a group or an individual plan, the policyholder's dependents, customarily the spouse and children, may also be covered for additional cost.

Indemnity Plans

Indemnity refers to protection against loss. Under an **indemnity plan,** the insurance company indemnifies the policyholder against the costs of medical services and procedures as listed on the benefits schedule. Patients choose the providers they wish to see. For each claim, four conditions must be met before the insurance company makes a payment:

1. The medical charge must be for medically necessary services and must be covered by the insured's health plan.
2. The premium payment must be up to date.
3. If the policy has a **deductible**—the amount that the insured must pay on covered services before benefits begin—the deductible must have been met. Deductibles range widely, usually from $200 to thousands of dollars annually. Higher deductibles generally mean lower premiums.
4. Any **coinsurance**—the percentage of each covered charge that the insured must pay—has to have been taken into account. The coinsurance rate shows the insurance company's percentage of payment for the charge followed by the insured's percentage, such as 80-20. This means that the payer pays 80 percent of the covered amount and the patient pays 20 percent after the premiums and deductibles are paid.

The formula is Charge − Deductible − Patient coinsurance = Health plan payment.

For example, a typical high-deductible plan might specify that the first $1,000 in covered annual medical fees is paid by the insured and that the coinsurance

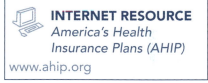

rate is 80-20. In this case, the patient with a first medical bill of $8,000 would owe the $1,000 deductible plus 20 percent of the remaining $7,000, or $1,400, for a total of $2,400. The insurance company payment is $5,600.

Managed Care Plans

Because they cost employers and patients less, managed care plans are the most popular insurance plans. More than 90 percent of all insured workers are enrolled in some type of managed care plan, and over two thousand different plan variations are offered by payers. The goal of managing care is to ensure the delivery of quality health care and at the same time control health care costs. To accomplish these goals, **managed care organizations (MCOs)** combine the financing and management of health care with the delivery of services. Managed care offers a more restricted choice of providers and treatments in exchange for lower premiums, deductibles, and other charges than traditional indemnity insurance.

Managed care organizations establish networks of providers, patients, and payers. Under managed care, the provider as well as the patient has an agreement with the insurance company. This arrangement gives the managed care plan more control over which services the provider performs and the fees that are charged for the services.

In addition to premiums, managed care plans usually require the policyholder to pay a specified charge called a **copayment (copay).** This payment is due at the time of service. In the hospital setting, copayments are usually collected before treatments are provided, unless the patient is admitted under emergency conditions.

The most popular type of managed care plan is a **preferred provider organization (PPO).** PPOs arrange discounted fees for services from the network of providers—hospitals and physicians—with which they have contracts. Plan members must use network providers to benefit from the reduced charges; visits with out-of-network providers cost members more. Unlike many managed care plans, a PPO does not require a primary care physician to oversee patients' care, and a referral from the patient's primary care physician is not required before the patient can see another physician. PPOs enroll almost 50 percent of the American workers who are insured through their employers.

Another main type of managed care plan is called a **health maintenance organization (HMO).** An HMO combines coverage of medical costs and delivery of health care for a prepaid premium. Over 20 percent of insured employees are enrolled in HMOs. The HMO creates a network of physicians, hospitals, and other providers by employing or negotiating contracts with them. Plan members must use only these providers in order to be covered; visits with out-of-network providers are not paid for. In an HMO, a primary care physician coordinates the patient's care. HMOs also require the use of referrals. Although HMOs are more restrictive than PPOs, premiums and copayments are lower than in PPO plans.

A third type of managed care plan is a **consumer-driven health plan (CDHP).** CDHPs combine two elements. The first element is a health plan, usually a PPO, that has a high deductible and low premiums. The second element is a special "savings account" that is used to pay medical bills before the deductible has been met. The savings account, similar to an individual retirement account (IRA), lets people put aside untaxed wages that they may use to cover their out-of-pocket medical expenses. Some employers contribute to employees' accounts as a benefit. Cost containment in consumer-driven health plans begins with consumerism—the idea that patients who themselves pay for health care services become more careful consumers.

FYI

Referrals

In some managed care plans, a *referral* from the patient's primary care physician is required before the patient can see any other physician. A referral authorizes the patient to see another specified physician for treatment. A referral is often a written document given to the patient to take to the other doctor or to the hospital; a referral number may also be assigned.

Medical Insurance Payers and Payment Methods

Nearly 250 million people in the United States have medical coverage through either private insurance plans or government programs. Another 47 million people have no medical insurance. Many of the uninsured people work for employers that either do not offer health benefits or do not cover certain employees, such as temporary workers or part-time employees. People who do not have insurance, or whose insurance does not cover procedures they are having, are categorized as self-paying patients or "self-pays." In some cases, hospitals and physicians who provide care for people who cannot pay for it—called "uncompensated care"—receive payment under a federal or state program.

Private Payers

A private payer is generally one of several large insurance companies that dominate the national market and offer all the leading types of insurance plans. The three largest are WellPoint, UnitedHealth Group, and Aetna. Other examples include Cigna, Humana, and Pacificare Health Systems. There are also a number of nonprofit organizations, such as Kaiser Permanente, which is the largest nonprofit HMO. Some entities, such as the Blue Cross and Blue Shield Association, have both for-profit and nonprofit components.

Private payers have contracts with businesses to provide benefits for their employees. These may be large-group or small-group health care plans. Payers may also offer individual insurance coverage.

Government-Sponsored Health Care Programs

A number of government-sponsored health care programs offer benefits for various groups of people who are eligible:

- Medicare is a 100 percent federally funded health plan that covers about 43 million people who are sixty-five and over, are disabled, or have permanent kidney failure (end-stage renal disease, or ESRD).

- Medicaid, a federal program that is jointly funded by federal and state governments, covers nearly 53 million low-income people who cannot afford medical care. Medicaid is administered by the states, which determine the program's qualifications and benefits under broad federal guidelines. States provide about 43 percent of the money for the program.

- TRICARE, a Department of Defense program, covers medical expenses for active-duty members of the uniformed services and their spouses, children, and other dependents; retired military personnel and their dependents; and family members of deceased active-duty personnel.

- CHAMPVA, the Civilian Health and Medical Program of the Department of Veterans Affairs, covers veterans with permanent service-related disabilities and their dependents. It also covers surviving spouses and dependent children of veterans who died from service-related disabilities.

Hospital Payment Methods

Payers determine the payments made under insurance plans in three major ways: cost-based reimbursement, per diem, and prospective payment.

$ $ Billing Tip $ $
Insurance Terms

In insurance terms, the facility or physician that provides medical services is the *first party*, and the patient (or policyholder) is the *second party*. The patient may have a policy with an insurance company, the *third party*, that agrees to carry the risk of paying for those services and therefore is called a *third-party payer*, commonly referred to as the *payer*.

Cost-Based Reimbursement

Cost-based reimbursement, also known as fee-for-service, is one method of paying for health care services. In this system, hospitals and payers sign contracts that state the fees the hospital will be paid for the various items that are used in treating a patient during a hospital stay. Often, hospitals' charges are subject to review, negotiations, and discounts by payers. For example, a hospital might normally charge $40 for a two-inch needle to administer a nerve block before surgery, but a PPO may negotiate a fee of $30 for their members for this service. This type of payment is often used for outpatient hospital services.

Per Diem

Under the **per diem** payment method, hospitals are paid a fixed amount for each day a patient is hospitalized. The per diem rate, which is negotiated by the provider and the payer in advance, covers all the costs for services and supplies that are associated with the patient's treatment, and no additional charges can be billed to the payer. Different categories of treatment are set up to compensate the hospital for the additional costs associated with special care categories, such as intensive care. This type of payment is used for inpatient hospital services.

Prospective Payment

The goal of the **prospective payment** method is to control costs for the payer. Under both the cost-based reimbursement and per diem methods, it is hard to control costs because payment is based on the services provided. The more services, the higher the bill. From the payer's point of view, this situation tends to reward inefficient providers. For example, if patients are hospitalized for seven days for appendectomies in one hospital, but another hospital releases similar patients in four days (with equally successful outcomes), the hospital that is releasing patients earlier is evaluated as providing more efficient care but is paid less. The prospective payment method pays each hospital the same amount for this service, rewarding the more efficient provider.

The prospective payment method, which was created by Medicare, determines national averages for hospital stays based on patients' diagnoses and pays each facility accordingly. The base rate of payment is fixed in advance—*prospectively*—and is adjusted by the payer to offset differences in factors that affect patients' outcomes, such as age and other health-related conditions. Chapter 5, "Payment Methods and Billing Compliance," covers the details of two prospective payment systems currently used by Medicare—the Medicare Inpatient Prospective Payment System (IPPS) and the Medicare Outpatient Prospective Payment System (OPPS). It also discusses private payer systems, most of which have adopted similar prospective payment methods.

Regulations and Accreditation

Hospitals and physicians are regulated by federal and state laws to ensure quality health care services. For example, all providers must be approved in order to treat Medicare beneficiaries. The contracts that hospitals and medical specialists have with managed care organizations to provide health care services to plan members are business relationships that are ruled by state laws. A number of nonprofit organizations rate how well each managed care organization provides its services. Hospital facilities are regularly surveyed to check whether their treatment of patients follows the health care industry's best practices for high-quality care.

Federal and State Regulation

The main federal government agency responsible for health care is the **Centers for Medicare and Medicaid Services (CMS),** formerly known as HCFA (pronounced hic-fuh), an abbreviation for Health Care Financing Administration. An agency of the Department of Health and Human Services (HHS), CMS administers the Medicare and Medicaid programs to more than 95 million Americans, undertaking many activities to ensure health care quality. For example, CMS:

- Regulates all laboratory testing other than research performed on humans
- Prevents discrimination based on health status for people buying health insurance
- Evaluates the quality of health care facilities and services
- Researches the effectiveness of various methods of health care management, treatment, and financing (such as by reviewing managed care plans that want to provide Medicare coverage)

Because of these activities, CMS policy is often the point of reference for private-sector payers. When government regulations change the way Medicare reimbursement is calculated, for example, insurance companies often adopt the same payment methods. The Medicare-required insurance claim form for hospital services has become the standard form for most private payers as well.

State legislatures, too, pass laws regulating the health care industry. States often regulate premium increases, require certain services to be covered, and gather medical data on illnesses or conditions of concern to public health officials.

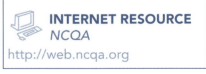

INTERNET RESOURCE
CMS Home Page
www.cms.hhs.gov

Accrediting Organizations

Several nonprofit organizations accredit health plans or focus on ensuring the quality of patient care in hospitals.

NCQA

The National Committee for Quality Assurance (NCQA) works with the health care industry to provide employers and consumers with information about the effectiveness of various managed care plans in preventing and treating disease, providing access to care, and obtaining member satisfaction with care. NCQA guidelines on the way plans select physicians and hospitals to join their networks, called credentialing, are an example of performance measures. NCQA requires a plan to review the credentials of all providers in the plan every two years to ensure that they remain professionally competent.

INTERNET RESOURCE
NCQA
http://web.ncqa.org

Joint Commission

Standards for many types of patient care are set and monitored by the Joint Commission (formerly known as the Joint Commission on Accreditation of Healthcare Organizations, or JCAHO). The Joint Commission's members are from the American College of Surgeons, the American College of Physicians, the American Medical Association, the American Hospital Association, and the American Dental Association. The Joint Commission verifies compliance with accreditation standards for hospitals and other health care facilities.

INTERNET RESOURCE
Joint Commission
www.jointcommission.org

URAC

The Utilization Review Accreditation Commission (URAC), also known as the American Accreditation Healthcare Commission, also establishes accreditation

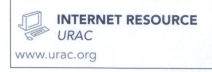
standards. URAC's central mission is to promote quality and accountability for health care organizations, especially organizations that provide managed care services. The accreditation process is designed to ensure that managed care organizations have addressed the issue of quality in both their structure and operations. Regulators in almost two-thirds of the states rely on URAC accreditation.

Standards for Business Conduct

Patient account specialists focus on gathering and processing correct, timely information so that insurance companies and patients make timely payments for services. Patient satisfaction with a facility's billing practices is extremely important.

Ensuring Fair Treatment of Patients

The way facilities charge patients must be without bias or discrimination. Patients need to know that they will receive straightforward answers to billing questions and that they can get the information they need to understand their financial responsibilities. To ensure that patients understand their bills and what they owe, facilities communicate information that is straightforward and easy for them to use. For example, Figure 1.3 shows a sample letter that a facility sends to patients before a hospital stay. It explains how the financial side of the patient's hospitalization will be handled. Figure 1.4 on page 15 is

Figure 1.3

Paying Your Hospital Bill

We are dedicated to the goal of providing the finest health care services to you. In order to do this, we must collect our accounts as promptly as possible. This letter explains how our staff will handle your claim with your insurance company(ies) and what your responsibility is.

Our staff will file a claim with your insurance company as soon as possible after your discharge. We will follow up the claim 30 days after submitting it. We will provide all necessary information to your insurance company to make a determination for payment. You will be expected to make full payment of the account balance if insurance fails to pay on time or denies payment. At the time of service, you are expected to pay any deductible and coinsurance amounts, and any charges not covered under your insurance.

If you do not have insurance, you will be expected to make a deposit or arrangements for payment before you register, unless the treatment is an emergency. Otherwise, your registration may be postponed in cooperation with your physician.

You may pay your bill by cash, check, Visa, Discover, Master Card, or American Express. We will help you apply for Medicaid and Uncompensated Care. Payment plans are only established on accounts confirming an inability to pay. To show an inability to pay, the patient must first apply for Medicaid and Charity. If denied, a credit application is taken and verified. Payments may be approved for a limited period of time. We will assist you in obtaining outside financing.

Our Financial Counselors are trained to assist you in resolving account payments; we will help you in working with a counselor if you wish this service. Please let us know of any other special needs with which we can assist you.

Figure 1.4

Bill Payment

We are committed...

to providing you with the best available healthcare along with convenient and reliable billing services. Our financial services office will gladly assist you in resolving any questions that you may have. You may phone them at (801) 555-5555 from 8:00 a.m. to 5:00 p.m. Monday through Friday. Correspondence regarding your bill should be mailed to Billing Department, 1200 E. 3900 South, Salt Lake City, UT 84124.

It is important to remember that your hospital bill covers services provided by the hospital: room, nursing care, meals, housekeeping and linen. It may also include services ordered by your physician: X-rays, laboratory tests, medical supplies and oxygen. The bill does not include charges for your personal physician, surgeon, anesthesiologist, pathologist, emergency physician, radiologist, or other physician assistants. You will receive separate bills from these physicians.

Our financial services office can resolve any questions that you may have. St. Mark's Hospital looks forward to serving you in the future.

Financial Procedures

- We verify your insurance coverage and determine the benefits the day following your admission to the hospital. We are then able to estimate your portion of the total bill.
- If your insurance carrier participates with us through a managed care program, we are able to give you a very accurate figure because the contracts usually allow a certain amount per day.
- If we are estimating you owe any portion of the bill, you will be asked to stop by the cashier's office upon discharge to set up monthly payments unless prior arrangements are made.
- To make your discharge easier, we highly recommend that a family member come to the cashier's office **before** the patient is actually leaving.
- If you do not have insurance, you will be able to speak to a financial advisor at the hospital. These advisors will fill out a worksheet and ask information about your finances. The worksheets are then reviewed and compared to our guidelines. If you meet the requirements, you may qualify for a 100% adjustment of your bill; if you do not qualify for the 100%, you may qualify for a partial adjustment if you agree to pay the remaining balance.

St. Mark's Hospital accepts the following Managed Care Plans. For information, call **801-268-7144.**

Altius
  Employees Choice Health Option (ECHO)
  HMO
  Indemnity
American Family Care
CIGNA HealthCare of Utah
Educator's Mutual
  Advantage
  Select care
First Health
Private Health Care Systems (PHCS)
Kemper National Services, Inc.
Regent Blue Cross Blue Shield (BCBS)
Premier Medical Network
  Mutual of Omaha Insurance Company
  United Omaha Life Insurance Company
Mailhandlers
Medicaid
Medicare
Union Pacific Railroad Employees Health System (UPREHS)
Utah Public Employees Health Program (PEHP)

Bill Payment Contacts

Customer Service Rep
Please send us an e-mail if you have any questions. This service is only available Monday-Friday, 8:00 a.m. to 5:00 p.m., excluding holidays.

an example of a website that offers patients billing information as well as many additional resources. Although billing and payment policies are not the same in every facility, the key is clearly explaining the rules to patients.

Patient account specialists follow their facilities' written billing guidelines, which provide procedures to:

- Ensure compliance with federal regulations, private payer policies, and internal procedures
- Provide the basis for honest, ethical processes and policies
- Encourage good relationships with patients as well as with representatives of private payers and government programs

Federal Health Care Regulation Under HIPAA

In addition to ensuring fair treatment of patients regarding billing procedures, patient account specialists must understand the importance of protecting the confidentiality of patients' personal information. Because they work with patients' medical records on a regular basis, patient account specialists must understand the laws that govern the use of medical records. The most important legislation regarding the confidentiality of patient information is contained in the **Health Insurance Portability and Accountability Act (HIPAA) of 1996.**

Initiated by Senators Edward Kennedy and Nancy L. Kassebaum, HIPAA began as a response to public concern about people who were denied health insurance when they changed jobs. The final version enacted by Congress, however, was much broader in its scope and its ongoing impact more than a decade after its passage. In addition to protecting the portability of health insurance, the law sets standards for the use of electronic technology by health care organizations. It establishes standards for protecting peoples' medical information during electronic exchange. HIPAA also imposes fines and possible prison terms for those who violate its provisions.

Patients' medical records are legal documents that belong to the provider who created them. But the provider cannot withhold the *information* in the records from patients unless providing it would be detrimental to the person's health. This information belongs to the patient. Patients control the amount and type of information that is released, except for the use of the data to treat them or to conduct normal business transactions. Under HIPAA, only patients or their legally appointed representatives have the authority to authorize the release of information to anyone not directly involved in their care.

Title II: Administrative Simplification

HIPAA, which became Public Law 104-191 on August 21, 1996, has two parts. Title I, health insurance reform, is the law related to the continuation of health insurance coverage when individuals change jobs. Title II, known as Administrative Simplification, affects individuals' private health information. This chapter focuses on Title II.

The U.S. Congress passed an act with provisions for **Administrative Simplification** because of concern over the rising costs of health care. A significant portion of every health care dollar spent in the United States goes to the overhead associated with administrative and financial transactions, such as filing claims for payment, checking patient eligibility for benefits, requesting authorization for services, and notifying providers of payments. It is generally agreed that the health care industry could achieve much greater efficiency if common business transactions were standardized and handled digitally.

The Administrative Simplification provisions encourage the use of **electronic data interchange (EDI)**. EDI is the computer-to-computer exchange of routine business information using publicly available standards. People working in allied health careers use EDI to exchange health information about patients among physicians and insurance companies.

Administrative Simplification Standards

INTERNET RESOURCE
Administrative Simplification Home Page
www.cms.hhs.gov/HIPAAGenInfo/

The Administrative Simplification provisions of Title II required the Department of Health and Human Services (HHS) to establish national standards for electronic health care transactions and national identifiers for providers, health plans, and employers. It also addressed the security and privacy of the health data that are exchanged electronically and the possible penalties that could result from failing to comply with HIPAA rules.

Since this umbrella act was passed, a number of HIPAA standards have been made into law. The three main HIPAA laws include:

- *The HIPAA Privacy Rule:* The privacy requirements cover patients' health information.

- *The HIPAA Security Rule:* The security requirements state the administrative, technical, and physical safeguards that are required to protect patients' health information.

- *The HIPAA Electronic Health Care Transaction and Code Sets Standards:* These standards require every provider who does business electronically to use the same health care transactions, code sets, and identifiers.

Because patient account specialists need to protect the information in patients' records, at times they need to know the following: What information can be released about patients' conditions and treatments. What information can be legally shared among providers and payers? What information must the patient specifically authorize to be released? The answers to these questions are based in the three HIPAA rules above.

Covered Entities: Complying with HIPAA

HIPAA TIP

Standards and Rules
A *standard* is a requirement, which is stated in a *rule*.

Before discussing the three HIPAA rules and their enforcement, it is important to understand who the covered entities are that are required by law to obey the HIPAA rules and regulations. Under HIPAA, a **covered entity** is an organization or a health care professional who provides health care in the normal course of business and electronically sends any information that is protected under HIPAA.

Under HIPAA, three types of covered entities must follow the regulations:

1. *Health plans:* The individual or group health insurance plans that provide or pay for medical care.

2. *Providers:* People or organizations that furnish, bill, or are paid for health care in the normal course of business, such as physicians and hospitals. Other organizations that work for the covered entities, called *business associates*, must also agree to follow the HIPAA rules.

3. *Clearinghouses:* Companies that help providers handle such electronic transactions as submitting claims and that manage electronic medical record systems. Clearinghouses process health information by converting it into a format that meets HIPAA standards.

FYI

Identifying Covered Entities
Most providers are covered entities under HIPAA. Excepted providers are only those that do not send any claims (or other HIPAA transactions) electronically *and* do not employ any other firm to send electronic claims for them. Since CMS requires providers to send Medicare claims electronically unless they employ fewer than ten full-time or equivalent employees, most providers have moved to EDI for the health claim processing.

The following types of insurance benefits are exempt from the HIPAA standards even when they are provided by a health plan:

- Accident or disability income insurance
- General and automotive liability insurance
- Workers' compensation
- Automobile medical payment insurance
- Coverage for onsite medical clinics

HIPAA Privacy Rule

The HIPAA Standards for Privacy of Individually Identifiable Health Information rule is known as the **HIPAA Privacy Rule.** It was the first comprehensive federal protection for the privacy of health information. Its national standards protect individuals' medical records and other personal health information. Before the HIPAA Privacy Rule became law, the personal information stored in hospitals, physician practices, and health plans was governed by a patchwork of federal and state laws. Some state laws were strict, but others were not.

The Privacy Rule says that covered entities must:

- Have privacy practices that are appropriate for its health care services
- Notify patients about their privacy rights and how their information can be used or disclosed
- Train employees so that they understand the privacy practices
- Appoint a privacy official responsible for seeing that the privacy practices are adopted and followed
- Safeguard patients' records

Protected Health Information

The HIPAA Privacy Rule covers the use and disclosure of patients' **protected health information (PHI).** PHI is defined as individually identifiable health information that is transmitted or maintained by electronic media, such as over the Internet, by computer modem, or on magnetic tape or compact disks. This information includes a person's:

- Name
- Address (including street address, city, county, and ZIP code)
- Relatives' and employers' names
- Birth date
- Telephone numbers
- Fax number
- E-mail address
- Social Security number
- Medical record number (MRN)
- Health plan beneficiary number
- Account number
- Certificate or license number
- Serial number of any vehicle or other device

- Website address
- Fingerprints or voiceprints
- Photographic images

Disclosure for Treatment, Payment, and Health Care Operations

Under HIPAA, patients' PHI can be used and disclosed by providers for treatment, payment, and health care operations. *Use of PHI* means sharing or analysis *within* the entity that holds the information. *Disclosure of PHI* means the release, transfer, provision of access to, or divulging of PHI *outside* the entity holding the information.

Both use and disclosure of PHI are necessary and permitted for patients' **treatment, payment, and health care operations (TPO).** *Treatment* means providing and coordinating the patient's medical care; *payment* refers to the exchange of information with health plans; and *health care operations* are the general business management functions. When using or disclosing protected health information, a covered entity must try to limit the information to the minimum amount of PHI necessary for the intended purpose. The **minimum necessary standard** means taking reasonable safeguards to protect PHI from incidental disclosure.

Examples of complying with HIPAA include the following:

- A medical coder does not disclose a patient's history of cancer on a workers' compensation claim for a sprained ankle. Only the information the recipient needs to know is given.
- A physician's assistant faxes only the appropriate patient cardiology test results before scheduled surgery at the hospital.
- A physician sends an e-mail message to another physician requesting a consultation on a patient's case.
- A patient's family member picks up medical supplies and a prescription.

Designated Record Set

A covered entity must disclose individuals' PHI to them (or to their personal representatives) when they request access to, or an accounting of disclosures of, their PHI. Patients' rights apply only to a *designated record set (DRS),* which does not include all items. For example, in a physician's office, the designated record set means the medical and billing records the provider maintains. It does not include appointment and surgery schedules, requests for lab tests, and birth and death records. It also does not include mental health information, psychotherapy notes, and genetic information.

Within this designated record set, patients have the right to:

- Access, copy, and inspect their PHI
- Request amendments to their health information
- Obtain accounting of most disclosures of their health information
- Receive communications from providers via other means, such as in Braille or in foreign languages
- Complain about alleged violations of the regulations and the provider's own information policies

HIPAA TIP

Health Care Providers and the Minimum Necessary Standard

The minimum necessary standard does not apply to any type of disclosure—oral, written, phone, fax, e-mail, or other—among health care providers for treatment purposes.

HIPAA TIP

Protecting PHI

Be careful not to discuss patients' cases with anyone not directly involved with their care, including family and friends. Avoid talking about cases, too, in any areas where other patients might hear. Close charts on desks when they are not being worked on. Position computer screens so that only the person working with a file can view it.

Authorizations

For use or disclosure other than for TPO, the covered entity must have the patient sign an authorization to release the information (see Figure 1.5 on page 21). Processing such requests for information involves careful checking and following the procedures on release of information.

Information about substance (alcohol and drug) abuse, sexually transmitted diseases (STDs) or human immunodeficiency virus (HIV), and behavioral/mental health services may not be released without a specific authorization from the patient. The authorization document must be in plain language and include the following:

- A description of the information to be used or disclosed
- The name or other specific identification of the person(s) authorized to use or disclose the information
- The name of the person(s) or group of people to whom the covered entity may make the use or disclosure
- A description of each purpose of the requested use or disclosure
- An expiration date
- The signature of the individual (or authorized representative) and the date

In addition, the rule states that a valid authorization must include:

- A statement of the individual's right to revoke the authorization in writing
- A statement about whether the covered entity is able to base the treatment, payment, enrollment, or eligibility for benefits on the authorization
- A statement that information used or disclosed after the authorization may be disclosed again by the recipient and may no longer be protected by the rule

Uses or disclosures for which the covered entity has received specific authorization from the patient do not have to follow the minimum necessary standard.

Exceptions

There are a number of exceptions to the usual rules for release:

- Court orders
- Workers' compensation cases
- Statutory reports
- Research

Although these types of disclosures do not require a release authorization, they must be logged, and the release information must be available to the patient who requests it.

De-Identified Health Information

There are no restrictions on disclosing **de-identified health information** that neither identifies nor provides a reasonable basis to identify an individual. To prepare this type of document, all identifiers must be removed, such as names, medical record numbers, health plan beneficiary numbers, device identifiers (such as pacemakers), and biometric identifiers, such as fingerprints and voiceprints. Such de-identified records are also called *blinded* or *redacted* documents.

Figure 1.5

Example of Authorization to Release or Disclose Information

Patient Name: _____

Health Record Number: _____

Date of Birth: _____

1. I authorize the use or disclosure of the above named individual's health information as described below.

2. The following individual(s) or organization(s) are authorized to make the disclosure: _____

3. The type of information to be used or disclosed is as follows (check the appropriate boxes and include other information where indicated)
❏ problem list
❏ medication list
❏ list of allergies
❏ immunization records
❏ most recent history
❏ most recent discharge summary
❏ lab results (please describe the dates or types of lab tests you would like disclosed): _____
❏ x-ray and imaging reports (please describe the dates or types of x-rays or images you would like disclosed): _____
❏ consultation reports from (please supply doctors' names): _____
❏ entire record
❏ other (please describe): _____

4. I understand that the information in my health record may include information relating to sexually transmitted disease, acquired immunodeficiency syndrome (AIDS), or human immunodeficiency virus (HIV). It may also include information about behavioral or mental health services, and treatment for alcohol and drug abuse.

5. The information identified above may be used by or disclosed to the following individuals or organization(s):

Name: _____

Address: _____

Name: _____

Address: _____

6. This information for which I'm authorizing disclosure will be used for the following purpose:
❏ my personal records
❏ sharing with other health care providers as needed/other (please describe): _____

7. I understand that I have a right to revoke this authorization at any time. I understand that if I revoke this authorization, I must do so in writing and present my written revocation to the health information management department. I understand that the revocation will not apply to information that has already been released in response to this authorization. I understand that the revocation will not apply to my insurance company when the law provides my insurer with the right to contest a claim under my policy.

8. This authorization will expire (insert date or event): _____

If I fail to specify an expiration date or event, this authorization will expire six months from the date on which it was signed.

9. I understand that once the above information is disclosed, it may be redisclosed by the recipient and the information may not be protected by federal privacy laws or regulations.

10. I understand authorizing the use or disclosure of the information identified above is voluntary. I need not sign this form to ensure healthcare treatment.

Signature of patient or legal representative: _____ Date: _____

If signed by legal representative, relationship to patient

Signature of witness: _____ Date: _____

Distribution of copies: Original to provider; copy to patient; copy to accompany use or disclosure

Note: This sample form was developed by the American Health Information Management Association for discussion purposes. It should not be used without review by the issuing organization's legal counsel to ensure compliance with other federal and state laws and regulations.

What specific information can be released

To whom

For what purpose

HIPAA Security Rule

The **HIPAA Security Rule** requires covered entities to establish safeguards to protect PHI. The Security Rule specifies how to secure such protected health information on computer networks, the Internet, and storage media such as CDs and flash drives. Security measures rely on *encryption,* the process of encoding information in such a way that only the person (or computer) with the key can decode it.

A number of other security measures help enforce the HIPAA Security Rule. These include:

- Access control, passwords, and log files to keep intruders out
- Backups to replace items after damage
- Security policies to handle violations that do occur

HIPAA Electronic Health Care Transactions and Code Sets

The **HIPAA Electronic Health Care Transactions and Code Sets (TCS)** standards require entities that do business electronically to use the same health care transactions, identifiers, and code sets. The goal of the rule is to improve the efficiency of the business of health care.

HIPAA Electronic Transactions and Identifiers

HIPAA-covered transactions include activities such as health care claims sent by physicians and hospitals to insurance companies, payments sent by the insurance companies in response, and employee enrollment information sent by employers to their insurance companies. Each standard is labeled with both a number and a name. Either the number (such as "the 837," which is the insurance claim form) or the name (such as the "HIPAA Claim") may be used to refer to the particular electronic document format.

Likewise, HIPAA national identifiers are being assigned to providers and employers, and in the future they will be assigned to health plans. *Identifiers* are numbers of predetermined length and structure. (Although it is not a HIPAA national identifier, a person's Social Security number is an example of an identifier.) The use of national identifiers in health care transactions is important because the identifiers can be used uniformly across the full span of transactions. For example, in the past hospitals used a separate provider identifier for each payer. Under HIPAA, a hospitals' National Provider Identifier is used to identify the hospital on all claims, regardless of the payer. These unique numbers replace the many different types of non-uniform numbers used in the past.

Standard Code Sets

Under HIPAA, a *code set* is any group of codes used for encoding data elements, such as tables of terms, medical concepts, medical diagnosis codes, or medical procedure codes. Of great importance for medical billing are the code sets HIPAA requires for diseases, for medical procedures, and for supplies. Details of these required code sets are covered in Chapter 4, "Medical Coding Basics."

HIPAA Enforcement

All Administrative Simplification provisions legislated under HIPAA are currently covered under a rule known as the *HIPAA Final Enforcement Rule,* which became law and was required to be implemented on March 16, 2006. The complete rule as published in the *Federal Register* is available through the HHS Office for Civil Rights HIPAA home page.

Enforcing HIPAA is the job of a number of government agencies. Which agency performs which task depends on the nature of the violation.

Office for Civil Rights

Civil violations of the HIPAA privacy standards are enforced by the Office for Civil Rights (OCR), an agency of the Department of Health and Human Services. The OCR is charged with enforcing the privacy standards because the right to privacy is considered a civil right. It is important to note, though, that individuals themselves do not have the right to sue a covered entity that may have disclosed their PHI inappropriately; action must be taken on individuals' behalf by the OCR.

Department of Justice

The *criminal* violations of HIPAA privacy standards are prosecuted by the federal government's Department of Justice (DOJ).

Centers for Medicare and Medicaid Services: Nonprivacy Standards

Nonprivacy standards are enforced separately from privacy standards by the Centers for Medicare and Medicaid Services. Also an agency of HHS, CMS is authorized by HHS to investigate complaints of noncompliance and enforce all of the following nonprivacy HIPAA standards:

- The Electronic Health Care Transactions and Code Sets (TCS) Rule
- The National Employer Identifier Number (EIN) Rule
- The Security Rule
- The National Provider Identifier Rule
- The National Plan Identifier Rule (currently under development)

Civil and Criminal Case Procedures

The enforcing agency must receive and then accept a complaint. If a complaint is accepted for investigation, the agency notifies the person who filed it as well as the covered entity that is named in the complaint as the violator. Both the filer and the covered entity are then asked to submit information. Covered entities are required by law to cooperate with complaint investigations. When the OCR or CMS investigates a complaint, the covered entity must provide access to its facilities, books, records, and systems, including relevant protected health information. The OCR also has the authority to issue subpoenas in investigations of alleged violations of the Privacy Rule.

The enforcing agency reviews the facts of the case. It may determine that the covered entity did not violate HIPAA requirements. If the evidence indicates that the covered entity was in violation, the agency attempts

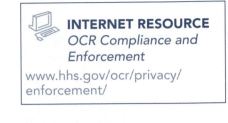

INTERNET RESOURCE
Final Enforcement Rule
www.hhs.gov/ocr/hipaa/

INTERNET RESOURCE
OCR Compliance and Enforcement
www.hhs.gov/ocr/privacy/enforcement/

FYI

Civil or Criminal?
Violations of HIPAA may be civil offenses, or they may be criminal in nature. A *civil violation* is based on civil law. These violations, which are handled in some kind of a legal court system, begin with a person entering a complaint against another person or entity and usually asking for some kind of remedy, such as a monetary payment. Examples of general civil cases are trespassing suits, divorce proceedings, and breach of contract proceedings. A *criminal violation*, on the other hand, is based on a branch of the law that defines crime—such as kidnapping, robbery, and arson—and provides for its punishment. A criminal violation is regarded as an offense committed against the public even though only one individual may have been wronged, and the wrongdoer is prosecuted by the government for the purpose of punishment, which may include financial penalties and prison sentences.

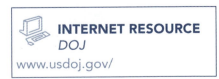

INTERNET RESOURCE
DOJ
www.usdoj.gov/

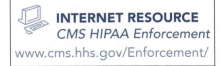

INTERNET RESOURCE
CMS HIPAA Enforcement
www.cms.hhs.gov/Enforcement/

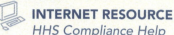
to resolve the case with the covered entity by obtaining voluntary compliance, corrective action, or other resolution. The chief weapon that the government has to encourage voluntary action is publicity. If an organization or physician is found to be out of compliance, HHS notifies the public as well as appropriate organizations and entities. Since bad publicity has a negative effect on patients' opinions of the covered entity, most covered entities take the necessary steps to avoid noncompliance. In keeping with this approach, HHS provides online help on compliant procedures to covered entities.

Most privacy complaints have been settled by voluntary compliance. But if the covered entity does not act to resolve the matter in a way that is satisfactory, the enforcing agency can impose *civil money penalties (CMPs)*. The Final Enforcement Rule establishes civil money penalties of not more than $100 for each violation and not more than $25,000 for all violations of an identical type during a single calendar year. The person who filed the complaint does not receive a portion of civil money penalties collected from covered entities; the penalties are deposited in the U.S. Treasury.

If the OCR or CMS receives a complaint that may lead to a criminal case, the agency will usually refer the complaint to the DOJ for investigation. For criminal cases, such as selling unique health identifiers for identity theft purposes, the following penalties can be imposed:

	Fine	*Prison*
Knowingly obtaining PHI in violation of HIPAA	$50,000	1 year
Offenses done under false pretenses	$100,000	5 years
Using PHI for profit, gain, or harm	$250,000	10 years

It is important to note that only covered entities—not employees or business associates—can be charged with HIPAA violations, and only the enforcing agencies—not individuals—can bring the charges. In the case of criminal violations, while HIPAA gives the government authority to prosecute covered entities for criminal violations, employees are not automatically covered by the law and may not be subject to criminal penalties. But depending on the facts of a particular case, certain employees may be directly liable under other laws, like corporate criminal liability laws.

Staying Up to Date

HIPAA rules will continue to be issued and updated. Patient account specialists and other allied health professionals stay up to date using a number of means. Professional articles, conferences, and continuing education are all important. Listed below are the most important sources for updated information.

Listserv

A *listserv* is an e-mail-based server that allows users to create, manage, and control electronic mailing lists on a network. Any user who signs up for a listserv may subscribe to lists, receive list postings, query the listserv, set up a new list, and access list archives.

To learn about the latest HIPAA outreach materials and events, the HIPAA outreach listserv is ideal. To sign up, go to the National Institute of Health (NIH) listserv home page, and under the Browse option select HIPAA-OUTREACH-L.

To learn about the latest developments in HIPAA regulations, the HIPAA-REGS listserv is recommended. To sign up, go to the same NIH listserv home page, and under the Browse option select HIPAA-REGS.

HHS Frequent Questions Home Page

The Department of Health and Human Services website contains a link to a Frequent Questions home page. Select the HIPAA category to display the home page for HIPAA—Frequent Questions (see Figure 1.6). This section provides answers to the most commonly asked questions about HIPAA.

INTERNET RESOURCE
NIH Listserv Home Page
https://list.nih.gov/

INTERNET RESOURCE
HIPAA—Frequent Questions Home Page
www.hhs.gov/hipaafaq

Figure 1.6

HIPAA—Frequent Questions Home Page on HHS Website

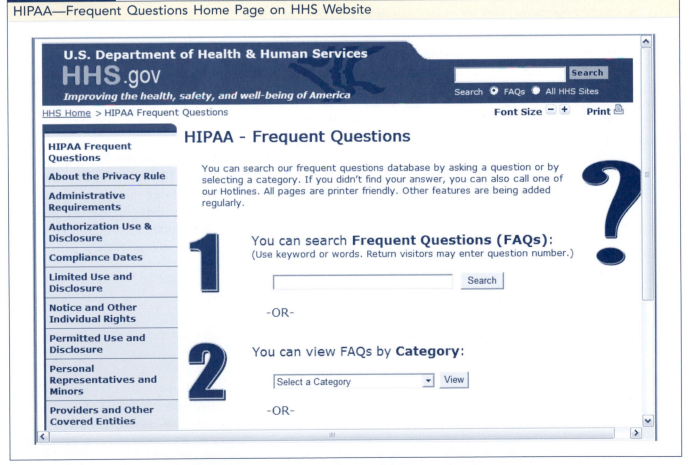

Other Resources

Table 1.1 lists Internet addresses for other HIPAA resources.

Table 1.1

HIPAA Resources

Resource	Internet Address
The National Committee on Vital and Health Statistics (NCVHS) is a public advisory board to the Secretary of Health and Human Services.	www.ncvhs.hhs.gov/
Accredited Standards Committee (ASC X12) is responsible for the development and maintenance of electronic data interchange (EDI) standards for many industries. The X12, or insurance, section of ASC X12 handles the EDI for the health insurance industry's administrative transactions. Under HIPAA, X12 standards have been adopted for most transactions between health plans and providers.	www.x12.org/
The National Council for Prescription Drug Programs (NCPDP) creates and promotes standards for the transfer of data to and from the pharmacy services sector of the health care industry. Under HIPAA, NCPDP standards were adopted for several retail pharmacy transactions.	www.ncpdp.org/
Designated Standard Maintenance Organizations (DSMOs) are organizations designated by HHS to maintain the standards adopted under HIPAA Administrative Simplification. The current organizations serving as DSMOs are Accredited Standards Committee X12, Dental Content Committee of the American Dental Association, Health Level Seven, National Council for Prescription Drug Programs, National Uniform Billing Committee, and National Uniform Claim Committee.	www.hipaa-dsmo.org/
X12 implementation guides are the specific technical instructions for implementing each of the adopted standards. The implementation guides are prepared by X12 (as the standard maintainer) and are made available to the public by the Washington Publishing Company for a modest fee.	www.wpc-edi.com/ hipaa
Workgroup for Electronic Data Interchange (WEDI) fosters widespread support for the adoption of electronic commerce in health care.	www.wedi.org/
Strategic national implementation process (SNIP) is a collaborative health care industry process for the implementation of the HIPAA standards. This website includes white papers on transactions, security, identifiers, and privacy.	www.wedi.org/snip/
Medicare Electronic Data Interchange (EDI) is the official Medicare website that contains important information about how providers can communicate electronically with the Medicare program. This website contains EDI formats and instructions, transaction mapping information, statistics, FAQs about Medicare EDI, and other valuable EDI data.	www.cms.hhs.gov/ ElectronicBillingEDITrans/ 01_overview.asp

CHAPTER SUMMARY

1. Higher health care costs and an aging population mean that medical providers are experiencing financial pressures and have an increasing need for knowledgeable patient account specialists.

2. Some important duties performed by patient account specialists are: (a) verifying patients' medical insurance coverage and other payment arrangements; (b) ensuring that government regulations are satisfied in all billing activities; (c) resolving problems so that pending claims can be sent; (d) completing insurance forms with technical accuracy; (e) following up on claims and bills that are denied or not paid; (f) answering questions about charges and payments; and (g) using interpersonal skills in dealing with insurance companies and patients.

3. Inpatient hospital services—offered by acute care facilities, skilled nursing homes, intermediate care facilities, and hospice centers— provide health care for patients whose conditions or treatments usually require overnight stays in the facility. Outpatient services— offered by some hospital departments (such as an emergency department), ambulatory surgical centers, clinics, and home health agencies—provide care for patients whose conditions or treatments do not require overnight stays in a facility.

4. Indemnity medical insurance plans reimburse beneficiaries according to the contract's schedule of benefits in exchange for payment of a specified premium, deductible, and coinsurance. Managed care plans, in contrast, have contracts with both beneficiaries and providers that control the delivery and the cost of health care services. In exchange for lower premiums and other cost reductions, plan members agree to a reduced choice of health care providers and tighter regulation of access to services.

5. Private-sector payers of medical insurance benefits are either for-profit or nonprofit organizations. Most private health insurance is employer-sponsored, and much of this business belongs to very large national companies. Government-sponsored health care programs include Medicare, Medicaid, TRICARE, and CHAMPVA.

6. Payers use three main methods to pay hospitals for services: (a) cost-based reimbursement, under which payments are based on the costs of treating the patient; (b) per diem, a set rate per day of hospitalization; and (c) prospective payment, under which the payer determines national averages in advance for hospital stays based on patients' diagnoses, taking into account factors that affect patients' outcomes.

7. Hospitals are regulated by the federal government and by state law. Several organizations also accredit them, providing information about patient satisfaction with their services.

8. Each facility has its own written guidelines regarding billing procedures that need to be followed to ensure compliance with

federal regulations, private payer policies, and internal procedures. These policies are based on building good working relationships with patients and payers.

9 The Administrative Simplification provisions of the Health Insurance Portability and Accountability Act of 1996 (HIPAA, Title II) were written because of concern over the rising cost of health care. To cut back on the overhead associated with administrative and financial transactions, Title II required the Department of Health and Human Services to establish national standards for electronic health care transactions and national identifiers for providers, health plans, and employers, resulting in the current HIPAA Electronic Health Care Transactions and Code Sets standards. Title II also addressed the need for security and privacy of the health data that are exchanged electronically. This concern resulted in the HIPAA Privacy Rule and the HIPAA Security Rule. Finally, to enforce all the Administrative Simplification provisions legislated under HIPAA, the HIPAA Final Enforcement Rule was enacted.

✔ CHECK YOUR UNDERSTANDING

Write *T* or *F* to indicate whether you think the statement is true or false.

_____ 1. Employment opportunities for patient account specialists are increasing because providers need skilled staff to maximize revenue and ensure patient satisfaction.

_____ 2. Skilled nursing facilities are classified as outpatient facilities.

_____ 3. Emergency care involves a life-threatening situation.

_____ 4. At-home care is considered outpatient care.

_____ 5. An inpatient is a patient who is usually hospitalized for more than twenty-three hours.

_____ 6. The third party to a medical insurance contract is the policyholder.

_____ 7. Under an indemnity plan, the premium, deductible, and coinsurance are taken into account before the payer reimburses the policyholder.

_____ 8. Cost-based reimbursement sets a fixed amount the hospital is paid for every day a patient is hospitalized.

_____ 9. Managed care organizations have contracts with both providers and patients.

_____ 10. The Centers for Medicare and Medicaid Services also administer the TRICARE program.

_____ 11. The Administrative Simplification provisions are contained in Title V of HIPAA.

_____ 12. There are no restrictions on disclosing health information that neither identifies nor provides a reasonable basis to identify an individual.

Choose the best answers.

13. Under a prospective payment system, payments for services are
- **a.** set in advance
- **b.** calculated based on the provider's fees
- **c.** based on a discount to the provider's fees
- **d.** none of the above

14. The abbreviation HHA stands for
- **a.** home health agency
- **b.** home hospice agenda
- **c.** home health hospice
- **d.** home health administration

15. In managed care insurance plans, what is collected at the time of service?
- **a.** coinsurance
- **b.** premium
- **c.** per diem
- **d.** copayment

16. An ASC provides only
- **a.** radiology services
- **b.** outpatient surgery services
- **c.** mammograms
- **d.** none of the above

17. NCQA and the Joint Commission are
- **a.** patient financial services
- **b.** accrediting organizations
- **c.** patient funding systems
- **d.** none of the above

18. Under HIPAA, a clearinghouse is an example of a
- **a.** business associate
- **b.** provider
- **c.** managed care plan
- **d.** covered entity

19. The HIPAA Administrative Simplification provisions encourage the use of
- **a.** primary care physicians
- **b.** electronic data interchange (EDI)
- **c.** hospice care
- **d.** consumer-driven health plans

20. CMS is authorized to investigate complaints of noncompliance and enforce all of the following HIPAA standards *except*
- **a.** the Health Care Transactions and Code Sets Rule
- **b.** the National Employer Identifier Number (EIN) Rule
- **c.** the Privacy Rule
- **d.** the Security Rule

Internet Applications

1. Investigate the websites of local hospitals. Note the information they provide patients about admissions and billing. Also examine the other types of information, such as patient education topics and career opportunities, they offer.

2. Patient account specialists, depending on their employment, often earn professional credentials. To do so, they pass competency tests and then meet annual requirements for continuing education. Visit the websites of the following associations, studying their membership, career ladders, and credentialing processes.

   - ACA International—The Association of Credit and Collection Professionals
   - American Academy of Professional Coders
   - American Association of Healthcare Administrative Management
   - American Health Information Management Association (AHIMA)
   - American Medical Billing Association
   - Association of Healthcare Administrative Management
   - Healthcare Billing and Management Association
   - Healthcare Financial Management Association
   - Professional Association of Health Care Office Management

The Hospital Billing Process

LEARNING OUTCOMES

After completing this chapter, you will be able to define the key terms and:

1 Describe the main steps in the hospital billing process.

2 List the items that are entered into the patient accounting system to establish the patient's account during preregistration or registration.

3 Compare and contrast routine charges and ancillary charges.

4 Discuss the content and purpose of the charge description master.

5 Identify the main causes of billing errors.

6 Identify the advantages and disadvantages of using information technology in the hospital billing process.

KEY TERMS

- accounts receivable (AR)
- adjustments
- admission
- aging
- ancillary charges
- appeal
- attending physician
- charge description master (CDM)
- charge explode
- charge slip
- compliance
- discharge
- DNFB (discharged/not final bill) list
- electronic health record (EHR) system
- encounter form
- explanation of benefits (EOB)
- guarantor
- inpatient-only procedures
- medical necessity
- precertification
- professional services
- Quality Improvement Organization (QIO)
- referring physician
- remittance advice (RA)
- routine charges
- uncollectible account
- utilization review (UR)

Chapter 2 introduces the hospital billing process. When patients visit a hospital, the facility's business staff works together with the clinical staff of physicians and nurses and with the support staff, such as housekeeping and food service, to make the encounters as satisfactory as possible. Clinicians plan and perform medical treatments and procedures. The business staff follows a process that helps ensure that all services are documented and reimbursed.

After patients are registered, the medical care provided to them is documented in their medical records. Also recorded is the cost of each service or supply that is billable to a patient's account. At the end of the inpatient hospitalization or outpatient visit, the charges are collected and entered in the patient accounting system. Patient account specialists use this system to prepare insurance claims and patients' bills. This work is done carefully to avoid billing errors that might lead to incorrect charges, unpaid bills, or late payments. The process continues with sending insurance claims to third-party payers and bills to patients, processing payments, and collecting overdue accounts.

The Billing Process

The business goal is to collect the facility's **accounts receivable (AR)**—the payments that are due from payers and patients—as quickly as possible. The billing process relates to the following landmarks:

- **Admission,** for beginning or updating the patient's medical record, verifying patient insurance coverage, securing consent for release of information to payers, and collecting time-of-service payments as appropriate
- Treatment, during which various clinical services are provided and charges generated
- **Discharge** from the hospital (in some cases, with a transfer to another facility or as a result of the death of the patient), at which point the patient's medical record is processed and claims and bills are sent out

Business Office Duties

Hospitals generally have large business staffs who are responsible for performing the major duties in the billing process. People specialize in:

- *Admissions (often also called registration or access):* Gathering the patient's personal and financial information when the patient enters the hospital, or shortly before entering
- *Insurance verification:* Checking with patients' health plans to confirm coverage, ascertain benefits, and meet plan requirements
- *Health information management (HIM):* Organizing and maintaining patients' medical records, and assigning diagnostic and procedure codes
- *Information systems (IS):* Supporting the computer hardware and software used by the facility to electronically record all information about patients, physicians, health plans, and services, including the patient accounting system
- *Patient accounting:* Insurance claim preparation and submission, posting payments, billing
- *Collections:* Collecting overdue payments

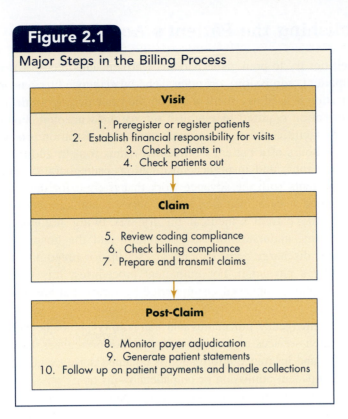

Figure 2.1

Major Steps in the Billing Process

Visit

1. Preregister or register patients
2. Establish financial responsibility for visits
3. Check patients in
4. Check patients out

Claim

5. Review coding compliance
6. Check billing compliance
7. Prepare and transmit claims

Post-Claim

8. Monitor payer adjudication
9. Generate patient statements
10. Follow up on patient payments and handle collections

Billing Process Steps

Business staff members are organized in a variety of ways. There are often separate departments for each function, but usually one management team directs them and coordinates the work. Teamwork is required throughout the billing process. Coordination and communication are essential, because work done at the front end—even before the patient arrives at the facility—helps reduce or eliminate problems after discharge, such as nonpayment of bills. The major steps in the billing process are shown in Figure 2.1.

Step 1　Preregister or Register Patients

The first step in the billing process is to preregister or register patients. Two main tasks are involved: scheduling appointments and establishing the patient's account.

Scheduling

The first step for either inpatients or outpatients is a physician's request for services. The order—the physician's diagnosis and treatment plan—may be sent to the facility by fax, letter, phone, or e-mail. A scheduling staff member, either in a central unit or in an individual department, schedules the service, such as an MRI or surgery. The **referring physician,** the patient, the appropriate department (such as surgery), and the **attending physician**—the doctor who is responsible for the patient's care during hospitalization—are notified of the appointment or admission.

Establishing the Patient's Account

Most facilities try to preregister patients who are scheduled for presurgical tests, inpatient admission, or other scheduled procedures or services. Preregistration is used to collect and enter the basic demographic and insurance information required to establish the patient's account. For inpatient stays, many facilities attempt to complete the preregistration process within twenty-four hours of a patient's scheduled admission. In addition to gathering demographic and insurance information, preregistration staff members help patients with the advance work that is done for their admission. A nurse called a case manager assists patients and family members in completing the patient's medical history, reviewing preoperative (pre-op) instructions, understanding the procedure and the hospital stay, and preparing for discharge care. Patients are set up for preadmission testing, if ordered by a physician. For outpatient procedures, this work may be handled in a phone conversation supported by forms that are mailed to the patient.

Although emergency procedures and admissions cannot be preregistered, most scheduled services are. If a patient does not preregister, then the basic demographic and insurance information is obtained during registration at the time of the inpatient admission or outpatient visit.

During preregistration or registration, the patient fills out an admission form similar to the one shown in Figure 2.2 on page 35. This information is then entered into the patient accounting system, which contains the following identifying data for the person:

- *Personal data:* Name, address, city, state, ZIP code, phone number, Social Security number, date of birth, and nearest relative or other emergency contact

- *Basic billing data:* Insurance and financial information, including employer, employer address and phone number, insurance company name, policy number, group number, and billing address

- *Medical information:* Referring physician's name, address, and phone number; patient's diagnosis and previous medical history; and the attending physician's name

- *Account number:* The patient account number assigned by the hospital for the current visit or hospitalization

- *Medical record number:* A number assigned to a new patient that is used to identify the patient's medical record, or chart; a returning patient's medical record number is already in the system

Correct and thorough work during the preregistration or registration process helps eliminate problems later in the process.

Step 2 Establish Financial Responsibility for Visits

The second step, determining financial responsibility for the visit, is important in the billing process because it helps ensure that patients will pay their bills when insurance benefits do not apply. This step involves two tasks: explaining the facility's payment policy to patients and verifying insurance coverage and precertification requirements.

Figure 2.2

Admission Form

ADMISSION FORM

611129 R1801

661129

PATIENT LAST NAME	FIRST NAME, INITIAL	MAIDEN	DOB	ADM DATE/TIME

PATIENT ADDRESS		PHONE NUMBER	MAR. STATUS

SOC. SEC. NO.	AGE	SEX	RACE	RELIGION	OCCUPATION

PATIENT'S EMPLOYER

PATIENT'S EMPLOYER ADDRESS	EMPLOYER TEL. NO.

PERSON TO NOTIFY #1	PERSON TO NOTIFY #2
HOME TEL. NO.	WORK TEL. NO.	HOME TEL. NO.	WORK TEL. NO.
STREET ADDRESS	CITY	STREET ADDRESS	CITY
STATE	ZIP	RELATIONSHIP	STATE	ZIP	RELATIONSHIP

HOSPITAL NUMBER ➜	MEDICAL RECORD NUMBER ➜	PREVIOUS NO.	MOTHER ACCT. NO.

CURRENT ADMISSION

ADM. SOURCE DESCRIPTION	ADM. PRIORITY	UNIT	ROOM/BED	TREATMENT CENTER
REFERRAL SOURCE DESCRIPTION	PATIENT TYPE DESCRIPTION	ADM. CLERK	COMMITTA;	IMPAIRMENT

ADMITTING DIAGNOSIS

ATTENDING PHYSICIAN	PRIMARY CARE PHYSICIAN
ADMITTING MD	INFANT MD	REFERRING PHYSICIAN

PATIENT INFORMATION:

INSURANCE INFORMATION

1
PAYOR NAME	PAYOR ADDRESS
POLICY NUMBER	CLAIM/GROUP NO.	GROUP NAME	INS. TEL. NO.
SUBSCRIBER NAME	SUBSCRIBER D.O.B.	TREATMENT AUTH. NO.	SOC. SEC. NO.

2
PAYOR NAME	PAYOR ADDRESS
POLICY NUMBER	CLAIM/GROUP NO.	GROUP NAME	INS. TEL. NO.
SUBSCRIBER NAME	SUBSCRIBER D.O.B.	TREATMENT AUTH. NO.	SOC. SEC. NO.

3
PAYOR NAME	PAYOR ADDRESS
POLICY NUMBER	CLAIM/GROUP NO.	GROUP NAME	INS. TEL. NO.
SUBSCRIBER NAME	SUBSCRIBER D.O.B.	TREATMENT AUTH. NO.	SOC. SEC. NO.

PATIENT ACCOUNT INFORMATION:

LIVING WILL	ORGAN DONOR

⬅ 1. Insert into ID bracelet
2. Tear off stub at perforation

MEDICAL RECORDS

⬅ 1. Insert into chart cover
2. Tear off stub at perforation

If patients must pay over time, a financial arrangement for a series of payments may be made. Such arrangements may be governed by specific laws in each state. If the payment policy of the facility covers adding finance charges on late accounts, it is acceptable to do so. The amount of the finance charge must comply with federal and state law.

COMPLIANCE GUIDE
Waivers for Uninsured and Underinsured Medicare Patients

Hospitals are able to provide discounts to uninsured and underinsured patients who cannot afford their hospital bills. They also may offer reductions or waivers of cost-sharing amounts for Medicare beneficiaries experiencing financial hardship. This means that a hospital may waive the copays and/or deductibles of Medicare beneficiaries at its own discretion, based on its own predetermined set of criteria. However, a hospital should understand that it will likely also be waiving its right to bill Medicare for any other services for that claim. As a general rule, no payer may be billed for any portion of a claim if copays and/or deductibles are waived. In addition to Medicare policy, most states also have rules to this effect.

Patient Payment Policy

Hospital stays can result in large bills. Educating patients about the billing process and their financial responsibilities helps create an environment in which they are more likely to pay for services promptly. Standard facility policy is to prepare patients for their financial obligations as early in the process as possible. This preparation reduces the amount due that must be billed or collected after the services have been performed.

Many facilities tell patients to contact their health plan to verify coverage and benefits before admission. This step causes patients to be aware of the bills they will incur. Facility staff members also examine the physician's order to determine the probable costs of the hospitalization. For example, some managed care organizations (MCOs) have contracts with hospitals that state the per diem allowance. Hospitalization costs for patients in these plans can be calculated quite accurately. Costs for other types of health plans that negotiate prospective payments are usually estimated when the patient is admitted and are updated after the insurance payment is received by the facility. If it is permitted by the particular plan, the balance due is billed to the patient.

Patient education, often handled by financial counseling staff members, includes:

- Reminding patients about their financial obligation to their health plans—copayments, deductibles, and coinsurance. In some cases, the patient's bill is the obligation of a **guarantor** rather than the patient. A guarantor—often a spouse, parent, or legal guardian—is a person other than the patient who has legal responsibility for the bill. For example, a patient might be covered by a spouse's employer-sponsored insurance plan.

- Informing patients that, after their insurer is contacted and the plan details checked, they will be given an estimate of the amount they will owe.

- Explaining to patients without insurance coverage that they are responsible for the complete payment.

- Asking patients scheduled for outpatient procedures to be prepared to pay the expected amount due at the time of service.

- Telling patients scheduled for inpatient services that they will be billed after discharge and after any insurance payments are received.

- Explaining that financial counseling services are available if the patient wishes to apply for financial assistance or to set up a payment plan.

- Going over the acceptable forms of payment—cash, check, or credit card.

Insurance Verification and Precertification Requirements

Insurance verification staff members contact patients' health plans and check their insurance benefits. They also check to be sure that the patient is currently eligible for the benefits. For example, if the health plan is a preferred provider organization (PPO), the facility must be in the plan's network for the patient to avoid higher costs. Most health care plans have automated systems, such as Internet-based or voice-activated response systems, to help facilities accomplish this task. Insurance verification staff members must also determine the first payer if more than one health plan covers the patient—this is the payer to whom the first claim will be sent. If Medicare is a payer, staff members must complete the MSP (Medicare as Secondary Payer) questionnaire to determine whether Medicare qualifies as the primary or secondary payer.

Precertification

Often **precertification**—also called preauthorization or authorization—is needed. A private-payer health plan that requires a "precert" has a policy that it must be notified several business days before a hospitalization or an elective surgical procedure. The notification allows the payer to authorize payment or recommend some other course of action. The Medicare program often requires a preadmission and preprocedure review as well. For certain surgical procedures and scheduled inpatient services, the conditions must be reviewed and approved before the services are provided. If the precertification policy is not followed, the payer may reduce benefits or deny payment.

Medical Necessity

Both private payers and Medicare, when examining requests for precertification, ask whether the planned procedure is medically necessary. The **medical necessity** of a procedure is defined by the HIAA (Health Insurance Institute of America) as "medical treatment that is appropriate and rendered in accordance with generally accepted standards of medical practice." Generally, the procedure must meet these conditions to be considered necessary:

- The procedure must be appropriate for the patient's diagnosis.
- The procedure is not elective (an elective procedure is not required by the physician to treat a condition but is elected to be done by the patient).
- The procedure is not experimental. The procedure must be approved by the appropriate federal regulatory agency, such as the Food and Drug Administration.
- The procedure is not performed for the convenience of the patient or the patient's family, rather than being essential for treatment.
- The procedure is furnished at an appropriate level. Straightforward diagnoses usually need uncomplicated procedures; complex or time-consuming procedures are reserved for complex conditions.

The medical necessity review is conducted because insurance plans cover only required procedures. Medicare hires state-based groups of physicians called **Quality Improvement Organizations (QIOs)** to conduct assessments of medical necessity. QIOs are paid by the government to review aspects of the Medicare program, including both quality and appropriateness of services provided and fees charged. Similarly, private payers hire **utilization review (UR)** companies that specialize in medical necessity reviews to monitor the necessity of admission and continued hospitalization during the patient's stay. Their onsite hospital reviewers may be called case managers or care coordinators.

Inpatient-Only Procedures

Medicare designates certain procedures as **inpatient-only procedures.** Based on the invasive nature of these procedures, Medicare has determined that a

$ $ **Billing Tip** $ $

Date and Time of Admission
Experienced patient account teams learn about billing rules related to the date and time of admission. For example, if patients have diagnostic tests at an outpatient department of the facility up to three days (seventy-two hours) before admission, Medicare requires those tests to be included on the hospital's inpatient bill. Registration staff members must ask about preadmission testing or other diagnostic services that have been done at a facility owned and operated by the hospital to comply with this rule.

$ $ **Billing Tip** $ $

Responsibility for the Inpatient-Only List
Generally the case management department has responsibility for keeping hospital staff aware of the inpatient-only list. During the registration process, case management staff members screen cases to determine whether a Medicare case involves an inpatient-only procedure. However, case management staff members should also educate scheduling and coding staff, as well as physicians, about the list to avoid mistakes. The list should be readily available and posted where staff members can quickly check it. Any procedures on the list that the hospital does not perform can be deleted to keep the list at a manageable size.

twenty-four-hour recovery time is required after surgery. The inpatient-only procedure list is reviewed and updated by CMS each year. Currently, the list contains over 1,700 codes. If one of these procedures is performed as an outpatient service, Medicare denies the entire stay, and the hospital must absorb the cost. For example, a case may involve an outpatient procedure; however, based on a subsequent finding, the physician performs a second inpatient-only procedure. The claim is denied because the patient was never admitted as an inpatient. Therefore, it is important for hospital staff to be aware of the inpatient-only list.

Step 3   Check Patients In

The third step is to check individuals in as patients of the facility. When patients arrive, detailed and complete demographic and medical information are verified at the registration desk, and outstanding procedures are taken care of. For example, the patient may bring a referral from a primary care physician that still needs to be processed. Both the front and back of insurance and other identification cards, such as drivers' licenses, are scanned or photocopied, and the copies are filed in the patient's record. If the health plan requires a copayment, the patient is told the correct amount. Copayments should always be collected at the time of service. Some practices collect copayments before services are received; others collect them afterward. If the patient owes a deductible, he or she should also be asked about paying the deductible at this time.

Patient Consent

At check-in, patients must give their consent in writing for planned procedures. Facilities use a standard form for this purpose. Also, when patients register, the HIPAA Privacy Rule requires patients to give their consent before the facility can disclose any information about their stay. The form used for this purpose is known as the HIPAA Privacy Disclosure. The patient registrar also gives the patient a copy of the hospital's Notice of Privacy Practices, which explains patient rights under HIPAA and provides examples of how the facility will use the information in the process of treatment, payment for services, and hospital operations (TPO).

Depending on the type of insurance the patient has, an assignment of benefits form may also be filled in at this point. On this form, the patient indicates whether any payment received from the insurance carrier should be sent directly to the provider.

Any other legal forms or waivers that apply are also secured at this time. Often advance directives, also called living wills, are filed. These written documents state how a patient wants medical decisions to be made on his or her behalf if he or she becomes incapacitated. Hospitals receiving Medicare and Medicaid funds are required by federal law to provide patients with information on advance directives before check-in.

Step 4   Check Patients Out

When an inpatient is discharged, the physician provides a discharge order or plan. Discharge planning recommendations are also prepared by a case-worker, social worker, or designated discharge planner who arranges the actual checkout for the patient. Copies of the discharge order and the discharge planning recommendations are filed in the patient's medical record. The time and date of the discharge are noted in the provider's ADT (admissions, discharges, and transfers) system. The time and date of discharge are important elements on an insurance claim as they determine the patient's length of stay.

For outpatient surgical procedures, patients usually spend time in a recovery room area until approved for discharge. If required, postdischarge care instructions are also provided. For other types of outpatient visits, such as for a routine mammography, there is no formal discharge procedure, but the date and time of the service received are entered in the facility's computer system by the department providing the service. This information is an important part of billing, as every service charge on an outpatient claim must be itemized and must include the date of service.

Step 5   Review Coding Compliance

After the patient is checked out, the patient's medical record is reviewed by the health information management (HIM) department. The HIM department staff review the documentation in the medical record and assign diagnosis and procedure codes. The diagnosis and procedure codes assigned must be compliant with official coding guidelines. **Compliance** means actions that satisfy official requirements. In the area of coding, compliance refers to following official coding guidelines. In addition, the codes should be logically connected so that the payer understands the medical necessity of the procedures. After diagnosis and procedure codes are selected, software programs check the codes for errors.

Reviewing coding compliance is an important step in the billing process; incorrect diagnosis and procedure codes usually lead to claim rejection, which holds up the payment process and may lead to lost revenue. The patient account specialist works closely with the HIM department to be sure that the specific information the health plan requires is documented in the medical record.

Patients' Records: Working with the HIM Department

Facilities are required to provide patient care at the appropriate medical and legal standard. To document that the appropriate level of care has been provided, facilities keep careful records of their work.

Standards for hospital patient medical records are set by the Joint Commission. The hospital's own bylaws and Medicare regulations also influence medical record standards. Each patient's record has a unique number. The record, in general, contains notes by the attending physician and other treating physicians; nurses' notes; pathology, radiology, operative, and laboratory reports; patient demographics; and a correspondence section with signed consent forms and other documents. The record shows whether the planned procedure was carried out or canceled, and the reason if it did not occur. As required by HIPAA, the confidentiality and security of patients' medical records are guarded by all hospital staff members.

Among the items that may be added to the record during the hospitalization are:

- History and physical examination, describing the physician's interview and examination of the patient, which should be completed within twenty-four hours of the patient's admission
- An operative report, describing surgery performed
- An anesthesia report, for the anesthesia during the surgery
- A pathology report, if tissue was removed and examined
- A recovery room record, describing the patient's condition after surgery and anesthesia
- The patient's medication records
- A discharge summary, including the reason for the admission, test findings, procedures done, response to treatments, condition at discharge, and follow-up care instructions

The health information management department is responsible for maintaining patients' medical records. It has three major tasks:

1. *Medical transcription:* Transcribing physicians' dictated reports about the treatments and procedures they performed
2. *Medical records:* Assembling and analyzing patients' medical records, making sure they are complete and accurate, and protecting them from unauthorized disclosure
3. *Medical coding:* Assigning codes to patients' diagnoses and procedures

These tasks are performed during a patient's hospitalization. For example, after surgery, the operative report and the anesthesia report are dictated by the physicians who did the operation, transcribed by medical transcriptionists, and signed by the dictating physicians. The last report—the discharge summary—must wait until the patient leaves the hospital.

Step 6   Check Billing Compliance

Checking billing compliance means applying knowledge of various payer guidelines in order to analyze what can be billed on the claim. Although there is a separate charge for each service a patient receives or supply item used during a hospital visit, not all services and supplies are billable as charged. For example, some payers "roll up," or include, charges for particular services or items in the payment for other services. Inpatient billing and outpatient billing also follow two different payment systems, each with its own set of rules for reporting charges on a claim. Following these rules when preparing claims results in billing compliance. Patient account specialists must use their knowledge of payer guidelines in preparing claims.

Charge Collection

The first step in checking billing compliance is to gather all the patient's charges. In fully automated systems, when a department enters the service code for a service into the computer, the charge for the service is automatically posted to the patient's bill. In this way, charges accumulate in the patient's account throughout the patient's stay. If a facility does not have a fully automated system, the charges need to be collected and entered as a separate step. Charge collection, also called charge capture, describes an important activity—gathering charges from a dozen or more hospital departments that may provide services to a patient. Hospital charges cover services such as:

- Room charges (for inpatients)
- Medications
- Related tests and procedures, such as laboratory workups and X-rays
- Supplies or equipment used during surgery or therapy
- The amount of time spent in an operating room, recovery room, or intensive care unit

Patients are charged according to the type of accommodations and services they receive. For example, the rate for a private room is higher than the rate for a semiprivate room, and intensive care unit or recovery room charges are higher than charges for standard rooms. When patients are transferred to these various services, this activity is tracked. In an outpatient or an emergency department encounter, there is no accommodation (room and board) charge; instead, there is a visit charge.

Routine Charges

Inpatient room and board charges and outpatient visits are **routine charges.** A routine charge is the total of the costs of all supplies that are customarily used to provide the service. For example, the inpatient room charge includes the use of bedding and other linens. Supplies such as those listed below are included in the routine charge and should not be billed separately:

- Admission kits and prep kits
- Lubricants
- Oxygen
- Irrigation solutions
- Drapes
- Gloves
- Reusable items such as microscopes and humidifiers

Ancillary Charges

In addition to routine charges, most patients receive other services, such as medications, during hospitalization. They incur **ancillary charges** for each specific service.

Ancillary charges include costs for:

- Operating room
- Anesthesia
- Blood products and administration
- Pharmacy
- Radiology services, such as X-rays, CT scans, MRIs, and PET scans
- Laboratory
- Medical, surgical, and central supplies (each item taken from inventory must be billed out)
- Physical, occupational, speech, and inhalation therapy

Charge Slips

The charge collection process involves posting charges from each appropriate department to the patient accounting system. Each department, whether inpatient or outpatient, has its own **charge slip** (also called an **encounter form** or charge ticket). Most hospitals have from ten to fifty different charge slips. Figure 2.3A and 2.3B on pages 43–44 shows a charge slip for a pediatric cost center.

The charge slip format lists the typical major services the department provides. The ordering physician or the technician who does the service checks off the general heading that describes the service. When this choice is posted, the patient accounting system—in a process called **charge explode**—automatically bills all the components of that major service. For example, the physician may select a particular laboratory test on the lab charge slip. When this service is posted, the bill reflects the original test and the materials associated with it—all the individual billable items of that service.

Hold Period

It is not possible to collect all the billing information for a patient's services at one time as different departments require different reporting times. Generally a hospital allows a hold period of from one to five days after an inpatient has been discharged for all inpatient charges to be reported by the various service departments. Charges for outpatient services are usually reported within seven to ten days.

Charge Description Master

When charges are posted to a patient's account, the details of each charge are picked up from a central file in the facility's patient accounting system called the **charge description master (CDM).** The CDM, also known as the chargemaster, is a computerized list of charge codes for all services or items that the hospital can bill to a patient, payer, or other provider. The CDM contains charge codes for all available hospital services. Each listing in the CDM contains a unique charge code (sometimes referred to as a service code or a hospital procedure code) that links it to the services listed on a hospital charge slip.

Some procedure codes are *hard-coded* in the computer system, so that whenever the procedure code from a charge slip is entered, the corresponding charge is posted to the patient's bill. Other procedure codes are *soft-coded,* meaning that the Health Information Management Department must select the appropriate procedure code for the service described in the patient's chart before the code can be entered into the computer and the charge posted to the patient's account.

In addition to a unique charge code, each listing in the CDM also contains a description of the service, a price for the service, and other data required for creating an insurance claim. Figure 2.4 on page 45 shows part of a typical CDM covering cardiac services. A CDM may contain many thousands of charges, since it is basically a menu of all the services and supplies that can be provided to patients by a facility.

The CDM database identifies the hospital department (such as radiology) and subcategory (such as nuclear medicine), the charge code for the service, the description, a medical code (when required), a standard claim form revenue code (RC), and the price. The department and subcategory

Figure 2.3A

Charge Slip

Encounter Form (F-3993 Rev. 8/07)

(Pediatric (94160)) — COST CENTER

Primary Care Center

Service Date:

Referring Provider: NPI:

Clinic: Select One Below

Primary Care   (Pedi ○ 4040) — SERVICE AREA

Evaluation and Management Services: (Provider)

New Patient	Level I	○ 1015	Initial Preventative	<1 yr	○ 0005
	Level II	○ 1016		1–4 yrs	○ 0006
	Level III	○ 1017 — CHARGE		5–11 yrs	○ 0007
	Level IV	○ 1018		12–17 yrs	○ 0008
	Level V	○ 1019		18–39 yrs	○ 0009
Established Patient	Level I	○ 1022	Estab. Preventative	<1 yr	○ 0010
	Level II	○ 1023		1–4 yrs	○ 0011
	Level III	○ 1024		5–11 yrs	○ 0012
	Level IV	○ 1025		12–17 yrs	○ 0013
	Level V	○ 1026		18–39 yrs	○ 0014
Consultation	Level I	○ 1028	Prevent Med, Indiv	15 min	○ 0015
	Level II	○ 1029		30 min	○ 0016
	Level III	○ 1030		45 min	○ 0017
	Level IV	○ 1031		60 min	○ 0018
	Level V	○ 1032			
			Prevent Med, Group	30 min	○ 0003
				60 min	○ 0004
No Charge Visit	Priv. OPS	○ 1020	Parent Child Assessment, New		○ 0001
	Hospital Clinic	○ 1021		Return	○ 0002

Immunizations:

Scheduled immunizations:

1st DTAP, 2 mos	○ 0101	1st HEPB, birth	○ 0116	Other Immunizations:		
2nd DTAP, 4 mos	○ 0102	2nd HEPB, 2 mos	○ 0117	Tetanus	○ 0130	
3rd DTAP, 6 mos	○ 0103	3rd HEPB, 3 mos	○ 0118	DT (under 7)	○ 0131	
4th DTAP, 12-18 mos	○ 0104	1st OPV, 2 mos	○ 0119	Td (under 7)	○ 0132	
5th DTAP, 4-6 yrs	○ 0105	2nd OPV, 2 mos	○ 0120	Influenza	○ 0133	
1st HIB, 2 mos	○ 0106	3rd OPV, 2 mos	○ 0121	Hepatitus A	○ 0134	
2nd HIB, 4 mos	○ 0107	4th OPV, 2 mos	○ 0122	Hep B, 11-12 yrs	○ 0135	
3rd HIB, 6 mos	○ 0108	1st IPV, 2 mos	○ 0123	Pneumococcal	○ 0136	
4th HIB, 12-15 mos	○ 0109	2nd IPV, 2 mos	○ 0124	Varicella>12 yrs	○ 0137	
		3rd IPV, 2 mos	○ 0125			
1st MMR, 12-15 mos	○ 0114	4th IPV, 2 mos	○ 0126			
2nd MMR, 4-6, 11-12 yrs	○ 0115	5th IPV, 2 mos	○ 0127			
		Varicella, 12-18 mos	○ 0128			
		Td, 11-16 yrs	○ 0129			

Performed by PCC:						
Blood Draw	○ 0138	Catheterization	○ 0151		EKG tracing	○ 0157
Complex Bld Draw	○ 0139	Colposcopy	○ 0152	70.21	Hearing Test	○ 0158
Blood Draw,<3 yrs	○ 0140	Incision&drainage	○ 0153	86.04	Infusion, 1st hour	○ 0159
Tine Test	○ 0141	Lumbar puncture	○ 0154	03.31	Infusion, each addl hr	○ 0160
Glucose Monitor	○ 0142	Remove imp. cerumen	○ 0155	96.52	Nebulization	○ 0161
Hemaque/POC	○ 0143	Acoustic reflex test	○ 0156		Peak Flow	○ 0162
Urine dip stick	○ 0144				Pulse oximetry	○ 0163
Pregnancy test	○ 0145				Injection Vaccines (state)	○ 0164
PPD	○ 0146				Procedure tray	○ 0165
Hemocult slide	○ 0147				Lead/POC	○ 0166
Wet mount	○ 0148				Injection, therapeutic (other)	○ 0168

Figure 2.3B

Charge Slip (continued)

Other Requested Services:

Education

_____	Asthma Education (V6549)
_____	Helmet Class Education (V6543)
_____	Bike Class Education (V6543)
_____	Breast Feeding (V201)

Diagnosis: Enter diagnosis as: 1 (primary), 2 (secondary), 3 (tertiary)

_____	314.01	ADHD	_____	279.3	Immune Deficiency
_____	285.9	Anemia	_____	684	Impetigo
_____	714.30	Arthritis (R/Juv)	_____	782.4	Jaundice
_____	493.90	Asthma	_____	V72.6	Laboratory Exam
_____	493.91	Asthma w/status	_____	984.0	Lead Poisoning (E86.15)
_____	493.92,	Asthma, w/acute	_____	V65.3	Nutrition Counseling
_____	493.0	Asthma, Extrinsic	_____	382.9	Otitis Media
_____	V58.3	Atten-dressing/suture	_____	462	Pharyngitis
_____	312.9	Behavioral Problems	_____	783.40	Physiological Dev., Uns.
_____	466.19	Bronchiolitis	_____	486	Pneumonia
_____	789.00	Colic	_____	V741	PPD Reading
_____	372.30	Conjunctivitis	_____	110.9	Ringworm
_____	783.42	Del. milestones	_____	133.0	Scabies
_____	692.9	Dermatitis/Eczema	_____	V62.3	School Problem
_____	110.9	Dermatophytosis	_____	780.39	Seizure Disorder
_____	691.0	Diaper Rash	_____	783.43	Short stature
_____	787.91	Diarrhea	_____	780.57	Sleep Apnea
_____	V65.3	Dietary Counsel	_____	378.9	Strabismus
_____	250.01	DM, Juvenile Onset	_____	112.0	Thrush/Oral
_____	692.9	Eczema	_____	465.9	URI
_____	V71.89	Eval/other spec cond	_____	599.0	UTI
_____	783.41	Failure to Thrive	_____	079.99	Viral Syndrome
_____	V61.9	Family Dysfunction	_____	V20.2	Well Child (Once per year—Do not use w/acute code)
_____	780.6	Fever			
_____	008.8	Gastroenteritis Viral			
_____	959.01	Head Trauma (CIS)			
_____	785.2	Heart Murmur			

Other Diagnoses:

_____

_____

_____

Next Appointment   **Length of Visit** _____ **20 Min.** _____ **40 Min.** _____ **OK to overbook**

Provider (If Different From Provider of Today's Visit) _____

Primary Provider Name (Today's Visit)

Print _____   Signature _____

Figure 2.4

Charge Description Master

DATE 02/04/09   CHARGE DESCRIPTION MASTER   SMS6517

CHARGES

DEPT. NO. 53601   CARDIAC LABORATORY

SERVICE DESCRIPTION	CHARGE CODE	SERVICE TYPE	CURRENT PRICE	POINT VALUE	PROF FEE FLAT AMT	CPT4 CODE	UB04 CODE	INS CODE	GL KEY	DATE INACTIVE
ETT LOW LEVEL	53601401-7	0	217.08	75.0000	0.00	93017	0481	41	585	00/00/00
ETT PERF LOW LEVEL	53061402-5	0	217.08	75.0000	0.00	93017	0481	41	585	00/00/00
ETT PHARM STRESS	53061403-3	0	217.08	75.0000	0.00	93017	0481	41	585	00/00/00
MYO PERF WALL MOT	53061404-1	0	107.97	13.0000	0.00	78478	0340	17	579	00/00/00
MYO PERF WALL EF	53061405-8	0	107.97	13.0000	0.00	78480	0340	17	579	00/00/00
ISOTOPE TC-99M	53061406-6	0	42.53	3.0000	0.00	A4641	0636	17	579	00/00/00
TCO S&I	53061410-8	0	1,937.96	30.0000	0.00	75894	0320	07	580	00/00/00
TRANS-CATH OCCL	53061411-6	0	2,832.63	300.0000	0.00	37204	0360	41	580	00/00/00
STENT FIRST	53061450-4	0	4,340.56	120.0000	0.00	92980	0481	41	580	00/00/00
STENT ADDL	53061451-2	0	4,340.56	120.0000	0.00	92981	0481	41	580	00/00/00
STENT C/C W/DS	53061453-8	0	2,730.00	1.0000	0.00	C1874	0278	07	580	00/00/00
STENT C/C W/O DS	53061455-3	0	2,730.00	1.0000	0.00	C1875	0278	07	580	00/00/00
STENT NC/NC W/DS	53601457-9	0	2,730.00	1.0000	0.00	C1876	0278	07	580	00/00/00
STENT NC/NC W/ODS	53601459-5	0	2,730.00	1.0000	0.00	C1877	0278	07	580	00/00/00
C&C, S&I R/L	53061500-6	0	257.63	22.0000	0.00	93555	0481	41	580	00/00/00
C&C, S&I OTH	53061501-4	0	391.27	34.0000	0.00	93556	0481	41	580	00/00/00
C&C, W/BYP, S&I R/L	53061502-2	0	252.27	29.0000	0.00	93555	0481	41	580	00/00/00
C&C, W/BYP, S&I OTH	53601503-0	0	383.15	43.0000	0.00	93556	0481	41	580	00/00/00
PEDI C&C/S&I R/L	53061504-8	0	252.47	10.0000	0.00	93555	0481	41	580	00/00/00
COR, S&I R/L	53061508-9	0	254.50	20.0000	0.00	93555	0481	41	580	00/00/00
COR, S&I OTH	53061509-7	0	386.52	30.0000	0.00	93556	0481	41	580	00/00/00
COR W/BYP, S&I R/L	53061510-5	0	262.69	26.0000	0.00	93555	0481	41	580	00/00/00
COR W/BYP, S&I OTH	53061511-3	0	398.95	39.0000	0.00	93556	0481	41	580	00/00/00
PEDI L THT/S&I R/L	53061512-1	0	209.83	13.0000	0.00	93555	0481	41	580	00/00/00
LVG, LH CATH	53061514-7	0	1,089.00	100.0000	0.00	93510	0481	41	580	00/00/00
LVG, S&I R/L	53061515-4	0	179.14	17.0000	0.00	93555	0481	41	580	00/00/00
AORTOG. LH CATH	53061516-2	0	903.19	157.0000	0.00	93510	0481	41	580	00/00/00
AORTOG, S&I OTH	53601517-0	0	225.63	39.0000	0.00	93556	0481	41	580	00/00/00
COR ONLY, LH CATH	53601518-8	0	1,110.05	138.0000	0.00	93510	0481	41	580	00/00/00
COR ONLY, S&I OTH	53601519-6	0	277.31	35.0000	0.00	93556	0481	41	580	00/00/00
2D,M-M COMPL ECHO	53601600-4	0	300.66	60.0000	0.00	93307	0481	41	584	00/00/00
IMAGING LIMITED	53601602-0	0	148.81	45.0000	0.00	93308	0481	41	584	00/00/00
DOPPLER COMPLETE	53601604-6	0	179.82	45.0000	0.00	93320	0481	41	584	00/00/00

codes and the charge code with its description are assigned by the facility. Often the department code is embedded in the charge code; for example, the first five digits of a charge code may indicate the department code (as seen in Figure 2.4). Following is a brief example of several lines taken from a CDM:

Department Code	Charge Code	Description	RC	CPT Code	Units	Price
10004 (Lab/Chemistry)	2122	Electrolyte	301	80051	1	$ 61.70
72560 (Radiology)	1601	Wrist, complete	320	73110	1	$118.00
10105 (Pharmacy)	3377	Aspirin Tab	250		1	$ 5.00

In the first entry, charge code 2122 is for an electrolyte panel that costs $61.70. This service is provided by the chemistry section of the laboratory department. In the second line, service code 1601 is performed by the radiology department and represents a complete X-ray of the wrist, with a charge of $118. In the third line, service code 3377 represents a pharmacy charge of $5.00 for an aspirin.

When reviewing a CDM, it is important to understand that the charge amount listed is not necessarily the amount that an insurance plan will agree to pay. The actual amount of reimbursement depends on the contractual agreement between the insurance plan and the hospital, whether the service is part of the patient's benefits, and whether the service is already paid for as part of another procedure and therefore not separately payable, among other factors. However, the charge listed in the CDM is the amount that is reported on an insurance claim. It becomes the basis for establishing the reimbursement amount.

Maintaining the Charge Description Master

Because the accuracy of hospital claims is tied directly to the accuracy of the codes contained in the CDM, hospitals maintain appropriate controls over the maintenance of the CDM. When procedure codes and revenue codes are added, changed, or deleted, a formal standardized process is followed. When a change is made to the CDM, the many departments that are affected must also be informed.

If possible, the CDM should be maintained on an ongoing basis. If it cannot be updated on a daily basis as needed, however, it should at least be updated quarterly. This is because some of the fields in the CDM contain medical procedure codes that are updated quarterly by CMS. These codes, called HCPCS and CPT codes, are used to identify outpatient nonsurgical services and tests. The codes are picked up from the CDM automatically, along with the charge codes, when an outpatient claim is created.

The CDM also contains insurance codes, known as revenue codes, that are picked up automatically when an insurance claim is created and that need to be updated regularly. (Revenue codes are a standard system used in hospital claims for indicating the department in which the service originated.) The incorrect use of HCPCS/CPT codes and revenue codes on a claim usually leads to claim rejection. Consistently using incorrect codes may also cause a hospital to be suspected of fraud. Therefore, maintenance of the CDM, which is a team effort among all the hospital service departments, the patient accounting department, medical coders, and the information systems department, is an important priority in the billing process.

After the account holding period for reporting charges ends, the patient account specialist can review the collected charges in the patient's account against the CDM and the patient's medical record to verify that all charges have been posted and that the details of the services are correct. If the patient has insurance coverage, the specialist verifies that the billing information is correct and sufficient based on a thorough knowledge of what payers require. An insurance claim for the account can then be created.

Step 7   Prepare and Transmit Claims

A major step in the billing process is the preparation of accurate, timely claims. A health care claim communicates information about the diagnosis, procedures, and charges to a payer. It is a request for reimbursement for services rendered. Patient account specialists use the facility's patient accounting system to prepare insurance claims and patients' bills. Although the computer systems are different in detail, in general their features are similar. They handle typical accounts receivable tasks, such as:

- Updating demographics (patient, guarantor, employer, and insurance information)
- Managing payer information, such as copayment, deductible, coinsurance, and other data
- Managing billing information, such as codes for patient type or account type
- Generating insurance claims and bills
- Posting payments, charges, adjustments, and comments to patient accounts

Timely Claims

Patient account specialists are knowledgeable about each payer's timeline for the submission of claims, and they monitor the release of claims to make sure they are within these guidelines.

Bills are generated and mailed to patients who do not have insurance coverage. Most facilities use a summary type of bill rather than a detailed bill. However, a patient may request a detailed bill, also called an itemized bill.

Many facilities use a separate software program called a claim editor or "scrubber" to test claims before sending them to payers. This program supplies feedback on problems with the various entries on the claim and their relationships to each other. For example, if the bill is for an outpatient, the claim should not have an accommodation charge. If a device such as a pacemaker is charged, it should match the procedure that was done. The patient account specialist reviews the program's results and investigates problems to create a correct claim.

Most hospital claims are sent electronically—that is, they are transmitted via computer—and a few are printed and mailed to the payer. Most facilities aim for bills and claims to "drop"—that is, to be created—within a specific period of time after patients are discharged.

Billing Errors

Billing errors are the source of two problems. First, billing errors lead to claims that insurance companies either do not pay or pay only partially. Second, billing errors can also be the cause of an even more serious situation— investigations by government regulators who suspect that the errors are not innocent mistakes, but instead are fraud. To avoid either situation, patient account specialists work to help avoid the following inaccuracies:

- Billing for services and supplies that are not documented in the patient's medical record

  EXAMPLE: The bill lists a cost for physical therapy, but the service is not mentioned in the record.

- Billing for services that are insufficiently documented in the patient's medical record

  EXAMPLE: The bill lists an antibiotic, but the physician did not document a condition that necessitated the drug.

- Billing twice for the same service (double billing)

  EXAMPLE: The bill lists two units of sodium serum, but only one was administered.

- Billing for medically unnecessary services

  EXAMPLE: Although the usual medical practice is to conduct four diagnostic tests for a particular condition, five were used. The fifth is considered unnecessary.

- Billing for services that are included in other charges

  EXAMPLE: The hospital's bill charged for bandages, which are a part of the routine charge and should not be additionally billed.

- Billing inaccurate information about providers or the wrong providers

  EXAMPLE: The physician tax identification numbers are incorrect.

Step 8 Monitor Payer Adjudication

After insurance claims have been transmitted, patient account specialists follow procedures to ensure that bills are paid on time and in full. The money due from health plans, as well as payments due from patients, add up to the hospital's accounts receivable—the money that is needed to run the facility.

Payers review claims by following a process known as *adjudication*. This term means that the payer puts a claim through a series of steps designed to judge whether it should be paid. What the payer decides about the claim—to pay it in full, to pay some of it, or to deny it—is explained on a report sent back to the hospital with the payment. When patients are covered by more than one health plan, the additional plans are then sent claims based on the amount still due. In most cases, the first plan forwards the claim to the second health plan automatically, together with its own report on how much it has paid and how much is still due. The patient account specialist must keep track of where each claim is in the adjudication process.

Claims Follow-up

When claims have not been paid, patient account specialists contact insurance companies. The timeline for follow-up is set by department practice. Typical policy is to follow up after thirty days, after which the payer has another thirty days to decide whether to pay the claim.

Often payers have questions about claims, and additional information must be supplied. For example, patient account specialists may need to obtain corrected insurance information from patients. Some payers request copies of medical records. Keeping good relationships with payers is very important in maintaining a smooth payment process.

Payment Processing

Payments from insurance companies are received, authenticated, and logged by the facility. A payment, which may be an electronic financial transfer directly to a facility's bank or a check, comes with a **remittance advice (RA),** often called a "remit." The RA is a report that explains each claim in detail, listing charges and the payer's actions. Patients automatically receive a printed copy of this report, which is called an **explanation of benefits (EOB).**

Payments sent electronically are automatically posted to the right bill using the patient accounting system. Check amounts are entered in the correct account in the system. The amount of the payment depends on the hospital's contract with the payer. Seldom do the hospital's fees and the payer's fees match exactly. Most payers have their own fee schedules for providers with whom they have contractual arrangements. The patient accounts specialist compares each payment with the claim to check that:

- All procedures that were listed on the claim also appear on the payment transaction
- Any unpaid charges are explained
- The codes on the payment transactions match those on the claim
- The payment listed for each procedure is correct according to the contract with the payer

When discrepancies are found and an incorrect payment is received, the patient account specialist investigates. The payer may have made a mistake or may have decided not to pay the claim in full. Often, payers reduce the amount of the payment based on the relationship between the diagnosis reported and the type of service received. In either case, a claim **appeal**— a written request for a review of reimbursement—may be sent by the facility. It is a formal way of asking the payer to reconsider its decision regarding a partially or fully denied claim. If a claim is denied, an appeal is the only recourse.

If a claim is rejected by an insurance carrier, as opposed to denied, it means that the claim may be corrected and resubmitted. If a claim has been rejected, for example, because of duplicate charges, a medical documentation error, nonbillable charges, or the like, the patient account specialist makes the necessary corrections, resubmits the claim, and again monitors the result.

Step 9   Generate Patient Statements

In most cases, payments from health plans do not fully pay bills, and patients must pay the balance. Therefore, after RAs are received and posted, patient statements (bills) are generated. Each statement shows the dates and services provided; any time-of-service payments made by the patient, such as copayments or deductibles; the insurance carrier payment; and the balance due. These statements are mailed periodically to patients with balances due.

Step 10   Follow up on Patient Payments and Handle Collections

Patient account specialists must analyze patient accounts regularly for overdue bills. When payments are later than permitted under the hospital's financial policy, a collection process may be started. The collection process really begins with effective communication with patients before treatments about their responsibility to pay for services. However, every facility has some patients who do not pay their bills when they receive their statements. Reasons for not paying range from forgetfulness or inability to pay to dissatisfaction with the services or charges.

Aging reports printed by the patient accounting system are the starting point for collections, since they show which payments are due or overdue (termed *past due*). The information systems staff sets up the computer program to print aging reports on a regular schedule, such as daily or weekly.

Aging begins based on the date of the bill. For each account, an aging report shows the name of the payer or patient, the last payment, and the amount of charges in categories such as:

- *Current:* 0 to 30 days
- *Past:* 31 to 60 days
- *Past:* 61 to 90 days
- *Past:* Over 91 days

Each facility sets its own procedures for the collection process. Large bills have priority over smaller ones. Usually, an automatic reminder notice and a second statement are mailed when a bill has not been paid thirty days after it was issued. Some facilities phone patients who have thirty-day overdue accounts. If the bill is not then paid, a series of collection letters is generated at intervals, each more stringent in its tone and more direct in its approach. An outside collection agency may be used to pursue large unpaid bills. The agency's fee is usually a percentage of the amount collected.

Collections from payers are considered business collections, but collections from patients are consumer collections and are regulated by federal and state law. The Fair Debt Collection Practices Act of 1977 and the Telephone Consumer Protection Act of 1991 regulate debt collections, forbidding unfair practices such as making threats and using any form of deception or violence to collect a debt. Hospital billing disputes involving individuals are covered by the dispute settlement procedures provided under the federal Fair Credit Billing Act (FCBA), which is enforced by the Federal Trade Commission. Dispute settlement procedures cover such problems as:

- Unauthorized charges
- Charges that list the wrong date or amount
- Charges for items that the patient did not accept or that were not provided
- Charges containing mathematical errors

Patients do not have to pay disputed charges while the hospital is investigating.

Writing Off Uncollectible Accounts

If no payment has been made after the collection process, the patient account specialist follows facility policy on bills that are not expected to be collected. Usually, if all collection attempts have been exhausted and the cost of continuing to pursue payment is higher than the amount to be collected, the process is ended. In this case, the amount is called an **uncollectible account** or bad debt and is written off (subtracted) from expected revenues.

Transactions should not be deleted in the patient accounting program, because deleting them could be interpreted by an auditor as a fraudulent act. Instead, corrections, changes, and write-offs are made with **adjustments** to existing transactions. The adjusting entries give both the facility office and the patient a history of events in case there is a billing inquiry or an audit.

The Hospital Billing Process and Information Technology

In 2004 the federal government announced a new initiative to create a seamless national health information system—including an electronic health record (EHR) for virtually every American—by the year 2014. Because of HIPAA requirements, which require the majority of hospital claims to be transmitted electronically, hospitals are already using patient accounting software to automate the claim preparation process—for managing patient accounts, for creating claims and transmitting them to payers, and for electronic reimbursement. The next major step in the information technology movement in health care management is the implementation of **electronic health record (EHR) systems** to replace paper files and the interfacing of these systems with current accounting systems. EHR systems capture and store each patient's clinical data electronically, including everything from laboratory tests to digital imaging records. While the startup cost for implementing an EHR system in a hospital is very high, EHR systems have many advantages:

- *Immediate access to health information:* The EHR is accessible from workstations in all the departments of the hospital as well as from remote sites such a physician's office. Retrieval of information from an EHR is almost immediate, which is critical in emergency situations.

- *Computerized management of physician orders:* Physicians can enter orders for medications, tests, and other services at any time. This information is then available throughout the patient's hospital visit.

- *Clinical decision support:* An EHR system can provide access to the latest medical research to facilitate medical decision making.

- *Automated alerts and reminders:* The system can provide medical alerts and reminders for staff members, ensuring that patients are scheduled for required tests or for regular preventive practices. Alerts can also be created to identify patient safety issues, such as possible drug interactions.

- *Electronic communication and connectivity:* An EHR system can provide easily accessible communication between physicians and staff members and, in some systems, between physicians and patients.

- *Patient support tools:* Some EHR programs offer tools that allow patients to access their health records and to request appointments electronically. The programs also offer patient education on health topics and instructions on preparing for common medical tests, such as HDL cholesterol tests.

- *Administrative reporting tools:* The EHR may include administrative tools including reporting systems that enable hospitals to comply with federal and state reporting requirements for clinical data.

- *Error reduction:* An EHR can decrease medical errors that are a result of illegible chart notes, as notes are no longer entered manually. The notes are entered electronically using a computer or a handheld device.

Similarly, an electronic encounter form contained in the handheld device or computer can be used by a physician to enter the services rendered during patient encounters, allowing for greater accuracy and consistency in reporting services rendered.

Many electronic devices and software programs for capturing patient information during the admissions process can be used with an EHR system. Some examples include:

- *Scanners:* Used to create digital images of patients' insurance cards or other forms of identification, such as driver's licenses, as well as physician orders during the admissions process
- *Electronic signature pads:* Electronic clipboard devices that capture legally binding signatures from patients, or electronic forms that incorporate electronic signatures, for use with consent and disclosure forms during check-in
- *Patient verification software:* Used to determine a patient's ability to pay and to verify a patient's billing address before services are received and to screen self-pay patients to determine whether they qualify for alternative funding sources such as Medicaid
- *Medical kiosks:* Self-serve preregistration kiosks in which patients enter demographic information themselves and possibly also check in, make payments, update information, and obtain patient education
- *Electronic insurance verification:* Web-based products that query the patient's payer and demographic information for insurance verification before services are received
- *Admission "scrubber" programs:* Used with electronic admission forms to screen each admission for errors that could cause denials or delays later in the billing process

In addition to the high cost involved, another obstacle to implementing an EHR system is the large learning curve for staff members to become proficient users of the new technology. EHR systems also raise confidentiality and security concerns. The storage of patient information on a computer and its transmission from one computer to another present significant risks. However, it is widely accepted that the increased use of information technology in health care management greatly improves the productivity and efficiency of the data that are collected and processed throughout the billing process.

1 The main steps in the hospital billing process are (a) preregister or register patients, including scheduling appointments and establishing the patient's account; (b) establish financial responsibility for visits by explaining the facility's payment policy to patients and verifying their insurance coverage and any precertification requirements; (c) check patients in by copying their insurance cards and other identification cards, collecting copays and/or deductibles, and obtaining the required consents forms, such as a HIPAA Privacy Disclosure and the hospital's Notice of Information Practices; (d) check patients out, providing them with postdischarge care instructions if required; (e) review coding compliance by checking the accuracy of the diagnosis and procedure codes recorded in the patient's medical record and verifying that they are logically connected; (f) check billing compliance by collecting the patient's charges accumulated during the hospital stay and verifying them against the charge description master, the patient's medical record, and knowledge of the payer's requirements; (g) prepare and transmit claims using the facility's patient accounting system, including the use of a scrubber to test claims before transmitting them; (h) monitor payer adjudication to ensure that bills are paid on time and in full, including claim follow-up and payment processing; (i) generate patient statements for remaining balances when health plan payments do not pay the bills in full and for self-pay patients; and (j) follow up on patient payments and handle collections, including writing off uncollectible accounts. The first four steps deal with the patient's visit, the next three steps with the patient's claim, and the final three steps with post-claim activities.

2 During preregistration or registration, the following information is gathered and entered into the patient accounting system to establish the patient's account: personal data, basic billing data, medical information, an account number, and a medical record number.

3 A routine charge is the total of the costs of all supplies that are customarily used to provide the service. An ancillary charge is made for each specific service that is used to treat the patient in addition to routine charges, such as for anesthesia and blood administration.

4 The charge description master (CDM) is a computerized list of charge codes and associated data for all services the facility offers. Each entry identifies the hospital department and subcategory, the charge code for the service, the description, a medical code (when required), a standard claim form revenue code (RC), and the price. When the codes for services from the various charge slips are entered into the patient accounting system, the code automatically posts the correct charge to the patient's bill.

5 Billing errors include (a) billing for services or supplies that are not documented in the patient's medical record; (b) billing for services that are insufficiently documented in the patient's medical record; (c) billing twice for the same service (double billing); (d) billing for medically unnecessary services; (e) billing for services that are included in other charges; and (f) billing inaccurate information about providers or the wrong providers.

6　The advantages of using information technology in the hospital billing process, such as electronic health record (EHR) systems and electronic input devices during the admissions process, are (a) immediate access to health information; (b) computerized management of physician orders; (c) access to research for decision-making processes; (d) automated alerts and reminders; (e) electronic communications and connectivity; (f) patient support tools such as patient education on health topics; (f) administrative reporting tools; and (g) error reduction. The biggest disadvantages are (a) the cost of implementing the system; (b) the large learning curve for staff in becoming proficient with the new technology; and (c) the potential risk to the confidentiality and security of patient data.

✔ CHECK YOUR UNDERSTANDING

Write *T* or *F* to indicate whether you think the statement is true or false.

_____ **1.** Transfer is one of the main steps in the hospital billing process.

_____ **2.** Charge collection means to gather and post charges for all services supplied to a patient.

_____ **3.** *Registration* and *access* are alternative terms for admission.

_____ **4.** The payments due from health plans and patients make up the hospital's accounts receivable—the money that is needed to run the facility.

_____ **5.** The health information management department is responsible for computer hardware and software, such as the patient accounting system.

_____ **6.** The referring physician is responsible for the patient's care during hospitalization.

_____ **7.** Facilities generally collect payments from patients as soon as possible; many collect at the time of admission.

_____ **8.** Precertification is required before a patient can be discharged.

_____ **9.** Patients' accounts are established when their charges are posted to the patient accounting system.

_____ **10.** The cost of medications ordered for patients is an example of an ancillary charge.

_____ **11.** The charge description master (CDM) is basically a menu of the services and supplies the facility can provide.

_____ **12.** The biggest obstacle to the implementation of electronic medical record systems is the lack of federal legislation promoting it.

Choose the best answers.

13. An overdue amount is written off because it has been judged to be

    a. an adjustment

    b. an uncollectible account

    c. an ancillary charge

    d. a routine charge

14. When a private-payer health plan must be notified several business days before a hospitalization or an elective surgical procedure, the plan is said to require

    a. precertification

    b. a QIO (Quality Improvement Organization)

    c. utilization review

    d. a hold period

15. What type of report is used to begin the collection process?

    a. aging

    b. remittance advice

    c. appeal

    d. explanation of benefits

16. Which of the following is a billing error?

    a. billing for documented services

    b. billing for medically necessary services

    c. accurate billing of providers

    d. none of the above

17. The charge description master (CDM) entry for a service has

    a. a unique charge code for the service

    b. a price for the service

    c. the department that supplies or performs the service

    d. all of the above

18. A bill for a patient with insurance coverage is generated

    a. before the remittance advice is received

    b. after the remittance advice is received

    c. after the ancillary charge is received

    d. none of the above

19. Corrections, changes, and _____ are made by entering adjustments to patients' accounts.

    a. routine charges

    b. authorizations

    c. discharge plans

    d. write-offs

20. In the process of _____, the patient accounting system automatically bills all the components of a major service when the unique charge code for the service is posted.

a. charge collection

b. charge explode

c. verification

d. adjudication

COMPUTER EXPLORATION

Internet Applications

1. The American Hospital Association (AHA) produces a report each year with the latest research and analysis of important and emerging trends in the hospital field. Visit the AHA website (www.aha.org) and locate the Health and Hospital Trends page. Compare two important trends in this year's report with two from last year. How do they compare?

2. The Certification Commission for Healthcare Information Technology (CCHIT) was created in 2004 as a voluntary private-sector organization to certify health information technology (HIT). Its goal is to accelerate the adoption of health information technology by creating an efficient, credible, and sustainable product certification program. Visit the CCHIT website (www.cchit.org) and investigate the group's progress in developing certification criteria for electronic medical record products. What are the benefits of having an electronic medical record product certified by CCHIT?

3. Go to the Medicare home page and locate the link for Quality Improvement Organizations (under the Quality Initiatives/Patient Assessment Instruments heading). Read the overview about Quality Improvement Organizations. What are three of the main functions performed by Quality Improvement Organizations?

Hospital Insurance

LEARNING OUTCOMES

After completing this chapter, you will be able to define the key terms and:

1. Compare primary, secondary, and supplemental insurance.
2. Describe the way in which an insurance company controls payment to a beneficiary who has more than one insurance plan.
3. Briefly describe the coverage that the two main parts of the Medicare program provide to beneficiaries.
4. Describe the purpose of the Medicare Secondary Payer program.
5. Discuss the eligibility requirements and coverage of the Medicaid, TRICARE, and CHAMPVA programs.
6. Discuss the purpose of workers' compensation.

KEY TERMS

- Advance Beneficiary Notice of Noncoverage (ABN)
- benefit period
- carriers
- cash deductible
- Civilian Health and Medical Program of the Veterans Administration (CHAMPVA)
- coinsurance days
- coordination of benefits (COB)
- covered days
- covered services
- durable medical equipment (DME)
- employer group health plans (EGHPs)
- end-stage renal disease (ESRD)
- excluded (noncovered) services
- fiscal intermediary (FI)
- Hospital-Issued Notice of Noncoverage (HINN)
- lifetime reserve days (LRDs)
- local coverage determinations (LCDs)
- Medicaid
- Medicare administrative contractor (MAC)
- Medicare Part A
- Medicare Part B
- Medicare Secondary Payer (MSP)
- Medicare Summary Notice (MSN)
- Medigap
- national coverage determinations (NCDs)
- primary insurance
- secondary insurance
- supplemental insurance
- TRICARE
- workers' compensation

Chapter 3 provides basic, essential information about hospital insurance. There are a number of different types of medical insurance coverage. Because one of the main jobs of a patient account specialist is to handle patients' questions about what their insurance has paid, how much money they owe, and why, an experienced patient account specialist needs to know the basic facts about medical insurance coverage.

Many patients have coverage through one of the **employer group health plans (EGHPs)** offered by their employers. Some patients—perhaps a third of acute care patients—have Medicare coverage. Other patients have medical insurance through another government-sponsored program. This chapter compares the coverage of the two parts of the Medicare program, Part A and Part B, and also discusses Medicaid, TRICARE, CHAMPVA, and workers' compensation.

Insurance companies restrict patient benefits to no more than 100 percent of a bill. The chapter describes the methods used to control payments to beneficiaries who have more than one insurance plan, whether they hold two private plans or Medicare and other coverage.

Patients' Insurance Coverage

To keep up to date, patient account specialists store the following information about popular plans in the patient accounting system's insurance database:

- Plan name and type—managed care organization (MCO), indemnity (fee-for-service), or other
- Payer contact information—where claims are to be sent and a contact for queries and follow-up
- Payer turnaround time (the number of days between claim receipt and payment) according to a contract or other rules
- **Covered services**—the types of services and prescription drugs that are covered, including **covered days**—the number of days of hospitalization the plan covers
- Eligibility verification contact
- Precertification and referral requirements
- Patient copayment, deductible, and/or coinsurance requirements

Primary Patient Coverage

Some patients have two or more plans, as these cases show:

- A person with insurance coverage from an employer who is also covered as a dependent under a spouse's insurance
- An employed person over sixty-five who is covered by both Medicare and an employer's plan
- A person who is insured by both an employer group health plan and a policy from union membership

When patients have more than one health care plan, the **primary insurance** must be determined by facility staff. Deciding which policy is primary is important, because that third-party payer receives the first claim. The **secondary insurance** is billed after the primary payer sends its remittance advice for the account. The secondary payer pays, according to its guidelines, any balance left over after the primary payer has paid.

Supplemental insurance may be purchased by people who want insurance to cover their financial responsibilities under their primary insurance. Supplemental plans are designed by insurance companies to pay for costs that the primary (or secondary) plan does not cover, such as coinsurance and deductibles.

$$ **Billing Tip** $$

Automatic Secondary Billing
Patient accounting software programs often have a secondary billing feature. With this feature, an electronically transmitted remittance advice automatically updates the account and creates the proper claim for the secondary insurance. This claim can then be checked by the patient account specialist and transmitted to the secondary payer.

Coordination of Benefits

Insurance policies contain a clause called **coordination of benefits (COB)**. The coordination of benefits rules state that when a patient is covered under more than one policy, benefits paid by all policies are limited to 100 percent of the charge. This clause prevents people from having a number of plans and collecting 100 percent from each one. For this reason, patients are required to list all their insurance plans during the admission process. If the facility is filing the claim for the patient, as is usually the case, it supplies the information about other insurance coverage on the claim sent to the primary payer.

Facility Participation and Assignment of Benefits

Many third-party payers establish networks of providers that their members are encouraged or required to use. Medicare also requires hospitals to be in its provider program in order to serve Medicare beneficiaries. To increase the number of patients who use their services, most facilities elect to join—to participate in—various health plans' networks of providers.

Participation requires the facility to follow the payer's rules in a number of areas, such as filing claims and billing. Many plans require facilities to submit claims on behalf of patients. For example, Medicare-participating hospitals agree to file claims for patients. Facilities often must limit what they charge patients. Under Medicare, for example, facilities agree not to charge patients extra for items and services that Medicare covers, even if the facility's costs are greater than the amount paid by Medicare.

To compensate providers for the work of filing claims and the limits they set on their charges, provider participation also offers the advantage of direct payments from third-party payers. Patients who receive services from participating facilities sign a form that authorizes the third-party payer to pay the provider directly for medical services, rather than sending a check to the patient who then pays the provider. This procedure reduces the amount of accounts receivable that facilities must collect from patients.

The Medicare Program

Medicare is a federal medical insurance program that was established in 1965 under Title XVIII of the Social Security Act. There are two main parts, Medicare Part A and Medicare Part B. To receive benefits, individuals must meet certain eligibility requirements. The Medicare program, managed by the Centers for Medicare and Medicaid Services (CMS) under the Department of Health and Human Services (HHS), has many rules and regulations that often set price controls. Generally, the same price controls are adopted by commercial carriers.

To receive benefits, individuals must be eligible under one of the following categories:

- Individuals sixty-five or older who have paid FICA taxes or Railroad Retirement taxes for at least forty calendar quarters
- Disabled adults who have been receiving Social Security disability benefits or Railroad Retirement Board disability benefits for more than two years; coverage begins five months after the two years of entitlement

- Spouses of deceased, disabled, or retired individuals who were or still are entitled to Medicare benefits

- Individuals disabled before age eighteen who meet the disability criteria of the Social Security Act

- Retired federal employees enrolled in the Civil Service Retirement System (CSRS) and their spouses

- Patients of any age who receive dialysis or renal transplants for **end-stage renal disease (ESRD).** Coverage typically begins on the first day of the month following the start of dialysis treatment. For a transplant case, entitlement begins the month the individual is hospitalized for the transplant, which must be completed within two months. The donor is covered for services related to the donation of the organ only.

Medicare Claim Processing

The federal government does not pay Medicare claims directly; instead, it hires insurance organizations to process its claims. Insurance companies that process facility claims such as hospital bills are known as **fiscal intermediaries (FIs).** Insurance companies that process claims for physicians, other providers, and suppliers are called **carriers.** These Medicare program contractors issue **local coverage determinations (LCDs)** that help hospitals and physicians understand current guidelines and regulations for services that are not governed by national policy. LCDs apply only within the contractor's geographical area.

Guidelines and regulations that are governed by national policy, known as **national coverage determinations (NCDs),** are available on the CMS website. There are over a hundred NCDs describing coverage criteria for services such as blood transfusion, intestinal bypass surgery, and MRIs. These determinations list diagnosis codes that support the medical necessity of a particular procedure or service. In some cases, NCDs also list diagnoses for which tests are not payable. If a screening is for a diagnosis of depression, for example, it may not be payable.

Medicare Part A

Medicare Part A pays for inpatient hospital care and skilled nursing facility care, and for home health, respite, and hospice care.

Coverage

Part A coverage includes:

- *Hospital stays:* Semiprivate room, meals, general nursing, and other hospital services and supplies. This includes care in critical access hospitals and inpatient mental health care. It does not include private duty nursing or a television or telephone in the room. It also does not include a private room unless medically necessary.

- *Skilled nursing facility (SNF) care:* Semiprivate room, meals, skilled nursing and rehabilitative services, and other services and supplies (following a related three-day hospital stay).

- *Home health care:* Intermittent skilled nursing care, physical therapy, occupational therapy, speech-language pathology, home health aid services, and **durable medical equipment (DME)** such as wheelchairs and oxygen, but not prescription drugs.

- *Psychiatric inpatient care.*

- *Hospice care:* Pain and symptom relief and supportive services from a Medicare-approved hospice for people with terminal illnesses.

- *Blood:* Pints of blood received in a hospital or skilled nursing facility during a covered stay (after a three-pint deductible).

Eligibility and Costs

Anyone who receives Social Security benefits is automatically enrolled in Part A as a beneficiary with no premium payment. People age sixty-five or older who are not eligible for Social Security benefits may enroll in Part A, but they must pay a premium for the coverage.

Services covered under Medicare Part A are measured in benefit periods. A **benefit period** begins when a patient first receives Medicare-covered inpatient hospital care and ends when that patient has been discharged from the hospital or SNF for sixty consecutive days. Beneficiaries have unlimited benefit periods, but must pay the following:

- An inpatient hospital deductible called the **cash deductible** once during each benefit period. The deductible amount changes annually. The 2008 deductible is $1,024.

- A coinsurance amount for the sixty-first through the ninetieth days of a hospital stay during a benefit period. These thirty days are referred to as **coinsurance days.** The 2008 coinsurance amount is $256 a day.

- A coinsurance amount for each **lifetime reserve day (LRD).** Lifetime reserve days are a total of sixty days of additional coverage under Medicare Part A. These days can be used when the patient is hospitalized for more than ninety days in one benefit period. The coinsurance rate for each lifetime reserve day in 2008 is $512.

- A blood deductible for the first three pints of unreplaced blood (subject to state rules).

- An inpatient coinsurance for the twenty-first through the hundredth days of a Medicare-covered stay in a SFN. The 2008 rate is $128 per day.

- Charges for **excluded (noncovered) services,** such as eye exams, foot care, eyeglasses, hearing aids, cosmetic surgery, custodial care, and personal comfort items.

Medicare Part B

Medicare Part B covers physicians' visits and procedures as well as supplies.

Coverage

Medicare Part B focuses on the following:

- Physicians' services other than routine physical exams

- Outpatient medical and surgical services and supplies, diagnostic tests, ambulatory surgery center facility fees for approved procedures, and durable medical equipment

- Second surgical opinions, outpatient mental health care, and outpatient physical and occupational therapy, including speech-language therapy

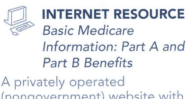

- Clinical laboratory services, such as blood tests, urinalysis, and more
- Home health care, including intermittent skilled nursing care, physical therapy, occupational therapy, speech-language pathology, home health aid services, and durable medical equipment
- Hospital services and supplies received as an outpatient as part of a physician's care
- Pints of blood given to outpatients or as part of a Part B covered service

Eligibility and Costs

Individuals entitled to Part A benefits automatically qualify for Part B benefits. U.S. citizens and also permanent residents over the age of sixty-five are eligible. Part B is a voluntary program; eligible persons must enroll for coverage. The premium is based on the income of the beneficiary. In 2008, depending on the beneficiary's income, Part B coverage costs between $96.40 and $238.40 per month. The patient's deductible for the year in 2008 is $135.00.

The Original Medicare Plan (OMP) is a fee-for-service plan. For its beneficiaries, Medicare pays 80 percent of approved charges after the patient has paid the deductible, and the patient or a secondary payer pays the remaining 20 percent. Other payment rules apply for people who enroll in one of the other Medicare plans, such as Medicare managed care plans.

Medicare managed care plans, called Medicare Advantage plans, are also known as Medicare Part C. These plans provide all Medicare-covered services, except hospice care, in return for a predetermined capitated payment. Private health insurance companies contract with CMS to offer Medicare Advantage plans as alternatives to the Original Medicare Plan.

The fourth part of Medicare, Medicare Part D, which was authorized under the Medicare Modernization Act of 2003, provides voluntary Medicare prescription drug plans that are open to people who are eligible for Medicare. Private companies provide the coverage, and beneficiaries choose the drug plan and pay a monthly premium.

Medicare Health Insurance Card

Each Medicare enrollee receives a health insurance card issued by the Social Security Administration (see Figure 3.1 on page 63). This card lists the beneficiary's name, sex, effective dates for Part A and Part B coverage, and Medicare number. The number is assigned by CMS and consists of nine digits (on older cards, this number is usually a Social Security number) followed by a numeric or alphanumeric suffix. The suffix indicates whether the benefits are drawn from the patient's work history or someone else's work history. Common suffixes are:

A	Primary wage earner (male or female)
B	Aged wife, first claimant (female)
B1	Husband, first claimant (male)
C1–C9	Child or grandchild, disabled/student
D	Aged widow, first claimant
T	Federal employee

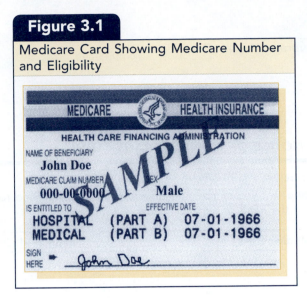

Figure 3.1

Medicare Card Showing Medicare Number and Eligibility

When the beneficiary's card shows a prefix (such as A, MA, WA, or WD), instead of a suffix, the patient is eligible for railroad retirement benefits, and claims must be submitted to the Railroad Medicare Part B claim office in Augusta, Georgia.

Advance Beneficiary Notices

Medicare does not pay for some services unless certain conditions are met. These conditions usually involve the relationship of the diagnosis and the service. For example, a vitamin B_{12} injection is covered only for patients with certain diagnoses, such as pernicious anemia, but not for a diagnosis of fatigue. If the patient does not have one of the specified diagnoses, the B_{12} injection is not covered because Medicare considers it not medically necessary. Local and national coverage determinations provide the details of what is covered for specific services and diagnoses.

Based on these determinations, when the facility judges that Medicare is not likely to pay for a planned service, an **Advance Beneficiary Notice of Noncoverage (ABN)** must be given to the patient for signature. In 2007, CMS revised the standard ABN form that has been in use since 2002. Figure 3.2 shows the revision that was available for testing at the time this text went to print. The changes to the form are designed to make it more user-friendly, while permitting customization for general as well as laboratory-specific use. The form shown in Figure 3.2 is customized for general use.

An ABN (also called a waiver of liability) explains why payment is likely to be denied by Medicare and includes a statement that the patient agrees to pay for the service when Medicare denies payment. A signed ABN is not required for services that are categorically excluded by Medicare—only for services that are noncovered under the given circumstances. A provider who could have been expected (by Medicare) to know that a service would not be covered and who performed the service without informing the patient could be liable for the charges.

ABN Modifiers

Procedure codes on insurance claims explain the details of the procedures the patient received. If a procedure is likely to be a noncovered Medicare service, a modifier may be appended to the procedure code to indicate to the payer

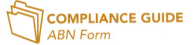

COMPLIANCE GUIDE
ABN Form

An ABN form must be signed and dated every time a patient receives a noncovered service.

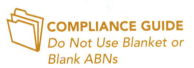

COMPLIANCE GUIDE
Do Not Use Blanket or Blank ABNs

- Medicare prohibits the use of blanket ABNs given routinely to all patients just to be sure of payment. The ABN must be specific to the service and date, signed and dated by the patient, and filed. It is a good practice to give the patient a copy of the signed document and to note this on the filed copy.

- Never have a patient sign a blank ABN for the physician to fill in later. The form must be filled in before the patient signs it.

Figure 3.2

Medicare Advance Beneficiary Notice of Noncoverage (ABN)—Draft Version

Notifier(s):

Patient Name: Identification Number:

ADVANCE BENEFICIARY NOTICE OF NONCOVERAGE (ABN)

NOTE: If Medicare doesn't pay for items or services below, you may have to pay.

Medicare does not pay for everything, even some care that you or your health care provider have good reason to think you need. We expect Medicare may not pay for the items or services below.

Items or Services:	Reason Medicare May Not Pay:	Estimated Cost:

WHAT YOU NEED TO DO NOW:

- Read this notice, so you can make an informed decision about your care.
- Ask us any questions that you may have after you finish reading.
- Choose an option below about whether to receive the items or services listed above.
    Note: If you choose Option 1 or 2, we may help you to use any other insurance that you might have, but Medicare cannot require us to do this.

OPTIONS: Check only one box. We cannot choose a box for you.

☐ **OPTION 1.** I want the items or services listed above. You may collect money from me now, but I also I want Medicare billed for an official decision on payment, which is sent to me on a Medicare Summary Notice (MSN). I understand that if Medicare doesn't pay, I am responsible for payment, but **I can appeal to Medicare** by following the directions on the MSN. If Medicare does pay, you will refund any payments I made to you, less co-pays or deductibles.

☐ **OPTION 2.** I want the items or services listed above, but do not bill Medicare. You may ask to be paid now as I am responsible for payment. **I cannot appeal if Medicare is not billed.**

☐ **OPTION 3.** I don't want the items or services listed above. I understand with this choice I am not responsible for payment, and I cannot appeal to see if Medicare would pay.

Additional Information:

This notice gives our opinion, not an official Medicare decision. If you have other questions on this notice or Medicare billing, call **1-800-MEDICARE** (1-800-633-4227/**TTY:** 1-877-486-2048).

Signing below means that you have received and understand this notice. You also receive a copy.

Signature:	Date:

According to the Paperwork Reduction Act of 1995, no persons are required to respond to a collection of information unless it displays a valid OMB control number. The valid OMB control number for this information collection is 0938-0566. The time required to complete this information collection is estimated to average 7 minutes per response, including the time to review instructions, search existing data resources, gather the data needed, and complete and review the information collection. If you have comments concerning the accuracy of the time estimate or suggestions for improving this form, please write to: CMS, 7500 Security Boulevard, Attn: PRA Reports Clearance Officer, Baltimore, Maryland 21244-1850.

Form CMS-R-131 (XX/07) - SAMPLE G   Form Approved OMB No. 0938-0566

whether an ABN is on file or needed. The modifier helps the payer determine who is responsible for the payment—the provider or the patient. Three modifiers used with ABNs are:

1. *GA:* Used when an item or service is expected to be denied as not reasonable or necessary and when a waiver of liability statement (ABN) is on file. This indicates that if the claim is not paid by Medicare, the patient is responsible for payment of the charges.

2. *GZ:* Used when an item or service is expected to be denied as not reasonable or necessary but the provider does not have a signed ABN from the patient. This might occur in an emergency care situation, or it might be used for a noncovered screening test or if a patient refuses to sign an ABN. This indicates that if the claim is not paid by Medicare, the patient cannot be billed for the service because no ABN was signed.

3. *GY:* This modifier is used to speed Medicare denials so the amount due can be collected from the patient (or a secondary payer if the patient is covered by two plans). It is used when an item or service is statutorily excluded or does not meet the definition of a Medicare benefit. This type of service, such as a routine physical or cosmetic surgery, is never covered by Medicare and therefore does not require an ABN.

Consent Forms

Patients must give their written consent to hospitals for a variety of reasons. Under the HIPAA Privacy Rule, a hospital must present a patient with a copy of its privacy practice at registration and have the patient sign an acknowledgment that he or she has received the notice. In addition, hospitals obtain the following other types of consent:

- Consent for medical treatments and procedures the patient will receive
- Acceptance of responsibility for payment
- Assignment of benefits
- Statement covering the conditions under which the facility is responsible for the patient's personal possessions
- Advance directives, also called living wills, or the appointing of a medical power of attorney

Medicare-Specific Consent Forms

In addition to these types of consent, hospitals must obtain written consent from Medicare inpatients, in particular, acknowledging that they have been informed of their Medicare rights. Hospitals must use a specially designated two-page CMS form called "Important Message from Medicare About Your Rights" (see Figure 3.3). Page 1 of the Important Message states the patient's rights as a hospital inpatient, as well as his or her appeal rights regarding hospital discharge. If a patient decides to appeal a discharge decision from the hospital, page 2 lists step-by-step instructions for calling the QIO and filing a discharge appeal. According to recent CMS regulations, the Important Message form must be presented to the beneficiary twice—once during admission and once before discharge. During admission, the hospital obtains the patient's acknowledgment of receipt at the bottom of page 1. During discharge, a copy of the signed form is presented again as a follow-up. Hospitals are expected to review the notices with beneficiaries, answer any

$ $ **Billing Tip** $ $

ABN Modifiers and Hospital Claims

Although ABN modifiers can be used on outpatient hospital claims (UB-04 forms), they are more frequently used on physician claims (CMS-1500 forms). For hospital claims, these modifiers are optional, as other condition and occurrence codes usually take precedence. For example, occurrence code 32 is used on hospital claims to indicate the date an ABN was signed.

On certain outpatient hospital bills, however, the use of the optional modifiers in combination with the required condition and occurrence codes provides more precise billing and may therefore reduce the risk of mistaken allegations of fraud and abuse. For example, occurrence code 32 is used to indicate the date an ABN was signed in connection with the bill; however, the code is not attached to a particular procedure. If other services provided on the same day must be billed on the same claim, modifier GA is used to identify the particular items or services for which an ABN was given.

Figure 3.3

Important Message from Medicare—Page 1

Patient Name:

Patient ID Number:

Physician:

DEPARTMENT OF HEALTH & HUMAN SERVICES
Centers for Medicare & Medicaid Services
OMB Approval No. 0938-0692

AN IMPORTANT MESSAGE FROM MEDICARE ABOUT YOUR RIGHTS

AS A HOSPITAL INPATIENT, YOU HAVE THE RIGHT TO:

- Receive Medicare covered services. This includes medically necessary hospital services and services you may need after you are discharged, if ordered by your doctor. You have a right to know about these services, who will pay for them, and where you can get them.
- Be involved in any decisions about your hospital stay, and know who will pay for it.
- Report any concerns you have about the quality of care you receive to the Quality Improvement Organization (QIO) listed here *MetaStar, (608) 274-1940 or toll-free at (800) 362-2320.*

YOUR MEDICARE DISCHARGE RIGHTS

Planning For Your Discharge: During your hospital stay, the hospital staff will be working with you to prepare for your safe discharge and arrange for services you may need after you leave the hospital. When you no longer need inpatient hospital care, your doctor or the hospital staff will inform you of your planned discharge date.

If you think you are being discharged too soon:

- You can talk to the hospital staff, your doctor and your managed care plan (if you belong to one) about your concerns.
- You also have the right to an appeal, that is, a review of your case by a Quality Improvement Organization (QIO). The QIO is an outside reviewer hired by Medicare to look at your case to decide whether you are ready to leave the hospital.
  - **If you want to appeal, you must contact the QIO no later than your planned discharge date and before you leave the hospital.**
  - If you do this, you will not have to pay for the services you receive during the appeal (except for charges like copays and deductibles).
- If you do not appeal, but decide to stay in the hospital past your planned discharge date, you may have to pay for any services you receive after that date.
- **Step by step instructions for calling the QIO and filing an appeal are on page 2.**

To speak with someone at the hospital about this notice, call _____.

Please sign and date here to show you received this notice and understand your rights.

_____   _____

Signature of Patient or Representative   Date

CMS-R-193 (approved 05/07)

questions, and help beneficiaries request review of a discharge decision by contacting a QIO if they decide to make an appeal.

Beneficiaries who choose to appeal a discharge decision will receive a second, more detailed notice entitled "Detailed Notice of Discharge," which explains why, based on Medicare coverage policies and the patient's medical condition, the hospital believes that the patient's inpatient hospital services should end. If the patient intends to stay in the hospital past the deadline to appeal, or past the discharge date determined by the appeal, the hospital may charge the patient for services received after these dates. The hospital then issues a HINN 12—Noncovered Continued Stay notice informing the patient of his or her responsibility for the continued stay together with the estimated cost. When patients sign the form, they are acknowledging that they are responsible for the charges of the continued stay.

HINN (Hospital-Issued Notice of Noncoverage)

The hospital provides a **Hospital-Issued Notice of Noncoverage (HINN)** to a beneficiary prior to admission, at admission, or at any point during an inpatient stay if the hospital determines that the care the beneficiary is receiving, or is about to receive, is not covered. The care is considered noncovered because it is not medically necessary, is not delivered in the most appropriate setting, or is custodial in nature. A HINN, sometime referred to as a hospital ABN, is used for noncovered inpatient stays the way an ABN is used for noncovered outpatient services.

Different versions of HINNs are used depending on the circumstances. When a Medicare beneficiary is planning to be hospitalized for services that Medicare usually pays for, but that are not considered to be reasonable and necessary in the particular situation, the hospital delivers a Preadmission/Admission HINN informing the patient of the cost of the noncovered stay. The HINN-12, a slightly different version of the same form, is used in association with a hospital discharge appeal notice as described above.

Medicare Secondary Payer Program

The **Medicare Secondary Payer (MSP)** program contains CMS guidelines about which insurance pays first when Medicare beneficiaries have additional plans. Many patients are classified as "MSP accounts" at registration. These patients are Medicare beneficiaries, but Medicare is the secondary payer. For example, Medicare requires automobile insurance companies to pay for patients' care after car accidents, no matter who is at fault. In these cases, the claim is sent first to the primary payer and then to Medicare with the remittance advice. Facilities must make every attempt to ensure that this claim sequence is followed for patients with insurance from a plan that is primary to Medicare—and almost all plans are primary to Medicare.

CMS supplies an MSP questionnaire that providers can use to determine the primary payer. It consists of six parts and lists questions to ask Medicare beneficiaries during each inpatient or outpatient admission. The questionnaire is used as a guide to help identify other payers that may be primary to Medicare. Facilities may also use their own version to gather the same information. Under the MSP program, every ninety days, hospitals have to ask Medicare beneficiaries about other insurance coverage they may have. For example, if a Medicare outpatient had surgery on October 1 and at that time reported only Medicare insurance, the admissions department would have to ask the patient about additional coverage for a subsequent procedure done in January.

INTERNET RESOURCE
MSP Questionnaire—
Part A: Other Insurer
Intake Tool
The MSP questionnaire may be downloaded from the CMS website: www.cms.hhs.gov/ProviderServices/Downloads/pro_othertool.pdf

Medigap Insurance

Medigap is private insurance that beneficiaries may buy to fill in some of the "gaps"—unpaid amounts—in Medicare coverage. These gaps include the annual deductible, any coinsurance that is required, and payment for some noncovered services. Even though private insurance carriers offer Medigap plans, coverage and standards are regulated by federal and state law. Medigap plans can legally be sold only to people who are covered by the Original Medicare Plan. Patients covered by a Medicare managed care plan or by Medicaid do not need Medigap policies.

A number of different options are available when choosing a Medigap policy. These plans are labeled A through J. The following benefits are common to all Medigap plans:

- Part A daily coinsurance amount for days sixty-one to ninety of hospitalization
- Part A daily coinsurance amount for each of Medicare's sixty lifetime reserve days
- 100 percent of covered hospital charges once all Medicare hospital benefits have been used
- Part B coinsurance amount (usually 20 percent of approved charges) after the deductible ($135 in 2008)
- First three pints of blood per calendar year

Plans B through J also pay the Part A hospital deductible for each hospitalization.

Medicare Summary Notice

At the same time the accounting department receives the Medicare remittance advice, the patient receives a **Medicare Summary Notice (MSN).** This document (see Figure 3.4 on page 69) replaces the previously issued Explanation of Your Medicare Part B Benefits (EOMB), the Medicare Benefit Notice (Part A), the Explanation of Medicare Benefits (Part A), and benefit denial letters.

The MSN tells patients what Medicare covered on claims sent on their behalf and what they are going to be billed. The facility then sends a bill for this balance. Patients also have the right to request an itemized bill from the facility. Patients often call after they compare the Medicare document and the facility bill. There are typically questions that patient account specialists must be prepared to answer or to research.

COMPLIANCE GUIDE
Medicare Fraud Watch

Under a special program, Medicare beneficiaries can earn rewards of up to $1,000 if they turn in providers who are proven to have committed fraud against the program. A Medicare beneficiary has the right to ask a provider for an itemized statement for any item or service for which Medicare has paid. The program instructs Medicare recipients to verify that they have received the services listed on the MSNs.

Medicaid

The **Medicaid** program was established under Title XIX of the Social Security Act of 1965 as an entitlement program to pay for the health care needs of low-income individuals and families. Medicaid is jointly funded by the federal government and state governments.

Eligibility

Individuals who apply for Medicaid benefits must meet minimum federal requirements and any additional requirements of the state in which they live.

Figure 3.4

Medicare Summary Notice

Medicare Summary Notice

① June 23, 2009

BENEFICIARY NAME ④
STREET ADDRESS
CITY, STATE, ZIP CODE

③ ⑤

HELP STOP FRAUD: Protect your Medicare
Numbers as you would a credit card number.

CUSTOMER SERVICE INFORMATION ②

➤ **Your Medicare Number: 111-11-1111A**

If you have questions, write or call:
    Medicare
    555 Medicare Blvd.
    Suite 200
    Medicare Building
    Medicare, US XXXXX-XXXX

Local: (XXX) XXX-XXXX
Toll-free: 1-800-XXX-XXXX
TTY for Hearing Impaired: 1-800-XXX-XXXX

This is a summary of claims processed from 5/15/2009 through 6/15/2009.

⑥

PART A HOSPITAL INSURANCE—INPATIENT CLAIMS

Dates of Service ⑦	Benefit Days Used ⑨	Non-Covered Charges ⑩	Deductible and Coinsurance ⑪	You May be Billed ⑫	See Notes Section ⑬
Claim number 12345–84956–84556–45621 ⑧ Care Hospital, 124 Sick Lane Dallas, TX 73555 ⑭ Referred by: Paul Jones, M.D. 6/1/09–6/15/09	14 days	$0.00	$776.00	$776.00	a, b

Explanation of numbered items:
1 The date the MSN was sent.
2 Patient's Medicare contact information.
3 Patient's Medicare number.
4 Patient's name and address.
5 Help Stop Fraud message.
6 Description of the services the patient received, and whether the service is Medicare Part A, Part B, or DME.
7 Dates of patient service.
8 Claim number assigned by Medicare.
9 Description of services provided.
10 Provider's charge for noncovered services as submitted to Medicare.
11 Patient's deductible and coinsurance responsibility.
12 Amount that the provider can bill the patient; it takes into account the deductibles, coinsurance, and noncovered services.
13 Reference to Notes about the claim.
14 Provider's name and address.

A person eligible in one state may be denied coverage in another state. Coverage also varies; each state determines coverage and coverage limits and sets payment rates, subject to the federal guidelines.

To receive federal matching funds, states must cover certain services, including inpatient and outpatient hospital services and emergency services. Some services covered under Medicaid require prior authorization before they are performed. If the provider does not obtain preauthorization, the plan may refuse to pay the claim. Rules regarding services not covered under Medicaid vary from state to state.

Medicaid Plans and Participation

In most states, Medicaid offers both fee-for-service and managed care plans. Medicaid clients enrolled in fee-for-service plans may be treated by the provider of their choice, as long as the provider accepts Medicaid. The provider submits the claim to the state Medicaid fiscal agent and is paid directly by Medicaid. Medicaid managed care plans restrict patients to a network of physicians, hospitals, and clinics. Providers in capitated managed care plans who are paid flat monthly fees must still file claims with the Medicaid payer, since the payer uses the claim data to assess utilization. Utilization reviews examine the necessity, appropriateness, and efficiency of services delivered.

Facilities participating in Medicaid sign a contract with the Department of Health and Human Services. They must agree to accept payment from Medicaid as payment in full for services; they may not bill patients for an additional amount. The difference must be entered into the billing system as a write-off. States may require a Medicaid recipient to make small payments in the form of a deductible, coinsurance, or copayment. These patient payments are referred to as *cost-sharing*. If Medicaid does not cover a service, the patient may be billed if certain conditions are met, such as prior notification that the bill would not be covered under the program.

Medicaid as the Payer of Last Resort

Before filing a claim with Medicaid, it is important to determine whether the patient has other insurance coverage. If the patient has coverage through any other insurance plan, or if the claim is covered by another program such as workers' compensation, the other plan is billed first, and the remittance advice from that primary payer is forwarded to Medicaid. For this reason, Medicaid is known as the payer of last resort, since it is always billed after another plan has been billed, if other coverage exists.

Medicare-Medicaid Crossover Claims

Some individuals are eligible for both Medicaid and Medicare (Medi-Medi) benefits. Claims for these patients are first submitted to Medicare. Then they are sent to Medicaid along with a copy of the Medicare remittance advice. Some Medicare carriers forward crossover claims to the state Medicaid payer automatically.

TRICARE

TRICARE is the Department of Defense health insurance plan for military personnel and their families. All military treatment facilities, including hospitals and clinics, are part of the TRICARE system. The TRICARE program brings the resources of military hospitals together with a network of civilian facilities and providers to offer increased access to health care services.

Information about patient eligibility is stored in the Defense Enrollment Eligibility Reporting System (DEERS). Sponsors may contact DEERS to verify eligibility; providers may not contact DEERS directly because the information is protected by the Privacy Act.

TRICARE Plans and Participation

TRICARE pays only for services rendered by authorized providers that are certified by TRICARE regional contractors. Participating providers agree to accept the TRICARE allowable charges as payment in full for services and to file claims on behalf of patients. Claims are submitted to the regional contractor based on the patient's home address, not the location of the facility. The regional TRICARE contractor sends payment directly to the provider, and the provider collects the patient's deductible and cost-share—the amount of the charges that are the responsibility of the patient.

TRICARE Standard

TRICARE Standard is a fee-for-service program that covers medical services provided by a military treatment facility (MTF). When an individual cannot be treated by a military treatment facility, the individual seeks treatment from a civilian provider, and TRICARE Standard benefits go into effect.

Formerly, if an individual lived near a military hospital that was unable to admit the patient, that hospital had to transmit a *nonavailability statement (NAS)* to the DEERS database before the patient could be covered for inpatient nonemergency care at a civilian hospital. Currently, under the 2002 National Defense Authorization Act, the requirement to obtain an NAS is eliminated, except for nonemergency inpatient mental health care services. However, some military treatment facilities have been given an exemption and may still require an NAS. Beneficiaries of TRICARE Standard, therefore, should be advised to check with the Beneficiary Counseling and Assistance Coordinator at the nearest military treatment facility.

Emergency services do not require a nonavailability statement. For outpatient services, TRICARE Standard does not require the statement other than for outpatient prenatal and postpartum maternity care. Many procedures, however, do require authorization.

TRICARE Prime

TRICARE Prime is a managed care plan. Each individual is assigned a primary care manager (PCM) who coordinates and manages that patient's medical care. Enrollees receive the majority of their health care services from military treatment facilities and receive priority at these facilities. A family member whose sponsor is not an active-duty service member must pay an annual enrollment fee. There is no deductible, and no payment is required for outpatient treatment at a military facility. All active-duty service

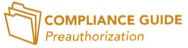

members are automatically enrolled in TRICARE Prime and do not have the option of choosing from among the additional TRICARE options.

TRICARE Extra

TRICARE Extra is an alternative managed care plan for individuals who want to receive services primarily from civilian facilities and physicians rather than from military facilities. Since TRICARE Extra is a managed care plan, individuals must receive health care services from a select network of health care professionals. TRICARE Extra is more expensive than TRICARE Prime, but less costly than TRICARE Standard. There is no enrollment fee, but there is an annual deductible.

TRICARE Reserve Select

Due to the large number of military reservists who have been called up for active duty, the Department of Defense implemented TRICARE Reserve Select (TRS). This program is a premium-based health plan available for purchase by certain members of the National Guard and Reserve activated on or after September 11, 2001. TRS provides comprehensive health care coverage similar to TRICARE Standard and TRICARE Extra for members and covered family members.

TRICARE for Life

TRICARE for Life is designed for individuals over age sixty-five who are eligible for both Medicare and TRICARE; it enables those who would like to continue to receive health care at a military treatment facility, rather than a civilian network facility, to do so. TRICARE for Life acts as a secondary payer to Medicare; Medicare pays first, and TRICARE pays for the remaining out-of-pocket expenses. All enrollees in TRICARE for Life must be enrolled in Medicare Parts A and B. (Individuals already enrolled in a Medicare HMO may not participate in TRICARE for Life.) Other than Medicare costs, TRICARE for Life beneficiaries pay no enrollment fees and no cost-share for inpatient or outpatient care at a military facility. Treatment at a civilian network facility requires a copayment at the time of service.

TRICARE and Other Insurance Plans

If the individual has other health insurance coverage that is primary to TRICARE, that insurance carrier must be billed first. TRICARE is a secondary payer in almost all circumstances with a few exceptions, such as Medicaid.

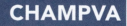

CHAMPVA

The **Civilian Health and Medical Program of the Veterans Administration (CHAMPVA)** is the government's health insurance program for veterans with 100 percent service-related disabilities and their families. Under the program, health care expenses are shared between the Department of Veterans Affairs (VA) and the beneficiary. Veterans with a 100 percent disability must be enrolled in the program to receive benefits.

CHAMPVA provides coverage for most medically necessary services, including inpatient services, room and board, hospital services, surgical procedures, physician services, anesthesia, and blood and blood products. Some procedures must be approved in advance. The patient, not the provider, is responsible for obtaining this preauthorization. CHAMPVA enrollees do not need to obtain nonavailability statements, since they are not eligible to receive service in military treatment facilities. A VA hospital is not considered a military treatment facility.

FYI

CHAMPVA Beneficiaries
The Department of Veterans Affairs is responsible for determining eligibility for the CHAMPVA program.

CHAMPVA Participation

For most services, CHAMPVA does not contract with providers. Beneficiaries may receive care from the providers they choose, as long as those providers are properly licensed to perform the services being delivered and are not on the Medicare exclusion list. Providers cannot charge more than the CHAMPVA allowable amounts. Providers agree to accept CHAMPVA payment and the patient's cost-share payment as payment in full for services. Most CHAMPVA claims are filed by the provider and sent to the centralized CHAMPVA claims processing center in Denver, Colorado.

CHAMPVA and Other Insurance Plans

When the individual has insurance benefits in addition to CHAMPVA, CHAMPVA is almost always the secondary payer. Two exceptions are Medicaid and supplementary insurance. Persons under age sixty-five who are eligible for Medicare benefits and who are enrolled in Medicare Parts A and B may also be enrolled in CHAMPVA.

CHAMPVA for Life

CHAMPVA for Life extends CHAMPVA benefits to enrollees who are age sixty-five and over. Similar to TRICARE for Life, CHAMPVA for Life benefits are payable after payment by Medicare or other third-party payers. Eligible beneficiaries must be sixty-five or older and must be enrolled in Medicare Parts A and B. For services not covered by Medicare, CHAMPVA acts as the primary payer.

Workers' Compensation

Workers' compensation is a government-supervised and employer-sponsored program for compensating employees for injury or disease in connection with employment, whether or not the employer was at fault. It provides employees who are injured while on the job with compensation for their injuries, and it protects employers against liability for employees' injuries. Workers' compensation insurance covers injuries, illnesses, and job-related deaths. Injuries are not limited to on-the-job occurrences; they may occur while performing an offsite service for the employer. Benefits include necessary medical and hospital services, medicines, transportation, equipment, nursing care, rehabilitation, and retraining.

INTERNET RESOURCE
Employment Standards Administration (ESA)

To locate programs administered by the OWCP, go to the Employment Standards Administration (ESA) home page on the Department of Labor website. www.dol.gov/esa/

HIPAA TIP

First Report of Injury Transaction Standard

The first report of injury transaction will be one of the HIPAA EDI standard transactions. The format and rules for the report must be HIPAA-compliant after the uniform transaction standard is mandated under federal law.

$ $ Billing Tip $ $

Turnaround Times

Track the date a workers' compensation claim is filed. Insurance carriers must pay workers' compensation claims within a specified amount of time, usually thirty to forty-five days, depending on the state. If the claim is not paid within the time specified, the claimant may be eligible for interest on the payment, or a late fee may apply.

Federal and State Programs

Work-related illnesses or injuries suffered by civilian employees of federal agencies are covered under various programs administered by the Office of Workers' Compensation Programs (OWCP) of the Department of Labor.

Each state administers its own workers' compensation program and has its own statutes governing workers' compensation, so coverage varies from state to state. However, all states provide two types of workers' compensation benefits. One type pays the employee's medical expenses that result from the work-related injury, and the other type pays the employee for lost wages while he or she is unable to return to work.

Handling Workers' Compensation Cases

Workers' compensation cases follow special procedures. When an employee is injured on the job, the injury must be reported to the employer within a certain time period. Most states require notification on a specific form. Once notified, the employer must notify the state workers' compensation office and the insurance carrier within a specified period of time. In some cases, the employee is given a medical service order to take to the physician who provides treatment.

When handling workers' compensation cases, facility staff members must be sure to collect the appropriate insurance information, employer information, the claim number assigned by the workers' compensation program, and the date of injury. In most cases, workers' compensation is primary to other plans.

1 Primary insurance is the first payer of a claim. Secondary insurance covers the balance due after the first-payer payment, based on the insurer's guidelines. Supplemental insurance is purchased to cover costs that primary and secondary insurance do not cover, such as deductible and coinsurance amounts.

2 When a beneficiary has more than one insurance plan, the coordination of benefits clause prohibits collecting more than 100 percent of the charges.

3 Medicare Part A covers inpatient hospital care, skilled nursing facility care, and home health, respite, and hospice care. Services covered under Medicare Part A are measured in benefit periods. A benefit period begins when a patient first receives Medicare-covered inpatient hospital care and ends when that patient has been discharged from the hospital or SNF for sixty consecutive days. Beneficiaries have unlimited benefit periods but are responsible for certain deductibles.

Medicare Part B covers physicians' visits and procedures as well as supplies. For Original Medicare Plan (OMP) beneficiaries, Medicare pays 80 percent of approved charges after the deductible is met, and the patient or a secondary payer pays the remaining 20 percent. For people who enroll in one of the other Medicare plans, such as the Medicare managed care plans, other payment rules apply. Medicare managed care plans, called Medicare Advantage plans, make up Medicare Part C. Medicare Part D provides voluntary Medicare prescription drug plans that are open to people who are eligible for Medicare.

4 The Medicare Secondary Payer program controls Medicare benefits when Medicare beneficiaries are covered by other plans. A claim is sent first to the primary payer and then to Medicare with the remittance advice.

5 Medicaid is an entitlement program that pays for the health care needs of individuals and families with low incomes and few resources. The program is jointly funded by the federal government and state governments. Individuals who apply for Medicaid benefits must meet minimum federal requirements and any additional requirements of the state in which they live. To receive federal matching funds, states must cover certain services, including inpatient and outpatient hospital services and emergency services.

TRICARE is the Department of Defense health insurance plan for military personnel and their families. All military treatment facilities, including hospitals and clinics, are part of the TRICARE system. TRICARE also contracts with civilian facilities and physicians to provide more extensive services to beneficiaries. TRICARE plans include Standard, Prime, Extra, Reserve Select, and TRICARE for Life.

CHAMPVA is the government's health insurance program for veterans with 100 percent service-related disabilities and their families. The Department of Veterans Affairs (VA) is responsible for determining eligibility for the CHAMPVA program. CHAMPVA provides coverage for most medically necessary services, including inpatient services, room and board, hospital services, surgical procedures, physician services, anesthesia, and blood and blood products.

⑥ Workers' compensation provides employees who are injured while on the job with a means of receiving compensation for their injuries, and it protects employers against liability for employees' injuries. Workers' compensation insurance covers injuries, illnesses, and job-related deaths.

✔CHECK YOUR UNDERSTANDING

Write *T* or *F* to indicate whether you think the statement is true or false.

_____ **1.** Patients usually buy secondary insurance and have supplemental insurance through their spouses.

_____ **2.** The primary insurance carrier is sent the first claim.

_____ **3.** Participating facilities can charge Medicare patients whatever the costs for their services are.

_____ **4.** Medicare is primarily a medical insurance plan for people over age sixty-five.

_____ **5.** Medicare Part A covers the work of physicians, such as surgeons or dermatologists.

_____ **6.** The Medicare Part A cash deductible is due once a year.

_____ **7.** The Medicare Modernization Act mandated that CMS replace the numerous LCDs and NCDs with Medicare administrative contractors (MACs).

_____ **8.** HINN, also known as a hospital ABN, stands for Hospital-Issued Notice of Noncoverage.

_____ **9.** The Medicare Secondary Payer program establishes the primary payer when the patient has another insurance plan.

_____ **10.** Medicaid coverage is provided to people with low income and few resources.

_____ **11.** CHAMPVA is coverage for active members of the uniformed services, whereas TRICARE is for disabled veterans.

_____ **12.** Workers' compensation covers injuries or illnesses associated with employment.

Choose the best answers.

13. The contractors hired by Medicare to process Part A claims are called
    a. either fiscal intermediaries or A/B MACs
    b. either carriers or A/B MACs
    c. LCDs
    d. DMEs

14. Under Medicare Part A, a benefit period ends when the patient has been discharged for
    a. twenty days
    b. sixty days
    c. sixty-one days
    d. ninety days

15. DME is defined as equipment that is
    a. designed to be disposable
    b. noncovered under Medicare Part B
    c. used in the home
    d. used in hospitals

16. What document do Medicare beneficiaries receive to explain their benefits?
    a. MSP
    b. LCD
    c. COB
    d. MSN

17. Which clause in insurance policies limits total payments to 100 percent of charges?
    a. COB
    b. MSP
    c. MSN
    d. none of the above

18. Medicare Part A beneficiaries are responsible for paying
    a. charges for excluded services
    b. cash deductibles
    c. coinsurance days
    d. all of the above

19. The Important Message from Medicare notice is given to Medicare inpatients
    a. to obtain consent for surgery
    b. to inform them of their Medicare rights
    c. for MSP development
    d. to establish advance directives

20. Eligible beneficiaries for the CHAMPVA for Life program must be

    a. enrolled in a prescription drug program

    b. age sixty-five or under

    c. enrolled in Medicare Part A and B

    d. active duty members of the armed forces

COMPUTER EXPLORATION

Internet Applications

1. Locate the Medicare fiscal intermediary (FI) or Medicare administrative contractor (MAC) for your state. Also locate the Part B carrier or Part B MAC.

2. On the website for your FI or MAC, locate a local medical review policy (LCD). What service or procedure does it describe? What diagnoses does it list that support the medical necessity for the service or procedure?

3. The deductible amounts required for Medicare Part A and Part B change annually. Visit the CMS website, and find this year's (a) Part A cash deductible and (b) coinsurance rate. How do these rates compare with last year's rates?

4. The MSP questionnaire may be downloaded from the CMS website at the following address: www.cms.hhs.gov/ProviderServices/Downloads/pro_othertool.pdf. Read through the form. How many pages does the form contain? What is the primary purpose of the form and how does the format of the questionnaire accomplish this purpose.

5. Locate the address and telephone number of the TRICARE regional contractor for your state.

Medical Coding Basics

LEARNING OUTCOMES

After completing this chapter, you will be able to define the key terms and:

1. Discuss the purpose of ICD-9-CM.
2. Describe the organization and content of Volumes 1, 2, and 3 of ICD-9-CM.
3. Understand the conventions that are followed in ICD-9-CM.
4. Identify the purpose and correct use of the present on admission (POA) indicator.
5. Discuss the purpose of the procedural codes in the HCPCS/CPT code sets.
6. Describe the structure and content of the index and the main text in CPT.
7. Describe the purpose and correct use of CPT modifiers
8. Describe the structure and content of HCPCS.
9. Describe the four-step process medical coders follow to assign correct ICD-9-CM and HCPCS/CPT codes.
10. Identify the code sets that are associated with inpatient and outpatient billing for hospital services.

KEY TERMS

- code set
- comorbidity
- complete procedure
- complication
- conventions
- crosswalk
- Current Procedural Terminology (CPT)
- diagnosis code
- E code
- Health Care Common Procedure Coding System (HCPCS)
- ICD-9-CM *Official Guidelines for Coding and Reporting*
- International Classification of Diseases, Ninth Revision, Clinical Modification (ICD-9-CM)
- manifestation
- modifier
- patient's reason for visit
- present on admission (POA)
- primary diagnosis
- principal diagnosis
- procedure code
- technical component (TC)
- Uniform Hospital Discharge Data Set (UHDDS)
- unlisted procedure code
- V code
- Volume 1 (Tabular List)
- Volume 2 (Alphabetic Index)
- Volume 3 (Procedures)

As a part of the medical billing process, medical coders in the health information management (HIM) department assign codes to patients' conditions and procedures. These codes are reported on claims to represent the services the facility provided for the patient and the medical necessity of those services. Clearly connecting what was done—the procedure code—with why it was done—the diagnosis code—is essential for maximum appropriate reimbursement. For this reason, patient account specialists need to understand the basics of the medical coding process.

As explained in Chapter 1, HIPAA mandates certain medical **code sets**—standardized alphabetic and/or numeric representations of data—for use in health care transactions. Table 4.1 summarizes the three classifications.

Diagnosis Coding: ICD-9-CM

Scientists and medical researchers have long gathered information from medical records about patients' illnesses and causes of death. To facilitate the data-gathering process, standardized codes have been developed to replace written descriptions of symptoms and conditions. Using these standardized codes provides an accurate way to collect statistics to keep people healthy and to plan for needed health care resources as well as to record morbidity (disease) and mortality (death) data. The diagnosis codes used in the United States are based on the **International Classification of Diseases** (ICD). The U.S. version of the ninth revision of the ICD (ICD-9), published in 1979, is called ICD-9 **Clinical Modification,** or **ICD-9-CM.**

An ICD-9-CM **diagnosis code** has three, four, or five digits plus a description. The system is built on categories for diseases, injuries, and symptoms. A category has three digits. Most categories have subcategories of four-digit codes. Some codes are further subclassified into five-digit codes.

EXAMPLE:
Category 415: Acute pulmonary heart disease (three digits)
  Subcategory 415.1: Pulmonary embolism and infarction (four digits)
    Subclassification: 415.11: Iatrogenic pulmonary embolism and infarction (five digits)

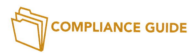

COMPLIANCE GUIDE

ICD-9-CM rules require the selection of the most specific code for the condition.

This structure enables a coder to assign the code representing the most specific diagnosis that is documented in the patient medical record. A fifth digit is more specific than a fourth digit, and a fourth digit is more specific than a three-digit code. When fourth and fifth digits are in ICD-9-CM, they are not optional; they must be used. For example, Centers for Medicare and Medicaid Services (CMS) rules state that a Medicare claim will be rejected when the most specific code available is not used.

Table 4.1

HIPAA Standard Code Sets for Diagnoses and Procedures

Purpose	Standard
Codes for diseases, injuries, impairments, and other health-related problems	International Classification of Diseases, Ninth Revision, Clinical Modification (ICD-9-CM), Volumes 1 and 2
Codes for procedures or other actions taken to prevent, diagnose, treat, or manage diseases, injuries, and impairments	Physicians' services: Current Procedural Terminology (CPT) Inpatient hospital services: International Classification of Diseases, Ninth Revision, Clinical Modification, Volume 3: Procedures
Codes for other medical services	Healthcare Common Procedure Coding System (HCPCS)

Codes are updated twice a year; new codes must be used as of the date they go into effect, and invalid (deleted) codes must not continue to be used. The U.S. Government Printing Office (GPO) publishes the official ICD-9-CM on the Internet and in CD-ROM format every year. Various commercial publishers include the updated codes in annual coding books that are printed soon after the July updates are released. Facilities must ensure that the current reference is available and that the current codes are in use.

INTERNET RESOURCE
ICD-9-CM Code Updates
www.cms.hhs.gov/
ICD9ProviderDiagnosticCodes

Organization of ICD-9-CM

ICD-9-CM has three parts:

1. *Diseases and injuries: **Tabular List—Volume 1:*** Volume 1, usually called the Tabular List, is made up of seventeen chapters of disease descriptions and codes with two supplementary classifications and appendixes.

2. *Diseases and injuries: **Alphabetic Index—Volume 2:*** Volume 2, usually called the Alphabetic Index, provides (a) an index of the disease descriptions in the Tabular List, (b) an index of drugs and chemicals that cause poisoning in table format, and (c) an index of external causes of injury, such as accidents.

3. *Procedures: Tabular List and Alphabetic Index—Volume 3:* This volume, called Volume 3 (Procedures), classifies inpatient procedures that are billed by hospitals.

The ICD-9-CM coding system is maintained by the National Center for Health Statistics (NCHS) and CMS, both of which are departments of the federal Department of Health and Human Services.

Alphabetic Index

Although the Tabular List and the Alphabetic Index are labeled Volume 1 and Volume 2, they are related like the parts of a book. First, the Alphabetic Index is used to find a code for a patient's condition or symptom. The index entry provides a pointer to the correct code number in the Tabular List. That code is then located in the Tabular List so that its correct use can be checked.

The Alphabetic Index contains all the medical terms in the Tabular List classifications. For some conditions, it also lists common terms that are not found in the Tabular List. The index is organized by the condition, not by the body part (anatomical site) in which the condition occurs. For example, the term *wrist fracture* is located by looking under *fracture* (the condition) and then, below it, *wrist* (the location), rather than under *wrist* to find *fracture*.

The assignment of the correct code begins with looking up the medical term that describes the patient's condition. Each main term relating to a patient's condition is printed in boldface type and is followed by its code number. For example, if the diagnostic statement is "the patient presents with blindness," the main term *blindness* is located in the Alphabetic Index. Additional terms relating to the condition also appear. Figure 4.1, on page 82, illustrates the format of the Alphabetic Index.

The Tabular List

The Tabular List received its name from the language of statistics; the word *tabulate* means to count, record, or list systematically. The diseases and injuries in the Tabular List are organized into chapters according to body system

Figure 4.1

Example of Alphabetic Index Entries

Blepharitis (eyelid) 373.00
 angularis 373.01
 ciliaris 373.00
  with ulcer 373.01
 marginal 373.00
  with ulcer 373.01
 scrofulous (*see also* Tuberculosis) 017.3
  [373.00]
 squamous 373.02
 ulcerative 373.01
Blepharochalasis 374.34
 congenital 743.62
Blepharocolonus 333.81
Blepharoconjunctivitis (*see also*
 Conjunctivitis) 372.20
 angular 372.21
 contact 372.22
Blepharophimosis (eyelid) 374.46
 congenital 743.62
Blepharoplegia 374.89
Blepharoptosis 374.30
 congenital 743.61
Blepharopyorrhea 098.49
Blepharospasm 333.81
 due to drugs 333.85

Blessig's cyst 362.62
Blighted ovum 631
Blind
 bronchus (congenital) 748.3
 eye—*see also* Blindness
  hypertensive 360.42
  hypotensive 360.41
 loop syndrome (postoperative) 579.2
 sac, fallopian tube (congenital) 752.19
 spot, enlarged 368.42
 tract or tube (congenital) NEC—*see* Atresia
Blindness (acquired) (congenital) (both eyes)
 369.00
 blast 921.3
  with nerve injury—*see* Injury, nerve, optic
 Bright's—*see* Uremia
 color (congenital) 368.59
  acquired 368.55
  blue 368.53
  green 368.52
  red 368.51
  total 368.54
 concussion 950.9
 cortical 377.75
 day 368.10

or type of condition. Supplementary codes cover other special situations. The organization of the Tabular List and the ranges of codes covered in each part are shown in Table 4.2 on page 83.

Each Tabular List chapter is divided into sections with titles that indicate the types of related diseases or conditions they cover. For example, Chapter 6 has six sections, one of which is "Diseases of the Ear and Mastoid Process" (380–389).

Within each section, there are three levels of codes: (1) categories, which are three-digit codes that cover a single disease or related condition, (2) subcategories, which are four-digit subdivisions, and (3) subclassifications, which are five-digit subdivisions of a subcategory. Figure 4.2 on page 83 illustrates the three levels of ICD codes for the section in Chapter 6 above. In this example, 380 is the category, 380.0 is the subcategory, and 380.00 through 380.03 are the five-digit subclassifications.

ICD-9-CM Conventions

Coding correctly requires understanding the **conventions**—the symbols, instructional notes, and punctuation marks—that appear in the Alphabetic Index and the Tabular List.

- *Symbol for fifth-digit requirement:* A symbol (such as ⑤ or √ 5th) may appear next to a chapter, a category, or a subcategory. This symbol means that for correct coding, a fifth digit is to be assigned.

- *Includes and excludes notes:* Notes headed by the word *includes* refine the content of the category or section appearing above them. Notes

---

$$ Billing Tip $$

Fifth-Digit Requirement

If ICD-9-CM indicates that a fifth digit is required, it must be included. But if it is not required, a zero or zeroes should not be added to the four-digit or three-digit code. The use of a fifth digit when it is not required makes the code invalid.

Table 4.2

ICD-9-CM Tabular List Organization

Chapter	Categories	Codes
	Classification of Diseases and Injuries	
1	Infectious and Parasitic Diseases	001–139
2	Neoplasms	140–239
3	Endocrine, Nutritional, and Metabolic Diseases, and Immunity Disorders	240–279
4	Diseases of the Blood and Blood-Forming Organs	280–289
5	Mental Disorders	290–319
6	Diseases of the Central Nervous System and Sense Organs	320–389
7	Diseases of the Circulatory System	390–459
8	Diseases of the Respiratory System	460–519
9	Diseases of the Digestive System	520–579
10	Diseases of the Genitourinary System	580–629
11	Complications of Pregnancy, Childbirth, and the Puerperium	630–677
12	Diseases of the Skin and Subcutaneous Tissue	680–709
13	Diseases of the Musculoskeletal System and Connective Tissue	710–739
14	Congenital Anomalies	740–759
15	Certain Conditions Originating in the Perinatal Period	760–779
16	Symptoms, Signs, and Ill-Defined Conditions	780–799
17	Injury and Poisoning	800–999
	Supplementary Classifications	
V Codes	Supplementary Classification of Factors Influencing Health Status and Contact with Health Services	V01–V83
E Codes	Supplementary Classification of External Causes of Injury and Poisoning	E800–E999

headed by the word *excludes* (which is boxed and italicized) indicate conditions that are not classifiable to the code above.

- *Requirement for two codes:* Some conditions may require two codes, one for the etiology and a second for the **manifestation,** the disease's typical signs or symptoms. This is the case when two codes, the second in brackets and italics, appear after a term in the Alphabetic Index:

EXAMPLE:
Phlebitis
    gouty 274.89 *[451.9]*

Figure 4.2

Example of Three Levels of ICD Codes

DISEASES OF THE EAR AND MASTOID PROCESS (380–389)

380 **Disorders of external ear**

√5th   380.0   Perichondritis and chondritis of pinna

            380.00   Perichondritis of pinna, unspecified

            380.01   Acute perichondritis of pinna

            380.02   Chronic perichondritis of pinna

            380.03   Chondritis of pinna

This entry indicates that the diagnostic statement "gouty phlebitis" requires two codes, one for the etiology (gout) and one for the manifestation (phlebitis). The use of italics for codes means that they cannot be used as primary codes; they are listed after the codes for the etiology.

- *Parentheses and brackets:* Parentheses ( ) are used around descriptions that do not affect the code. Brackets < > are used around synonyms, alternative wordings, or explanations.

- *Braces:* A brace } encloses a series of terms that is attached to the statement that appears to the right of the brace. It is an alternate format for a long list after a colon and also indicates incomplete terms.

- *NEC and NOS:* NEC, not elsewhere classified, means that no code matches the diagnosis. Another abbreviation, NOS, or not otherwise specified, means unspecified. This term or abbreviation indicates that the code above it should be used when a condition is not completely described in the medical record.

- *New and revised codes:* Many publishers use a bullet (•) at a code or a line of text to show that the entry is new. A single triangle (▲) or facing triangles (▶◀) are also often used to mean a new or revised description.

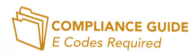
V Codes and E Codes

Two supplementary classifications follow the chapters of the Tabular List:

- **V codes** identify encounters for reasons other than illness or injury.
- **E codes** identify the external causes of injuries and poisoning.

Both V and E codes are alphanumeric; they contain letters followed by numbers. For example, the code for a complete physical examination of an adult is V70.0. The code for a fall from a ladder is E881.0.

Assigning ICD-9-CM Diagnosis Codes

The correct procedure for assigning accurate diagnosis codes has four steps.

Identify the Diagnosis (Diagnoses) to Be Coded

The first step the medical coder takes is to identify the diagnosis or diagnoses to be coded. For inpatient cases, the **principal diagnosis** is determined. It is defined under the **Uniform Hospital Discharge Data Set (UHDDS),** the minimum data set established for inpatient claims, as the condition established after study to be chiefly responsible for occasioning the admission of the patient to the hospital. Also identified are any other conditions that affect the patient's care during the hospital stay. A patient's other conditions at admission that affect care during the hospitalization are called **comorbidities,** meaning coexisting conditions. Conditions that develop as problems related to surgery or other treatments are coded as **complications.** Comorbidities and complications are shown in the patient medical record with the initials *CC*.

Table 4.3 on page 85 shows the elements required to be recorded at the discharge of an inpatient, representing the complete UHDDS data set.

Table 4.3

Uniform Hospital Discharge Data Set Definitions*

Data Element	Description
Personal identification	A unique number identifying the patient, applicable to the individual regardless of health care source or third-party arrangement
Date of birth	Month, day, year
Sex	Male or female
Race and ethnicity	Race
	(1) American Indian/Eskimo/Aleut
	(2) Asian or Pacific Islander
	(3) Black
	(4) White
	(5) Other race
	(6) Unknown
	Ethnicity
	(1) Spanish/Hispanic origin
	(2) Not of Spanish/Hispanic origin
	(3) Unknown
Residence	Usual residence, full address, and ZIP code; nine-digit ZIP code if available
Hospital identification	National Provider Identifier (NPI)* (a unique institutional number across data systems)
Admission date	Month, day, and year of admission
Type of admission	Scheduled: an arrangement with the admissions office at least 24 hours before the admission
	Unscheduled: all other admissions
Discharge date	Month, day, and year of discharge
Physician identification—attending	NPI*
Physician identification—operating	NPI* for the clinician who performed the principal procedure
Other diagnoses	All conditions that coexist at the time of admission, or develop subsequently, that affect the treatment received and/or the length of stay; diagnoses that relate to an earlier episode that have no bearing on the current hospital stay are to be excluded. Code conditions that affect patient care in terms of requiring:
	• Clinical evaluation
	• Therapeutic treatment
	• Diagnostic procedures
	• Extended length of hospital stay
	• Increased nursing care
	• Monitoring
External causes of injury code	The ICD–9-CM code for the external cause of an injury, poisoning, or adverse effect
Birth weigh of newborns	The specific birth weight of the newborn, preferably recorded in grams
Procedures and dates	All significant procedures are to be reported. A significant procedure is one that:
	(1) Is surgical in nature
	(2) Carries a procedural risk
	(3) Carries an anesthetic risk
	(4) Requires specialized training
	Surgery includes incision, excision, amputation, introduction, endoscopy, repair, destruction, suture, and manipulation.

UPIN has been updated to NPI to reflect current practice.

Table 4.3

Uniform Hospital Discharge Data Set Definitions *continued*

Data Element	Description
	The date must be reported for each significant procedure.
	When more than one procedure is reported, the principal procedure is to be designated. In determining which of several procedures is principal, the following criteria apply: The principal procedure is one that was performed for definitive treatment rather than for diagnostic or exploratory purposes, or was necessary to take care of a complication. If two procedures appear to be principal, the one most related to the principal diagnosis should be selected as the principal procedure.
Disposition of patient	Home, nursing facility, other health care facility, left against medical advice, expired.
Expected sources of payment	Primary source: the primary source that is expected to be responsible for the largest percentage of the patient's current bill
	Other source(s): other sources, if any, that are expected to be responsible for a portion of the patient's current bill; more than one can be identified
Total charges	All charges billed by the hospital for this hospitalization; professional charges for individual patient care by physicians are excluded

Source: www.cdc.gov/nchs/data/ncvhs/nchvs92.pdf.

HIPAA TIP

The Official Guidelines

HIPAA also mandates following the *Official Guidelines* to ensure consistent coding. They are available at www.cdc.gov/nchs/data/icd9/icdguide.pdf.

$ $ Billing Tip $ $

POA Mandate

The federal requirement to report POA indicators so that Medicare does not pay hospitals for conditions the hospital caused or allowed to develop during an inpatient stay was established in the Deficit Reduction Act of 2005. The *Official Guidelines* added the reporting requirements on POA to Appendix I in the version effective November 15, 2006, to take effect the following year. The payment impact is effective October 1, 2008.

For outpatient cases, because the diagnostic process may not be completed during the encounter, the **primary diagnosis** is coded—this is the code representing the patient's reason for the encounter. If the encounter was unscheduled—such as an emergency department visit—the **patient's reason for visit** is coded.

Locate the Diagnosis (Diagnoses) in the Alphabetic Index

The second step is to research each diagnosis in the Alphabetic Index and identify probable codes to be checked. The coder follows the conventions and rules of ICD-9-CM during this process.

Verify the Diagnosis Code(s) in the Tabular List

The third step is to verify the possible codes in the Tabular List, making sure that the selection is accurate. The coder reads all surrounding notes and instructions.

Sequence Multiple Diagnosis Codes

The fourth step applies when the patient has more than a single diagnosis. In this situation, the chosen codes are placed in the correct sequence for reporting on claims. The reporting order is governed by the **ICD-9-CM** *Official Guidelines for Coding and Reporting,* which are written by NCHS and CMS and approved by the American Hospital Association (AHA)**,** the American Health Information Management Association (AHIMA), CMS, and NCHS.

Present on Admission (POA) Guidelines

Once the diagnosis codes have been assigned and sequenced, the medical coder in the inpatient setting must also determine whether each principal and secondary diagnosis, as well as external cause of injury, was **present on admission (POA).** *Present on admission* means present at the time the

Table 4.4

Present on Admission (POA) Indicators

Indicator	Meaning	Definition
Y	Yes	Present at the time of inpatient admission
N	No	Not present at the time of inpatient admission
U	Unknown	Documentation is insufficient to determine whether condition was present on admission
W	Clinically undetermined	Provider is unable to clinically determine whether condition was present on admission
____ (blank) or 1	Unreported/ not used	If the diagnosis code for the condition is on the list of exempt codes, the field is left blank or a 1 is reported

INTERNET RESOURCE
Official Guidelines: POA Reporting
POA reporting guidelines begin on page 92. www.cdc.gov/nchs/datawh/ftpserv/ftpicd9/icdguide07.pdf This version of the *Official Guidelines* is effective October 1, 2007.

$ $ Billing Tip $ $

Returned Claims When POA Missing

For discharges as of April 1, 2008, Medicare will return claims lacking POA indicators for resubmission with the correct assignment of POA indicators. POA indicators must be assigned to the principal diagnosis field and the secondary diagnosis fields, including an E code if reported as a secondary diagnosis.

$ $ Billing Tip $ $

Types of Conditions That Will Not Be Paid Unless POA

Among the conditions that are not reimbursed by Medicare if they are hospital-stay-generated are pressure ulcers; injuries caused by falls; and infections resulting from the prolonged use of catheters in blood vessels or the bladder. Also noted are "serious preventable events" like leaving a sponge or other object in a patient during surgery and providing a patient with incompatible blood or blood products.

order for inpatient admission occurs. Conditions that develop during an outpatient encounter that leads to admission—including in the emergency department, during observation, or during outpatient surgery—are considered present on admission. Whether the condition was present on admission is reported by the use of an indicator, as shown in Table 4.4. The indicator is placed next to each ICD-9-CM diagnosis code reported on a hospital health care claim.

Notice that indicators U and W refer to documentation issues, or knowledge about whether a condition was present that the provider was unable to clinically determine. Issues related to inconsistent, missing, conflicting, or unclear documentation must be resolved by the provider.

Leaving the POA field blank (on paper claims), or reporting the number 1 (on Medicare claims and all electronic claims) is appropriate when an ICD-9-CM diagnosis code that is listed on the POA exempt from reporting list is assigned. The use of this indicator either represents a condition that is always present on admission or one that does not represent a current disease or injury. For example, normal delivery codes represent conditions that are always present on admission, whereas screening codes and the palliative care code do not represent current diseases. POA indicator 1 or a blank POA field would be used in each of these situations.

New Version: ICD-10-CM

The tenth edition of the ICD was published by the World Health Organization in 1990. In the United States, the new Clinical Modification (ICD-10-CM) data set is being reviewed by health care professionals, and ICD-10-CM is expected to be adopted as the mandatory U.S. diagnosis code set soon. (Other countries, such as Australia and Canada, already use their own modifications of ICD-10.) The major changes are as follows:

- ICD-10 contains more than two thousand categories of diseases, many more than ICD-9. This creates more codes to permit more-specific reporting of diseases and newly recognized conditions.

- Codes are alphanumeric, each containing a letter followed by up to five numbers.

- A sixth digit is added to capture clinical details. For example, all codes that relate to pregnancy, labor, and childbirth include a digit that indicates the patient's trimester.

- Codes are added to show which side of the body is affected for a disease or condition that can be involved with the right side, the left side, or bilaterally. For example, separate codes are listed for a malignant neoplasm of right upper-inner quadrant of the female breast and for a malignant neoplasm of left upper-inner quadrant of the female breast.

When ICD-10-CM is mandated for use, a **crosswalk** will also be available. A crosswalk is a printed or computerized resource that connects two sets of data. The crosswalk will relate ICD-10-CM to ICD-9-CM. In anticipation of the adoption of ICD-10-CM, the claim formats (the 837I and the paper UB-04 claim) have already been revised to accept the longer codes.

Procedural Coding: ICD Volume 3 and HCPCS/CPT

Procedural coding is done using two different sources. ICD Volume 3 is used for coding inpatient hospital procedures, and HCPCS/CPT codes are used for coding outpatient hospital procedures.

Procedure codes, like diagnosis codes, are an important part of the billing process. Facilities and physicians use standard procedure codes to report the medical, surgical, and diagnostic services they provide. Accurate procedural coding ensures that providers receive the maximum appropriate reimbursement. Correct codes also help establish guidelines for the delivery of the best possible care for patients. Medical researchers track various treatment plans for patients with similar diagnoses and evaluate patients' outcomes. The results are shared with providers and payers so that best practices can be implemented. For example, this type of analysis has shown that a patient who has had a heart attack can reduce the risk of another heart attack by taking a class of drugs called beta blockers.

ICD-9-CM Volume 3

Volume 3 (Procedures) of ICD-9-CM classifies procedures performed in the hospital inpatient setting, and the codes are used only by facilities. To payers, the Volume 3 codes report that the hospital used resources such as a surgical suite or a room in the delivery of services. Volume 3 codes are maintained and updated by CMS.

Volume 3 contains both an Alphabetic Index to Procedures and a Tabular List of Procedures. The Alphabetic Index to Procedures is formatted alphabetically by type of procedure, eponym (a procedure named after a person), or operation. Once a code has been located in the Alphabetic Index to Procedures, the code is verified in the Tabular List of Procedures (see Table 4.5 on page 89). The format of the Volume 3 Tabular List is similar to the format of the Volume 1 Tabular List of Diseases and Injuries. Volume 3 procedure codes contain three or four digits, with two characters placed to the left of the decimal point. Coding to the highest level of specificity is required, meaning that the code must include the most digits available.

Table 4.5

ICD-9-CM Volume 3 Tabular List Organization

Classifications of Operations

Chapter		Codes
1	Operations on the Nervous System	01–05
2	Operations on the Endocrine System	06–07
3	Operations on the Eye	08–17
4	Operations on the Ear	18–20
5	Operations on the Nose, Mouth, and Pharynx	21–29
6	Operations on the Respiratory System	30–34
7	Operations on the Cardiovascular System	35–39
8	Operations on the Hemic and Lymphatic System	40–41
9	Operations on the Digestive System	42–54
10	Operations on the Urinary System	55–59
11	Operations on the Male Genital Organs	60–64
12	Operations on the Female Genital Organs	65–71
13	Obstetrical Procedures	72–75
14	Operations on the Musculoskeletal System	76–84
15	Operations on the Integumentary System	85–86
16	Miscellaneous Diagnostic and Therapeutic Procedures	87–99

Healthcare Common Procedure Code Set (HCPCS)

The **Healthcare Common Procedure Code Set (HCPCS,** pronounced hic-pix), is the HIPAA code set for physicians' services and supplies and for outpatient facility billing. HCPCS has two parts. Officially, CPT procedure codes make up the first part (called Level I) of HCPCS, and supply codes are the second part (Level II). Most people, though, refer to the codes in the CPT book as *CPT codes* and the Level II codes as *HCPCS codes*.

CPT Codes

CPT codes are selected from the **Current Procedural Terminology** data set, called **CPT,** which is owned and maintained by the American Medical Association (AMA). CPT lists the procedures and services that are commonly performed by physicians across the country.

There are three categories of CPT codes:

1. CPT Category I codes—which are the most numerous—have five digits (with no decimals). Each code is listed with its descriptor, which is a brief explanation of the procedure. Although the codes are grouped into sections, such as Surgery, codes from all sections can be used by all types of physicians. For example, a family practitioner might use codes from the Surgery section to describe an office procedure such as the incision and drainage of an abscess.

2. Category II codes are used to track performance measures for a medical goal such as reducing tobacco use. These codes, which have alphabetic characters for the fifth digit, are optional; they are not paid by insurance carriers.

> **HIPAA TIP**
>
> *Mandated Code Set*
> CPT is the mandated code set for physician procedures and services under HIPAA Electronic Health Care Transactions and Code Sets. Codes must be current as of the date of service.

3. Category III codes are temporary codes for emerging technology, services, and procedures. These codes also have alphabetic characters for the fifth digit.

CPT is a proprietary code set, meaning that it is not available to the public for free. Instead, the information must be purchased, either in print or electronic format, from the AMA, which publishes the revised CPT codes. The annual changes for Category I codes are released by the AMA on October 1 and are in effect for procedures and services provided after January 1 of the following year. The codebooks can be purchased in different formats, which range from a basic listing to an enhanced edition. The AMA also reports the new codes on its website. Category II and III codes are prereleased on the AMA website every six months. These codes can be used on their implementation date even before they appear in the printed books.

Organization of CPT

The manual is made up of the main text—sections of codes—followed by appendixes and an index. The main text has the following six sections of Category I procedure codes:

Section	*Codes*
Evaluation and Management	99201–99499
Anesthesia	00100–01999
Surgery	10021–69990
Radiology	70010–79999
Pathology and Laboratory	80048–89356
Medicine	90281–99602

Table 4.6 on page 91 summarizes the types of codes, organization, and guidelines of the six main sections.

The Index

The assignment of a correct procedure code begins with review of the physician's statements in the patient's medical record to determine the service, procedure, or treatment that was performed. Then the index entry is located, which provides a pointer to the correct code range in the main text. Using the CPT index makes the process of selecting procedure codes more efficient. The index contains the descriptive terms that are listed in the sections of codes in CPT.

The Main Text

After the index is used to point to a possible code or code range, the main text is read to verify the selection of the code. To save space in the book, CPT uses a semicolon and indentions when a common part of a main entry applies to entries that follow. For example, in the entries listed below, the procedure "partial laryngectomy (hemilaryngectomy)" is the common descriptor. This same descriptor applies to the four unique descriptors after the

Table 4.6

CPT Category I Code Sections

Section	Definition of Codes	Structure	Key Guidelines
Evaluation and Management	Physicians' services that are performed to determine the best course for patient care	Organized by place and/or type of service	New/established patients; other definitions Unlisted services, special reports Selecting an E/M service level
Anesthesia	Anesthesia services by or supervised by a physician; includes general, regional, and local anesthesia	Organized by body site	Time-based Services covered (bundled) in codes Unlisted services/special reports Qualifying circumstances codes
Surgery	Surgical procedures performed by physicians	Organized by body system and then body site, followed by procedural groups	Surgical package definition Follow-up care definition Add-on codes Separate procedures Subsection notes Unlisted services/special reports
Radiology	Radiology services by or supervised by a physician	Organized by type of procedure followed by body site	Unlisted services/special reports Supervision and interpretation (professional and technical components)
Pathology and Laboratory	Pathology and laboratory services by physicians or by physician-supervised technicians	Organized by type of procedure	Complete procedure Panels Unlisted services/special reports
Medicine	Evaluation, therapeutic, and diagnostic procedures by or supervised by a physician	Organized by type of service or procedure	Subsection notes Multiple procedures reported separately Add-on codes Separate procedures Unlisted services/special reports

semicolon—horizontal, laterovertical, anterovertical, and antero-latero-vertical. Note that the common descriptor begins with a capital letter, but the unique descriptors after the semicolon do not. Also note that after the first listing, the second, third, and fourth descriptors are indented. Indenting visually reinforces the relationship between the entries and the common descriptor.

EXAMPLE:

31370 Partial laryngectomy (hemilaryngectomy); horizontal
31375   laterovertical
31380   anterovertical
31382   antero-latero-vertical

This method shows the relationships among the entries without repeating the common word or words.

Each section begins with guidelines for the use of its codes. The guidelines cover definitions and items unique to the section. They also include special notes about the structure of the section or the rules for its use. The guidelines must be carefully studied and followed in order to correctly use the codes in the section.

Each of the six sections then lists procedure codes and descriptions under subsection headings. These headings group procedures or services, such as

Figure 4.3

Example of CPT Codes

Digestive System

Lips

(For procedures on skin of lips, see 10040 et seq)

EXCISION

40490	Biopsy of lip
40500	Vermilionectomy (lip shave), with mucosal advancement
40510	Excision of lip; transverse wedge excision with primary closure
40520	V-excision with primary direct linear closure

(For excision of mucous lesions, see 40810-40816)

40525	full thickness, reconstruction with local flap (eg, Estlander or fan)
40527	full thickness, reconstruction with cross lip flap (Abbe-Estlander)
40530	Resection of lip, more than one-fourth, without reconstruction

(For reconstruction, see 13131 et seq)

Therapeutic or Diagnostic Injections; body systems, such as Digestive System; anatomical sites, such as Abdomen; and tests and examinations, such as Complete Blood Count (CBC). Following these headings are additional subgroups of procedures, systems, or sites. The section, subsection, and code number range on a page are shown at the top of the page, making it easier to locate a code. Figure 4.3 shows the digestive system subsection from the surgery section of the CPT.

Unlisted Procedures

Most sections' guidelines give **unlisted procedure codes** for procedures or services not completely described by any code in the section. For example, in the Evaluation and Management section, two unlisted codes are provided:

EXAMPLE:
99429 Unlisted preventive medicine service
99499 Unlisted evaluation and management service

Unlisted procedure codes are used for new services or procedures that have not yet been assigned either Category I or III codes in CPT. When an unlisted code is reported to a payer, documentation of the procedure should accompany the claim. Often the operative report or a letter from the physician describing the procedure meets this need.

Complete Procedures

Many surgical codes, as explained in the CPT Surgery section guidelines, represent groups of procedures that include all routine elements. This combination of services is called a **complete procedure** or a surgical package. One code covers a visit before the surgery, local anesthesia, the operation itself, and routine follow-up care.

$ $ **Billing Tip** $ $

Unlisted Procedure Codes

Unlisted procedures require special reports, which delay claims because they must be processed manually. Check with the payer to find out if a temporary code or Category III code has been assigned. If so, that code should be used. If not, use the unlisted code, and supply the payer-required documentation.

CPT Conventions

These symbols have the following meanings when they appear next to CPT codes:

•	A bullet (a black circle) indicates a new procedure code. The symbol appears next to the code only in the year that it is added.
▲	A triangle indicates that the code's descriptor has changed. It, too, appears only in the year the descriptor is revised.
►◄	Facing triangles (two triangles that face each other) enclose new or revised text other than the code's descriptor.
+	A plus sign next to a code in the main text indicates an add-on code. Add-on codes describe secondary procedures that are commonly carried out in addition to a primary procedure.
⊙	A bullet inside a circle next to a code means that conscious sedation is part of the procedure that the surgeon performs. This means that, for compliant coding, conscious sedation is not billed in addition to the code. Conscious sedation is a moderate, drug-induced depression of consciousness during which the patient can respond to verbal commands. This type of sedation is typically used with procedures such as bronchoscopies.
⊘	A circle with a backslash inside indicates that the code cannot be modified with a −51 modifier to indicate multiple procedures because the code already includes a multiple descriptor (modifiers are discussed below).
⚡	Also used is the symbol for a lightning bolt, which indicates vaccine codes that have been submitted to the Federal Drug Administration (FDA) and are expected to be approved for use soon. The codes cannot be used until approved, at which point this symbol is removed.

CPT Modifiers

A CPT modifier is a two-digit number that may be attached to most five-digit procedure codes. **Modifiers** show that some special circumstance applies to the service or procedure the physician performed. Because the service or procedure has been modified, it is different than its description in CPT, but not enough to require another code. Modifiers are often used to indicate that:

- A service or procedure has been performed more than once, by more than one physician, and/or in more than one location
- A service or procedure has been increased or reduced
- Only part of a procedure has been done
- A bilateral or multiple procedure has been performed
- Unusual difficulties occurred during the procedure

For example, the CPT modifier −62 indicates that two surgeons worked together, each performing part of a surgical procedure, during an operation. Each physician will be paid part of the amount normally reimbursed for that procedure code. Likewise, modifier −80 indicates that the services of a surgical assistant were used and that this person's fees are part of the claim. A modifier usually affects the normal level of reimbursement for the code to which it is attached.

> **$ $ Billing Tip $ $**
>
> **Professional Component Modifier −26**
>
> The professional component modifier tells the payer that the physician did not perform all the work, just the professional part, so only part of the fee is due. The other part of the fee is paid to the technician.

Although hospitals use certain CPT modifiers in the outpatient setting, most modifiers apply to physician billing only. For this reason, CPT coding books usually list modifiers that are approved for hospital outpatient use separately on the inside cover for quick reference. An example of a modifier used in the hospital outpatient setting is –27 (Multiple outpatient hospital E/M encounters on the same date).

Evaluation and Management Codes

INTERNET RESOURCE
Evaluation and Management Documentation Guidelines
1995 Guidelines: www.cms.hhs.gov/MLNProducts/ Downloads/1995dg.pdf
1997 Guidelines: www.cms.hhs.gov/MLNProducts/ Downloads/MASTER1.pdf

The Evaluation and Management (E/M) section is a unique section in CPT that lists codes used to report evaluation and management services provided during hospital visits, in the physician's office, or in an outpatient facility. These codes are used specifically to report physician visits. Depending on the visit, E/M codes may be used alone on a claim or they may result in specific diagnostic or therapeutic services reported by other codes in CPT.

E/M codes are assigned based on the extent of documentation with regard to the patient history, the physical exam, and the level of medical decision making that occurs during the visit. The place of service, type of service and patient status help determine the range of the code selected.

For example, if a patient is seen in the emergency department by the ED physician, a code from the series 99281–99285 would be assigned. On the other hand, if a patient was an established patient seen in the physician's office, a code from the series 99211–99215 would be assigned.

Documentation is reviewed to determine the extent of each key component in order to assign a specific code. Medicare publishes guidelines known as the Evaluation and Management Documentation Guidelines that provide specific details on E/M code assignment. Review of these guidelines is essential in assigning accurate E/M codes. Currently two versions are used—the 1995 and the 1997 guidelines. A physician can use either version; however, both versions cannot be used together. One set or the other must be followed consistently.

Assigning CPT Procedure Codes

The correct process for assigning accurate procedural codes has four steps:

1. The first step is to identify the procedures to be coded.

2. The second step is to research each procedure in the CPT Index.

3. The third step is to verify the possible codes in the main text, making sure the selection is accurate, and to assign modifiers if needed.

4. The fourth step is to rank the codes to be reported for each day's services in order of highest to lowest rate of reimbursement. The actual order in which they were performed on a particular day is not important. For services on multiple dates, the earliest day is listed first, followed by subsequent dates of service.

EXAMPLE:

Date	Procedure	Charge
11/17/2008	**99204**	$202
11/20/2008	**43215**	$355
11/20/2008	**74235**	$ 75

HCPCS Codes

The national codes for products, supplies, and those services not included in CPT are in the HCPCS Level II code set, which was set up to give health care providers a coding system that describes specific products, supplies, and services that patients receive. HCPCS codes provide uniformity in medical services reporting and enable the collection of statistical data on medical procedures, products, and services.

CMS is responsible for maintaining the HCPCS code set, which is public. Information about the codes and updates is located on the CMS HCPCS website. Many publishers also print easy-to-use HCPCS reference books.

A Level II code is made up of five characters beginning with a letter followed by four numbers, such as J7630. The HCPCS Tabular list of codes has more than twenty sections, each of which covers a related group of items (see Table 4.7). HCPCS Level II codes can be used in conjunction with CPT codes on claims for Medicare, Medicaid, and other payers. As with CPT codes, reporting HCPCS codes does not guarantee payment. Each payer's coverage and payment decisions apply. Also, decisions regarding the addition, deletion, and revision of HCPCS codes are made independent of the adjudication process.

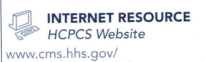
INTERNET RESOURCE
HCPCS Website
www.cms.hhs.gov/
MedHCPCSGenInfo/

Table 4.7

HCPCS Sections

Section	Codes
Transport Services Including Ambulance	A0000–A0999
Medical and Surgical Supplies	A4000–A8999
Administrative, Miscellaneous, and Investigational	A9000–A9999
Enteral and Parenteral Therapy	B4000–B9999
C Codes (for use only under the hospital Outpatient Prospective Payment System; not to be used to report other services; updated quarterly by CMS)	C1000–C9999
Dental Procedures (copyrighted by the American Dental Association and not included in the general HCPCS coding text)	D0000–D9999
Durable Medical Equipment (DME)	E0100–E9999
Procedures/Professional Services (temporary) and Assigned by CMS (on temporary basis)	G0000–G9999
Alcohol and/or Drug Services	H0001–H1005
Drugs Other Than Chemotherapy	J0100–J8999
Chemotherapy Drugs	J9000–J9999
K Codes for Durable Medical Equipment (temporary codes assigned by CMS for the exclusive use of Durable Medical Equipment Regional Carriers)	K0000–K9999
Orthotic Procedures	L0100–L4999
Prosthetic Procedures	L5000–L9999
Medical Services	M0000–M0399
Pathology and Laboratory Services	P0000–P2999
Temporary Codes	Q0000–Q9999
Diagnostic Radiology Services	R0000–R5999
Temporary National Codes (non-Medicare)	S0009–S9999
National T Codes for State Medicaid Agencies (not valid for Medicare)	T1000–T9999
Vision Services	V0000–V2999
Hearing Services	V5000–V5299

To assign HCPCS Level II codes, first look up the name of the supply or item in the index. The index is arranged alphabetically, with the main term in bold print followed by the HCPCS Level II code. Verify the code selection in the appropriate Tabular List section of the HCPCS Level II codebook.

Assigning HCPCS Drug Codes

Assigning drug codes is made easier by the Table of Drugs in Appendix 1 of the HCPCS codebook. It presents drugs in alphabetical order, followed by the dosage, the way the drug is administered (such as intravenously), and the HCPCS code.

EXAMPLE:

Adenosine 30 mg	IV	J0152
Adenosine 6 mg	IV	J0150
Adrenalin 1 mg	IM, IV, SC	J0170

In the Tabular List section of the codebook, the code is listed first, followed by the name of the drug, the method of administration, and then the dosage. The dosage is described in appropriate quantities, such as milligrams (mg) or milliliters (ml).

EXAMPLE:

J7506   Prednisone, oral, per 5 mg

If a patient's dosage of Prednisone is 10 mg, the code to report is J7506 X2. On the claim form, the HCPCS code would be followed by the quantity 2 in the units column. If the patient had been administered 12 mg, the unit indicator would be 3, since this drug comes in 5 mg doses. It is important to make this distinction between the amount the patient receives and the unit amount. The unit amount of a drug (the number of doses), not the amount in milligrams or milliliters the patient has actually received, is reported when the insurance claim is prepared, because the unit amount reflects the actual cost.

HCPCS Modifiers

Like CPT, HCPCS Level II uses modifiers to provide additional information about services, supplies, and procedures. For example, a –UE modifier is used when an item identified by a HCPCS code is used equipment, and an –NU modifier is used for new equipment. Similar to CPT modifiers, there are a limited number of HCPCS modifiers that are approved for hospital outpatient use. This list is limited largely to location modifiers, such as –LT (Left side), –RT (Right side), or F6 (Right hand, second digit).

HCPCS Level II modifiers are made up of either one letter and one number or two letters.

EXAMPLES:

–F5	Right hand, thumb
–GA	Waiver of liability on file
–RC	Right coronary artery

The HCPCS modifier –TC is used when a procedure has two parts—a **technical component (TC)** performed by a facility technician, such as a radiologist, and a professional component (PC) that the physician performs, usually the interpretation and reporting of the results. The facility appends the HCPCS modifier –TC to the CPT procedure code to indicate the technical portion of the procedure. Coders must follow specific guidelines when applying modifiers, as not all modifiers are available for use with all codes. For example, a HCPCS modifier can be used with a CPT or HCPCS code; however, a CPT modifier can only be used with a CPT code.

CHAPTER SUMMARY

1 ICD-9-CM is the Clinical Modification of the World Health Organization's International Classification of Diseases used for diagnostic coding in the United States. ICD-9-CM codes are required under HIPAA for reporting patients' conditions in both the inpatient and outpatient settings. Codes are made up of three, four, or five numbers and a description.

2 Two volumes of ICD-9-CM are used for diagnostic coding: the Tabular List (Volume 1) and the Alphabetic Index (Volume 2). The Alphabetic Index is used first in the process of finding a code. It contains an index of all the diseases that are classified in the Tabular List. The codes themselves are organized into seventeen chapters according to etiology or body system and are listed in numerical order in the Tabular List. A code category consists of a three-digit grouping of a single disease or a related condition. Subcategories have four digits to show the disease's etiology, site, or manifestation. Further clinical detail is supplied by fifth-digit subclassifications. V codes and E codes are supplementary classifications for encounters for reasons other than illness or injury and for the external causes of illnesses or conditions. Volume 3 of ICD-9-CM classifies inpatient procedures that are billed by hospitals.

3 The conventions used in ICD-9-CM must be observed to correctly select codes. Notes provide details about conditions that are either excluded or included under the code. A symbol is used to show a fifth-digit requirement. The abbreviation NOS (not otherwise specified or unspecified) indicates the code to use when a condition is not completely described. The abbreviation NEC (not elsewhere classified) indicates the code to use when the diagnosis does not match any other available code. Parentheses and brackets indicate supplementary terms. Colons and braces indicate that one or more words after the punctuation must appear in the diagnostic statement for the code to be applicable. Codes that are not used as primary appear in italics and are usually followed by instructions to code first underlying disease or use an additional code.

4 Once ICD-9-CM codes for inpatient stays have been assigned and sequenced, each code must be assigned an indicator that identifies whether the condition was present on admission (POA). Y (for yes) is reported if the condition was present. Other indicators are N (no) if the condition was not present on admission, U if the presence of the condition on admission is unknown, and W if the presence of the condition on admission is clinically undetermined. Some codes, mostly V and E codes, are exempt from reporting the present on admission indicator, and the indicator is 1 or left blank (on paper claims).

5 HCPCS is the overall title of the two HIPAA-mandated outpatient procedural code sets, Level I (CPT) and Level II (HCPCS). CPT, a publication of the American Medical Association, contains the most widely used system of codes for outpatient medical, diagnostic, and procedural services. CPT codes have five digits and a description. HCPCS codes are supply codes made up of five characters beginning with a letter followed by four numbers. Updated HCPCS/CPT codes are released annually; current codes must be used.

6 CPT contains six sections of Category I codes, Evaluation and Management, Anesthesia, Surgery, Radiology, Pathology and Laboratory, and Medicine, followed by the Category II and Category III codes, nine appendixes, and an index. The index is used first in the process of selecting a code; it contains alphabetic descriptive terms for the procedures and services contained in the main text. The codes themselves are listed in the main text and are generally grouped by body system or site or by type of procedure.

Each coding section begins with section guidelines, which discuss definitions and rules for the use of codes, such as for unlisted codes, special reports, and notes for specific subsections. When a main entry has more than one code, a semicolon follows the common part of a descriptor in the main entry, and the unique descriptors that are related to the common description are indented below it. Seven symbols are used in the main text: (a) • (a bullet or black circle) indicates a new procedure code; (b) ▲ (a triangle) indicates that the code's descriptor has changed; (c) ▶◀ (facing triangles) enclose new or revised text other than the code's descriptor; (d) + (a plus sign) before a code indicates an add-on code that is used only along with other codes for primary procedures; (e) the symbol ⊙ next to a code means that conscious sedation is a part of the procedure that the surgeon performs; (f) a ⊘ indicates that the code cannot be modified with a –51 modifier; and (g) a ⁄ is used for codes for vaccines that are pending FDA approval.

7 A CPT modifier is a two-digit number that may be attached to most five-digit procedure codes to indicate that the procedure is different from the listed descriptor, but not in a way that changes the definition or requires a different code. HCPCS modifiers are a different set of modifiers that contain either two letters or a letter with a number. Like CPT modifiers, they provide additional information about services, supplies, or procedures. Only a limited number of CPT and HCPCS modifiers are approved for hospital outpatient use.

8 HCPCS has an index and a listing of codes by alphabetic chapter. Chapters cover various supplies, such as durable medical equipment and drugs.

9 The basic four-step process medical coders follow to assign correct ICD-9-CM and HCPCS/CPT codes is (a) identify the diagnosis (diagnoses) and/or procedures to be coded; (b) locate the term in the index of the code set; (c) verify the code selection in the main listings of the code set; and (d) sequence multiple codes for correct billing.

10 The code sets that are associated with inpatient versus outpatient billing for hospital services are:

	Hospital Inpatient	Hospital Outpatient
Diagnosis codes	ICD-9-CM Volumes 1 & 2	ICD-9-CM Volumes 1 & 2
Procedure codes	ICD-9-CM Volume 3	HCPCS/CPT

✔ CHECK YOUR UNDERSTANDING

Write *T* or *F* to indicate whether you think the statement is true or false.

_____ **1.** The ICD-9-CM coding system is used to assign codes to patients' diagnoses.

_____ **2.** The third volume of ICD-9-CM is used to code hospital inpatient procedures.

_____ **3.** Medical coders have the option of choosing three-, four-, or five-digit ICD-9-CM diagnosis codes.

_____ **4.** A POA code indicates the type of admission.

_____ **5.** CPT is published by the American Medical Association.

_____ **6.** Both ICD-9-CM and CPT codes are updated every year.

_____ **7.** CPT modifiers may contain two letters or one letter and one number.

_____ **8.** The technical component of a CPT code refers to the physician's work, such as a surgery.

_____ **9.** CPT is the mandated code set for physician procedures and services under HIPAA Electronic Health Care Transactions and Code Sets.

_____ **10.** HCPCS Level II codes have five characters.

_____ **11.** A modifier is used to indicate that only part of a procedure was done.

_____ **12.** Procedure codes are listed in the order in which they were performed on a particular day.

Choose the best answer.

13. A complete procedure in CPT terminology means
   a. a procedure that was completed by one physician
   b. a procedure code that represents all routine elements of a service
   c. a procedure that is too new to be included in CPT
   d. a Level II code

14. Which of the following is not a step in the process of assigning correct procedure codes?
   a. identify the procedures to be coded
   b. locate the term in the index of the code set
   c. assign a POA indicator
   d. sequence multiple codes for correct billing

15. All of the following codes are valid POA indicators except
   a. Y (yes)
   b. W (clinically undetermined)
   c. N (no)
   d. NA (not applicable)

16. V codes are reported to identify
   a. complete routine physical examinations
   b. accidents
   c. unlisted procedures
   d. surgical procedures

17. The principal diagnosis code is a condition that
   a. develops as a problem related to surgery or treatment
   b. can be defined by an E code
   c. is chiefly responsible for the patient's admission to the hospital
   d. is present on admission

18. Which of the following contains the data elements recorded at an inpatient's discharge?
   a. ICD-9-CM   **c.** ICD-10-CM
   b. UHDDS   **d.** HCPCS

19. The listing for Pepcid in the HCPCS Table of Drugs is: Pepcid, 20 mg, IV, S0028. A patient receives 30 mg. How should the amount be reported for billing purposes?
   a. S0028, 30 mg   **c.** S0028 ×2
   b. S0028, 30 units **d.** S0028 ×30

20. An E code indicates
   a. an emergency department procedure
   b. an external cause of injury
   c. a comorbidity
   d. a complication

COMPUTER EXPLORATION

Internet Application

1. Access the website of CMS, and research the topic ICD-9-CM to locate the ICD-9-CM Provider and Diagnostic Codes Overview home page. Find a listing of the current year's new, revised, or deleted ICD-9-CM codes, which is called the Addenda. Locate five new codes in the Tabular Addenda.

2. Access the website of the National Center for Health Statistics at www.cdc.gov/nchs/icd9.htm. Preview the status of ICD-10-CM. Research current changes to the ICD-9-CM *Official Guidelines*.

3. Visit the website of the American Medical Association at www.ama-assn.org. Under the heading CPT Codes and Resources, read the information on the CPT process, and report on how new CPT codes are approved.

Payment Methods and Billing Compliance

LEARNING OUTCOMES

After completing this chapter, you will be able to define the key terms and:

1. Describe the purpose and use of the Medicare Inpatient Prospective Payment System.
2. Explain how a DRG is assigned.
3. Compare and contrast MCC, CC, and non-CC.
4. List the eight conditions that will not be considered for assigning a DRG unless they are documented as existing when the patient was admitted.
5. Discuss the types of errors that are detected by the Medicare Code Editor.
6. Describe the purpose and use of the Medicare Outpatient Prospective Payment System.
7. Explain how an APC is assigned.
8. List the three types of CCI edits.
9. Discuss fraud and abuse in the hospital billing setting.
10. Describe the parts of a compliance plan.
11. Explain the purpose of a pay-for-performance program.

KEY TERMS

- abuse
- ambulatory payment classifications (APCs)
- base rate
- benchmark
- case mix index (CMI)
- CCI column 1/column 2 code pair edits
- CCI mutually exclusive edits
- CC and MCC lists
- compliance plan
- compliance program guidance
- Correct Coding Initiative (CCI)
- diagnosis-related groups (DRGs)
- DRG weight
- external audit
- *Federal Register*
- fraud
- hospital-acquired condition
- Inpatient Prospective Payment System (IPPS)
- internal audits
- major CC (MCC)
- major diagnostic category (MDC)
- Medicare Common Working File (CWF)

- Medicare Code Editor (MCE)
- Medicare-Severity DRGs (MS-DRGs)
- MS Grouper
- non-CC
- Office of the Inspector General (OIG)
- outlier payment
- Outpatient Code Editor (OCE)
- Outpatient Prospective Payment System (OPPS)
- pay-for-performance programs
- quality measures
- status indicator (SI)
- triggered reviews

When patients have medical insurance, patient account specialists must take the payer's billing requirements into account. In the inpatient setting, there are hospital charges associated with ICD-9-CM codes; in the outpatient setting, charges are related to HCPCS/CPT procedure codes. Although charges are related to all the codes reported on hospital claims, each code is not necessarily payable; payment depends on the payer's rules and the terms of the contract with the provider. Following these rules and terms when preparing claims results in billing compliance. Compliant billing avoids even a remote suggestion of fraudulent or abusive behavior and ensures the maximum appropriate reimbursement for the hospital.

The Medicare Inpatient Prospective Payment System

$ $ **Billing Tip** $ $

Other Payers' Use of the PPS

Many state Medicaid programs, Blue Cross plans, and commercial payers use some version of the Medicare IPPS as the payment system for their non-Medicare hospital patients.

Medicare, by far the largest health plan for hospital reimbursement, is authorized under Section 1886(d) of the Social Security Act to pay for acute care inpatient visits under the Medicare **Inpatient Prospective Payment System (IPPS).** This system is called *prospective* because rather than paying for each service based on what the hospital charges, the rate has been set in advance. Rates are established based on Medicare's analysis of how long people are hospitalized, on average, for similar conditions, and the average cost incurred. The length of stay (LOS) is a good predictor of the average use of the hospital's resources, and thus of the cost of care.

DRGs

Medicare analyzes and updates a study of all ICD-9-CM codes—both diagnosis and procedure codes—that are reported for care during a period of time. Medicare then designs a payment system based on **major diagnostic categories (MDCs),** which are then further divided into **diagnosis-related groups (DRGs).**

At discharge, a patient is assigned a single DRG, which is based on these elements of the UHDDS (Uniform Hospital Discharge Data Set):

- The principal diagnosis is used to determine the major diagnostic category.

- Other diagnoses, significant procedures (like surgery), and the patient's age, sex, and discharge status refine the major diagnostic category and are used to assign the DRG.

Each DRG has a national relative **DRG weight,** which represents the average resources required to care for cases in that particular DRG relative to the average resources used to treat cases in all DRGs. The greater the weight assigned to a DRG, the more resource-intensive it is. To figure what a hospital will be paid for a particular DRG, the DRG weight is multiplied by the hospital's **base rate,** which is calculated based on its costs, wage index, and location. In other words, the weight for the assigned DRG multiplied by the hospital rate equals the DRG payment for that discharge: hospital base rate × DRG weight = hospital payment.

The DRG weights and rates are updated annually and are published in the *Federal Register*. Hospitals receive this predetermined amount regardless of the actual cost of care, although adjustments may be made in some cases.

A DRG can be calculated manually using decision trees. However, Medicare and hospitals use the **MS Grouper**—a software program—to assign the DRG. The program follows the logic of the DRG decision tree to factor together the principal diagnosis, additional diagnoses, and the procedures performed, plus the patient's age, gender, and other discharge data, to calculate the DRG along with the payment.

The MS Grouper is offered for sale by the National Technical Information Service, part of the federal Department of Commerce. Hospitals use the grouper program to assign DRGs to estimate revenue and check claims before they are released. The DRG ultimately assigned by Medicare during its adjudication process, however, determines the payment.

Medicare-Severity DRGs

In 2008, Medicare replaced the former CMS DRG system with the current **Medicare-Severity DRGs (MS-DRGs)** system. MS-DRGs account for the different severities of illness among patients with the same diagnosis. The system was changed to better recognize these differences; the corresponding higher cost of treating Medicare patients with more complex conditions is offset in the MS-DRGs system by decreasing payments for other, less severely ill patients.

Under the MS-DRG system, there are twenty-five major diagnostic categories, as shown in Table 5.1 (on page 104), and 745 DRGs. Each diagnosis code in the ICD-9-CM (more than thirteen thousand codes!) is covered in one of the DRGs.

Secondary Conditions: The CC Factor

The MS-DRG system increases the importance of documenting and coding secondary conditions because when patients have or develop them, the payment for the hospital stay may be increased. Such secondary conditions are those that affect patient care by requiring at least one of the following:

- Clinical evaluation
- Therapeutic treatment
- Diagnostic procedures
- Extended length of hospital stay
- Increased nursing care and/or monitoring

Secondary conditions are either comorbidities or complications, known as the CCs. Comorbidities represent secondary conditions that patients have at admission that affect treatment. They are usually either chronic conditions that affect a patient's recovery, such as diabetes mellitus, or other acute illnesses or injuries. Complications are conditions that happen after admission and that affect care. Such complications affect the patient's recovery, so the length of the hospital stay is increased, logically increasing payment. The

$$ \$\$ \text{ Billing Tip } \$\$ $$
Use the Correct Version
Billing must be based on the current version of the MS Grouper. A new version is released annually to accompany the IPPS changes that are announced by CMS.

FYI

Major Diagnostic Categories 14 and 15
The DRGs in the major diagnostic categories 14 (pregnancy, childbirth, and puerperium) and 15 (newborns and other neonates) are not subject to the severity adjustment because the severity adjustment focuses on the Medicare population, which typically does not fall into these categories.

Table 5.1

Major Diagnostic Categories (MDCs)

1	Diseases and Disorders of the Nervous System
2	Diseases and Disorders of the Eye
3	Diseases and Disorders of the Ear, Nose, Mouth, and Throat
4	Diseases and Disorders of the Respiratory System
5	Diseases and Disorders of the Circulatory System
6	Diseases and Disorders of the Digestive System
7	Diseases and Disorders of the Hepatobiliary System and Pancreas
8	Diseases and Disorders of the Musculoskeletal System and Connective Tissue
9	Diseases and Disorders of the Skin, Subcutaneous Tissue, and Breast
10	Endocrine, Nutritional, and Metabolic Diseases and Disorders
11	Diseases and Disorders of the Kidney and Urinary Tract
12	Diseases and Disorders of the Male Reproductive System
13	Diseases and Disorders of the Female Reproductive System
14	Pregnancy, Childbirth, and the Puerperium
15	Newborns and Other Neonates with Conditions Originating in the Perinatal Period
16	Diseases and Disorders of the Blood and Blood-Forming Organs and Immunological Disorders
17	Myeloproliferative Diseases and Disorders and Poorly Differentiated Neoplasms
18	Infectious and Parasitic Diseases (Systemic or Unspecified Sites)
19	Mental Diseases and Disorders
20	Alcohol/Drug Use and Alcohol/Drug-Induced Organic Mental Disorders
21	Injuries, Poisonings, and Toxic Effects of Drugs
22	Burns
23	Factors Influencing Health Status and Other Contacts with Health Services
24	Multiple Significant Trauma
25	Human Immunodeficiency Virus Infections

CCs are not just additional illnesses a patient has; they are conditions and illnesses that affect the patient's level of care during the hospital stay.

Three Levels of Severity

To build DRG clusters, every diagnosis code was assigned to one of three levels of severity:

1. *Major CC (MCC):* Diagnosis codes that are classified as MCCs reflect a higher level of severity. Generally a major CC requires double the additional resources of a normal CC.

2. *CC:* A CC is a regular or normal level of severity of illness and thus of resource use. CCs can include acute exacerbations of chronic conditions (level 3) that, when documented and coded correctly, are classified to this level with the higher-paying DRG.

3. *Non-CC:* The non-CC category has chronic conditions that do not require staff members to expend additional resources to the patient portion of the stay.

Possible combinations of a principal diagnosis code and secondary codes are then grouped into DRG clusters, such as:

EXAMPLE:
DRG 154: nasal trauma and deformity with major CC (MCC)
DRG 155: nasal trauma and deformity with CC
DRG 156: nasal trauma and deformity without CC or MCC

Based on this example, a patient whose diagnosis is nasal trauma and deformity who has another condition that is a major CC is "grouped" to DRG 154. The same diagnosis with another condition that affects the hospital stay goes to DRG 155. In the third case, a patient with this diagnosis but with no CCs, major or regular, goes to DRG 156. Consider another example:

EXAMPLE:
DRG 485: knee procedure with principal diagnosis of infection with MCC
DRG 486: knee procedure with principal diagnosis of infection with CC
DRG 487: knee procedure with principal diagnosis of infection without CC
DRG 488: knee procedure *without* principal diagnosis of infection with CC or MCC
DRG 489: knee procedure *without* principal diagnosis of infection without CC

In this example, the first major difference is whether infection was present; then the DRGs are organized by the presence of one of the three levels of secondary conditions.

The Medicare CC and MCC Lists

The Medicare **CC and MCC lists** contain the ICD-9-CM codes for the secondary diagnoses that are considered significant acute diseases, acute exacerbations of significant chronic diseases, or other chronic conditions that have an effect on the use of hospital resources and can therefore be assigned as CCs or MCCs. If a secondary diagnosis code is not on the CC or MCC list, that condition is not counted in arriving at the DRG.

Related Payment Issues

Relating CCs/MCCs and the POA Indicators

The Deficit Reduction Act (DRA) requires CMS to reduce payment in cases where patients develop a **hospital-acquired condition** that would move them from a lower-paying to a higher-paying DRG. Under the law, CMS does not assign a higher paying DRG to patients who have/suffer from the following eight hospital-acquired conditions unless they are documented as present on admission:

1. Serious preventable event—object left in surgery
2. Serious preventable event—air embolism
3. Serious preventable event—blood incompatibility
4. Catheter-associated urinary tract infections
5. Pressure ulcers (decubitus ulcers)
6. Vascular catheter-associated infection
7. Surgical site infection—mediastinitis after coronary artery bypass graft (CABG) surgery
8. Falls

These conditions lose their CC/MCC status if they happened during the admission (POA designated as N, no).

Case Mix Index

An average of the DRG weights for all discharged patients during a certain time period is a hospital's Medicare **case mix index (CMI).** Based on the

When a limited number of codes can be reported, such as on the UB-04 claim, correctly sequencing those codes is very important for reimbursement for patients whose conditions are extremely complex.

value of 1.0, the hospital can determine whether its case mix index is above or below the norm. For example, a case mix index of 1.2345 indicates that a hospital treats patients with more-severe illnesses than does a hospital with a case mix index of 0.9999.

Medical cases have average weights that are lower than surgical cases, so the proportion of medical to surgical cases is a factor in the case mix index calculation. However, a low CMI may indicate that the hospital's DRG assignments do not adequately reflect the resources used to treat Medicare patients. The hospital may then focus attention on improving the medical record documentation so that all appropriate secondary conditions are properly identified and coded.

Outlier Payments

In addition to the base payment for the DRGs, Medicare must make a supplemental payment called an **outlier payment** to a hospital if its costs for treating a particular case exceed the usual Medicare payment for that case by a set threshold.

Transfer Payments

Hospitals receive adjusted payments if Medicare patients are transferred to other PPS acute care facilities. The hospital that transfers the patient, the first hospital, is paid a per diem (per day) rate for the specific DRG instead of the full DRG payment. (The per diem rate is the DRG rate divided by the average length of stay for that DRG. At a maximum, the DRG payment is paid if the length of stay is beyond the DRG mean length of stay). The receiving facility, the second hospital, gets the full DRG payment.

On the other hand, when the patient is transferred from a PPS hospital to a post-acute-care facility such as a skilled nursing facility (SNF), home health agency (HHA), or some other PPS-exempt facility, the first hospital usually receives the full DRG payment. The second hospital is paid according to its fee schedule, for example, an inpatient rehabilitation facility rate or a long-term-care hospital rate. A few hospitals and states do not follow this policy.

Transfer Payments and Discharge Status Codes

There are many DRGs for which Medicare pays an adjusted amount if the patient either engages a home health agency within three days of inpatient discharge or enters a nursing home within fourteen days of discharge. For these DRGs, if the patient's discharge status code indicates either of these transfers, the hospital does not receive the full DRG amount.

Even if the hospital receives the full DRG payment because the patient does not need HHA or SNF services at the time of discharge and is discharged to home at first, if Medicare receives a claim from a home health care agency or a nursing home indicating that the patient ended up requiring these services, Medicare takes back the original DRG payment. The hospital must then submit a new claim with the corrected discharge status code indicating the transfer to home with the help of home health care or a transfer to a nursing home, and a lesser payment is made.

To ensure that Medicare payments are correct, special edits were added into the CMS Common Working File, Medicare's master patient/procedural database.

Because different discharge status codes have different effects on the DRG payment hospitals receive, this code must be carefully checked for each discharge. Chapter 8 discusses patient discharge status codes and how they are reported on hospital bills.

FYI

Common Working File: Medicare Beneficiaries' Histories

The **Medicare Common Working File (CWF)** is a series of computer databases that maintain Medicare beneficiaries' claim and clinical histories. CMS established the CWF program to help the FIs and the Medicare carriers (for Part B claims) handle Medicare claims. The beneficiary history is used by these payers to check for patient eligibility, coordination of benefits—which manages and collects information for each Medicare recipient to determine the correct order of payers if a beneficiary has more than one health plan—and other claims issues. CMS has set up nine regional CWF sectors.

Medicare Code Editor

When claims are processed by Medicare, a patient's diagnosis, procedure, discharge status, and demographic information are analyzed by a software program called the **Medicare Code Editor (MCE).** The MCE is used to detect and report errors in coding before the data are run through the MS Grouper and a DRG is assigned.

The MCE identifies and indicates the nature of the error, but it does not correct the error. A particular error condition is associated with each type of coding error identified by MCE. When MCE identifies an error in a medical claim, it prints a summary of the claim information along with the error message identifying the problem. These cases require further review before a DRG is assigned. Once the questionable information is updated or the necessary information is supplied, the case is classified into the appropriate DRG by the MS Grouper. The MCE, like the MS Grouper, is offered for sale by the National Technical Information Service, part of the federal Department of Commerce.

The MCE software detects the following kinds of errors:

- The code is not in the ICD-9-CM code set.
- The code does not include the required fourth or fifth digit.
- An E code is listed as the principal diagnosis.
- Entries are duplicated.
- The age or gender of patient does not match the coding.
- The code is not an acceptable principal diagnosis.
- The discharge status code is not valid.
- The operating room procedure is nonspecific or noncovered by Medicare.
- The coded services have limited Medicare coverage.

INTERNET RESOURCE

National Technical Information Service: Medicare Code Editor
www.ntis.gov/products/families/cms/grouper.asp

$ $ Billing Tip $ $

Purchasing Medicare Code Editor

As is the case with the Medicare Grouper, hospitals can purchase the Medicare Code Editor software to be sure their claims are clean and will be paid promptly.

$ $ Billing Tip $ $

Medicare Pricer

After the cases are screened through the MCE and assigned to a DRG by the MS Grouper, a third software program called a *pricer* calculates the payment for the case based on the DRG relative weight and additional factors associated with the billing hospital.

The Medicare Outpatient Prospective Payment System

The Medicare **Outpatient Prospective Payment System (OPPS)** is used to pay hospitals for services to Medicare patients that are provided on an outpatient basis. These services include most Medicare Part B services, such as same-day surgery, radiology services, pathology work, and any other procedures that do not require hospital admission. Some hospital outpatient services, however, are not paid for under OPPS. These include physician services, outpatient laboratory, ambulance transport, durable medical equipment, orthotic and prosthetic devices, and physical, occupational, and speech-language therapies, as these services are paid for under other fee schedules or payment systems. In addition to hospital outpatient services, the OPPS covers partial hospitalization services furnished by community mental health centers.

Certain types of hospitals are exempt from the OPPS, including critical access hospitals, certain hospitals in Maryland that are paid under Maryland waiver provisions, and hospitals outside the fifty states.

Ambulatory Payment Classifications

Mirroring the DRGs for the IPPS, the OPPS is based on a prospective payment system that uses a pricing unit called the **ambulatory payment classification (APC).** CMS was authorized to begin using APCs on August 1, 2000, under the Balanced Budget Act of 1997. Prior to this date, CMS used a traditional cost-based system for hospital outpatient services.

APC Payment Rates

Like the inpatient system based on DRGs, each APC has a preestablished prospective payment amount associated with it. However, unlike the inpatient system that assigns a patient to a single DRG, multiple APCs can be assigned to one outpatient record. If a patient receives multiple outpatient services during a single visit, the total payment for the visit is computed as the sum of the individual APC payments for each service.

The APC system establishes groups of covered services so that the services within each group are comparable clinically and with respect to the use of resources. Just as rates are established for DRGs based on Medicare's analysis of how long people are hospitalized, on average, for similar conditions and on the average cost incurred, rates for APCs are calculated based on Medicare's analysis of the national median cost for outpatient procedures.

The rate for an APC is determined using a basic formula that takes into consideration the relative weight assigned to the APC and a conversion factor, reflecting the cost of inflation, that translates the relative weight into a national payment rate for the APC group. Geographical differences are factored into the conversion factor using a hospital wage index. The basic formula is relative weight × conversion factor = APC payment.

The APC payment is the amount the hospital will receive for a given procedure. Medicare's portion of the APC payment is equal to the APC payment amount minus the patient's coinsurance (also referred to by CMS as the patient's copayment). The patient's portion, or coinsurance, is also determined by several factors, including the national median charge that hospitals have used in previous years and a labor wage index. Although CMS anticipates that, in time, the national unadjusted copayment for each APC will equal 20 percent of the allowable APC payment amount, in reality the coinsurance rate can represent up to 40 percent of the APC payment.

APC payment levels are intended to cover all parts of a procedure, including anesthesia, some drugs, implantable medical devices such as pacemakers, and recovery room services. Since one of the goals of a prospective payment system is to minimize reimbursement by bundling services, future changes to the OPPS will likely call for more bundling in APCs.

APC Structure

Under the APC classification system, all CPT/HCPCS codes are linked to an APC code (unless, like laboratory services, they are reimbursed under a different method). The four-digit APC code represents a group of services. The services within each group are clinically similar and require comparable resources, such as recovery room time or hours of observation after an operation.

Each APC code is assigned a relative weight based on its usual cost, a payment rate, a status indicator, a national unadjusted copayment amount, and a minimum unadjusted copayment amount. Each CPT/HCPCS code assigned to the APC group has the same relative weight, payment rate, and other information. In 2007, more than eight thousand outpatient services were classified into nearly 350 APCs.

Each APC group can also be classified into one of several large payment groups. Payment groups have similar service categories. The APC system contains payment groups for significant procedures, surgical procedures, ancillary services, and medical visits. Additional APC payment groups have been established for partial hospitalization and for transitional pass-through items. Pass-through items are services, drugs, or devices too new to have been included in APCs, so providers are permitted to charge for them separately based on transitional pass-through APCs.

Addenda to the OPPS Final Rule

Each year, updates to the APC system, including APC payment rates for each CPT/HCPCS code, are published in the *Federal Register* as addenda to the OPPS final rule. These updates are effective January 1 of the year following the year in which they appear. Quarterly updates to the addenda are posted on the CMS website. Hospitals must rely on the information in the addenda for many purposes. Following are descriptions of Addenda B, D-1, and E.

Addendum B: Master List of CPT/HCPCS Codes

Addendum B, which is published by the *Federal Register* once a year, contains a master list of CPT/HCPCS codes with corresponding APC codes and payment rates. It is formatted as a Microsoft Excel file and was 227 pages long in 2007. Table 5.2 shows six lines as a sample. As seen in Table 5.2, Addendum B lists the following information for each CPT/HCPCS code:

- CPT/HCPCS code number
- Description
- Status indicator (SI)
- APC code
- Relative weight
- National payment rate
- National coinsurance rate, labeled "National Unadjusted Copayment"
- Minimum coinsurance rate, labeled "Minimum Unadjusted Copayment"

Addendum D-1: Status Indicators

In the APC system, every CPT/HCPCS code is assigned a status indicator. A **status indicator (SI)** is a single-digit code that explains how a procedure is paid. The status indicator may indicate that the full APC amount is due, that a discounted amount is due, or that no payment is due for the service under OPPS. Addendum D-1 lists the definitions of the each status indicator.

Table 5.2

Sample from Addendum B—January 2007

CPT/HCPCS	Description	CI	SI	APC	Relative Weight	Payment Rate	National Unadjusted Copayment	Minimum Unadjusted Copayment
31395	Reconstruct larynx & pharynx		C	—	—	—	—	—
31400	Revision of larynx		T	0256	38.1991	2348.02		469.60
31420	Removal of epiglottis		T	0256	38.1991	2348.02		469.60
31500	Insert emergency airway		S	0094	2.4233	148.96	46.29	29.79
31502	Change of windpipe airway		T	0121	2.3587	144.98	43.80	29.00
31505	Diagnostic laryngoscopy		T	0071	0.7698	47.32	11.20	9.46

$ $ Billing Tip $ $

Packaged Services and HCPCS Codes

Some packaged services have HCPCS codes. These services have a status indicator of N or Q to indicate they are packaged. N indicates that the services are always packaged; Q indicates services, such as observation services, that are usually packaged but may be separately paid under certain circumstances.

Other packaged services, such as surgical and pharmacy supplies, do not have HCPCS codes. When a covered item or service listed on an outpatient claim has no corresponding HCPCS code, it should be considered packaged. These services do not require HCPCS codes, as no separate payment is being requested. For cost reporting purposes, however, it is recommended that hospitals report all services rendered.

EXAMPLES:

Status indicator A   Assigned to services that are not paid under OPPS because they are paid by fiscal intermediaries under a fee schedule or payment system other than OPPS; used for procedures such as ambulance services, laboratory services, or physical, occupational, and speech therapy, which are paid under other payment systems.

Status indicator T   Assigned to surgical procedures where a multiple procedure reduction applies. If two surgical procedures with a status indicator of T are performed during the same operative session, the first procedure will be paid the full APC payment amount, but the second (and third, fourth, etc.) procedure will only be paid 50 percent of the APC amount.

Status indicator S   Assigned to a surgical procedure where multiple procedures are not discounted. If this surgical procedure is performed during the same operative session with another status S procedure, both services are paid 100 percent of the APC payment.

Status indicator N   Assigned to packaged services. Packaged services do not receive a separate payment because payment for them is considered to be "packaged" into other separately payable services.

Addendum E: Inpatient-Only Procedures

As discussed in Chapter 3, Medicare regards some surgical procedures payable only if they are performed in an inpatient setting. Medicare determines whether a procedure falls into this category based on the invasive nature of procedure and the need for an overnight recovery period. Addendum E contains a list of more than 1,700 inpatient-only procedure codes. Hospital personnel must be aware of procedures that are included on the inpatient-only procedure list so that they do not mistakenly perform them in an outpatient setting, thereby foregoing payment. CMS reviews and updates the inpatient-only procedure list in Addendum E each year. Surgical procedures that are inpatient-only procedures are assigned status indicator C.

APC Grouper

Typically hospitals have a software program called an APC grouper or OPPS grouper. The program uses information about the outpatient services to assign the appropriate APC payment group to each service on a claim and calculate reimbursement before the claim is sent to a payer. The grouper works on a line-item basis, as outpatient claims are required to list each service received on a separate line. Although the grouper can estimate APC reimbursement, the APC rules that Medicare applies when it processes the claim ultimately determine the actual reimbursement.

The Medicare Outpatient Code Editor

Just as the Medicare Code Editor edits inpatient claims, the Medicare **Outpatient Code Editor (OCE)** detects and reports errors in the coding in outpatient hospital claims. The OCE also assigns the APC codes for the claims.

Functions of the OCE

Prior to OPPS, the OCE software focused simply on editing claims. It did not specify any action to take when an edit occurred, nor did it compute any information for payment purposes. Since the implementation of the OPPS, the functionality of the OCE has changed to incorporate both capabilities. Currently the OCE performs three major functions:

1. It edits the data to identify errors and returns a series of edit flags.
2. It assigns an APC number for each service covered under OPPS and returns information to be used as input to a pricer program.
3. It assigns an ambulatory surgical center (ASC) payment group for services on claims from certain non-OPPS hospitals.

The computerized edits are performed on claims to identify problems such as coding errors, issues involving medical necessity, and data inconsistencies (for example, male- or female-specific procedures that conflict with the patient's gender). The OCE not only identifies individual errors, but also returns a list of edit numbers to indicate what actions should be taken and the reasons that these actions are necessary.

Table 5.3 shows a sample of OCE edits. The OCE edit numbers are listed in the left column, followed by a description of the edit, and the claim's

Table 5.3

Sample of OCE Edits

Edit #	Description	Non-OPPS Hospitals	Disposition
1	Invalid diagnosis code	Y	RTP
2	Diagnosis and age conflict	Y	RTP
3	Diagnosis and sex conflict	Y	RTP
4	Medicare secondary payer alert		Suspend
5	E-diagnosis code cannot be used as principal diagnosis	Y	RTP
6	Invalid procedure code	Y	RTP
7	Procedure and age conflict (not activated)		RTP
8	Procedure and sex conflict	Y	RTP
9	Noncovered for reasons other than statute	Y (NCL)	Line item denial
10	Service submitted for denial (condition code 21)	Y (new)	Claim denial
11	Service submitted for FI review (condition code 20)	Y (new)	Suspend
12	Questionable covered service	Y	Suspend
13	Separate payment for services is not provided by Medicare		Line item rejection
14	Code indicates a site of service not included in OPPS		Claim RTP
15	Service unit out of range for procedure	Y (new)	RTP
16	Multiple bilateral procedures without modifier −50 (see Appendix A)		RTP
17	Inappropriate specification of bilateral procedure (see Appendix A)	Y (new)	RTP
18	Inpatient procedure		Line item denial
19	Mutually exclusive procedure that is not allowed by NCCI even if appropriate modifier is present		Line item rejection
20	Code 2 of a code pair that is not allowed by NCCI even if appropriate modifier is present		Line item rejection
21	Medical visit on same day as a type "T" or "S" procedure without modifier −25 (see Appendix B)		Line item rejection
22	Invalid modifier	Y (new)	RTP
23	Invalid date	Y	RTP
24	Date out of OCE range	Y	Suspend
25	Invalid age	Y	RTP
26	Invalid sex	Y	RTP

Source: www.cms.hhs.gov/OutpatientCodeEdit/Downloads/EditClaimReasons.pdf.

current disposition as a result of the edit. The "Non-OPPS Hospitals" column indicates whether the edit applies to claims from non-OPPS hospitals. Claims with edit numbers require further review before APCs are assigned. The edit numbers and corresponding information are designed to help the provider understand how to correct the claim. RTP in the disposition column, for example, stands for "return to provider." When a claim receives an RTP edit, the claim is returned to the provider and the provider is allowed to correct the claim and resubmit it.

The occurrence of an edit can result in one of six different dispositions in the disposition column:

- *Claim Rejection:* One or more edits present cause the whole claim to be rejected; the provider can correct and resubmit the claim but cannot appeal the claim rejection.

- *Claim Denial:* One or more edits present cause the whole claim to be denied; the provider cannot resubmit the claim but can appeal the claim denial.

- *Claim Return to Provider (RTP):* One or more edits present cause the whole claim to be returned to the provider; the provider can resubmit the claim once the problems are corrected.

- *Claim Suspension:* One or more edits present cause the whole claim to be suspended; the claim is not returned to the provider, but it is also not processed for payment until the FI makes a determination or obtains further information.

- *Line Item Rejection:* One or more edits present cause one or more individual line items to be rejected; the claim can be processed for payment with some line items rejected for payment. The line item can be corrected and resubmitted but cannot be appealed.

- *Line Item Denials:* One or more edits present cause once or more individual line items to be denied; the claim can be processed for payment with some line times denied for payment. The line item cannot be resubmitted but can be appealed.

After the edits for the claim are resolved, the OCE assigns an APC number for each service on the claim. The OCE also assigns status indicators, computes discounts, determines whether packaging is applicable, calculates payment adjustments if applicable, and performs other functions related to payment. The program then generates the required information to be used as input to a pricer program.

The pricer program calculates the final APC rates, coinsurance, and deductibles. Although the OCE cannot perform all these functions on non-OPPS claims, it does assign specific edit numbers for line items on non-OPPS hospital claims, as shown in Table 5.3.

The OCE and the National Correct Coding Initiative Edits

In addition to the Medicare edits that are built into the OCE, the OCE also contains National Correct Coding Initiative edits. The **Correct Coding Initiative (CCI)** is Medicare's national policy on correct CPT coding. The CCI is an ongoing process to control improper coding that would lead to inappropriate payment for Medicare Part B claims. The CCI list contains more than ninety thousand CPT code combinations used by Medicare to check physician claims for improper coding.

The CCI was initially implemented by Medicare carriers, which process claims for physicians, other providers, and suppliers. Subsequently, the CCI was also implemented by fiscal intermediaries, which incorporated a subset of the CCI edits into the OCE. The CCI edits contained in the OCE are specifically for use in processing hospital outpatient services under the hospital OPPS.

The two main types of CCI edits contained in the OCE are the **CCI column 1/ column 2 code pair edits** and the **CCI mutually exclusive edits.** Both types of edits are designed to edit out combinations of codes that do not match Medicare's payment rules. These edits represent the procedure and service combinations that cannot be billed together for the same patient on the same day of service.

Column 1/Column 2 Code Pair Edits

In this group, the first column of codes contains the comprehensive code, and the second column shows the component code or codes. According to the CCI, the comprehensive code includes all the services that are described by the component code. Therefore, the component code cannot be billed together with the comprehensive code for the same patient on the same day of service unless an appropriate modifier is attached that explains why the service was necessary.

EXAMPLE:

Column 1	Column 2
27370	20610, 76000

If 27370 (Injection procedure for knee arthrography) is billed, neither 20610 (Injection; major joint or bursa) nor 76000 (Fluoroscopy—separate procedure) should be billed with it because the payment for each of these codes is already included in the column 1 code. Medicare edits out the column 2 code, as it is considered bundled into the column 1 code, and pays for the column 1 code only.

Mutually Exclusive Edits

This group also lists codes in two columns. According to CMS regulations, the services represented by these codes could not have both reasonably been done during a single patient encounter, so they cannot be billed together.

EXAMPLE:

Column 1	Column 2
50021	49061, 50020

In this example, a biller cannot report either 49061 (Drainage of retroperitoneal abscess; percutaneous) or 50020 (Drainage of perirenal or renal abscess; open) when reporting 50021 (Drainage of perirenal or renal abscess; percutaneous). If the provider reports both codes from both column 1 and column 2 for a patient on the same day, Medicare will reimburse the lower paid code only (column 1).

Medically Unlikely Edits

A third set of edits developed by CCI, which are also included in the OCE, are known as the medically unlikely edits (MUEs). These edits do not involve incorrect code combinations. Rather the MUEs are unit-of-service edits that are used to determine the maximum allowed number of services for certain CPT/HCPCS codes. Currently there are two types of MUEs—anatomical

Edits for Covered/Noncovered Services

CCI edits incorporated into the OCE also include logic that identifies whether services are covered by Medicare. For example, a facelift is typically not a covered service for Medicare patients, and the claim would be denied.

edits and typographical error edits. Claims with MUE edits contain service unit amounts that are highly medically unlikely. Medicare considers the units in excess of the MUE limit to be excess charges and therefore will not pay for them.

For example, under the MUEs, if a line item on a claim listed more than one service unit for a hysterectomy, the claim would be returned with an RTP (return-to-provider) message, as the service unit amount is medically unlikely. Similarly, an extremely high service unit may be assumed to be a typographical error, and the claim will be returned. On receiving an RTP message, the provider fixes the service units for the line item involved and resubmits the claim.

The Effect of Modifiers on CCI Edits

Modifiers created by the AMA or CMS have been designated specifically for use with the column 1/column 2 code pair and mutually exclusive edits. These NCCI-associated modifiers include:

- Anatomical modifiers:
  E1–E4 (eyelids)
  FA–F9 (fingers)
  LC, LD, and RC (arteries)
  LT and RT (left and right sides)
  TA–T9 (toes)

- Global surgery modifiers:
  25 (significant, separately identifiable E/M service)
  58 (staged or related procedure)
  78 (related procedure)
  79 (unrelated procedure or service)

- Other modifiers:
  59 (distinct procedural services)
  91 (repeat lab test)

When one of these modifiers is used, it identifies the circumstances for which both services rendered to the same beneficiary, on the same date of service, by the same provider should be allowed separately because one service was performed at a different site, in a different session, or as a distinct service or involved separate specimens.

Under certain circumstances, these modifiers may be appended to a component code or a mutually exclusive code (the column 2 code) to "break," or bypass, the NCCI edit. Under most circumstances, however, a modifier cannot be used to bypass the CCI edit. To be clear when a CCI-associated modifier may be used to override a CCI edit, a modifier status indicator is assigned to each set of CCI code pairs in the code pair tables. Using 1 in the status indicator column indicates that a CCI-associated modifier can be used to bypass the edit under appropriate circumstances. Using 0 indicates that a CCI-associated modifier cannot be used to bypass the edit. To avoid compliance problems, it is very important that CCI-associated modifiers be used only when appropriate. In the case of the MUEs, modifiers do not apply, as currently there are no modifiers that bypass MUEs.

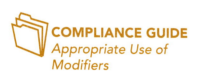

COMPLIANCE GUIDE
Appropriate Use of Modifiers

Only certain modifiers are intended to bypass CCI edits and only when the clinical circumstances justify doing so. Inappropriate use of modifiers to override CCI edits, or for any other purpose, can result in overpayments that could be perceived as fraud.

INTERNET RESOURCE
National Technical Information Service: Hospital OPPS CCI Edits
www.ntis.gov/products/families/hoppscciedits.asp

Purchasing the Hospital OPPS CCI Edits

Hospitals and other providers purchase the hospital OPPS CCI policies and edits from the National Technical Information Services (NTIS). They may also be downloaded from the CMS website. The CCI manual contains both correct coding policies and correct coding edits and is updated quarterly.

Although the policies and edits are available from commercial services, CMS regards the CMS website and NTIS as the official sources.

It is important to note that the CCI edits incorporated into the OCE are a subset of the complete CCI edits that are used in physician billing. The OCE does not include CCI edits for anesthesiology, evaluation and management, and mental health services. The CCI-associated modifiers and coding pairs included in the OCE may also differ from those in the physician version because of differences between facility and physician services.

INTERNET RESOURCE
CMS Website: Hospital OPPS CCI Edits
www.cms.hhs.gov/ NationalCorrectCodInitEd/ NCCIEHOPPS/list.asp# TopOf Page

Billing Compliance

Although almost everyone involved in the delivery of health care is trustworthy and is devoted to patients' welfare, some are not. Health care fraud and abuse laws help control cheating in the health care system. Are the laws really necessary? The evidence says that they are. Cases filed under federal fraud laws resulted in court judgments and settlements of nearly $3.2 billion in 2006.

Fraud and Abuse Defined

Fraud is an act of deception used to take advantage of another person. For example, misrepresenting professional credentials and forging another person's signature on a check are fraudulent. Pretending to be a physician and treating patients without a valid medical license is also fraudulent. Fraudulent acts are intentional; the individual expects an illegal or unauthorized benefit to result.

Claim fraud occurs when health care providers or others falsely report charges to payers. A provider may bill for services that were not performed, overcharge for services, or fail to provide complete services under a contract. A patient may exaggerate an injury to get a settlement from an insurance company.

In federal law, **abuse** means an action that misuses money that the government has allocated, such as Medicare funds. Abuse is illegal because taxpayers' dollars are misspent. An example of abuse is an ambulance service that billed Medicare for transporting a patient to the hospital when the patient did not need ambulance service. This abuse—billing for services that were not medically necessary—resulted in improper payment to the ambulance company. Abuse is not necessarily intentional. It may be the result of ignorance of a billing rule or of inaccurate coding.

$ $ **Billing Tip** $ $
Fraud Versus Abuse
To bill when the task was not done is fraud; to bill when it was not necessary is abuse. Remember the rule: in the view of the payer, a service that was not documented was not done and cannot be coded and billed. To bill for undocumented services is fraudulent.

Fraud and Abuse Laws

The following are the major laws that address fraud and abuse:

- The Health Care Fraud and Abuse Control Program, created under HIPAA and enforced by the HHS **Office of the Inspector General (OIG),** has the task of detecting health care fraud and abuse and enforcing all laws relating to them. The OIG works with the U.S. Department of Justice (DOJ), which includes the Federal Bureau of Investigation (FBI), under the direction of the U.S. attorney general to prosecute those suspected of medical fraud and abuse.

- The federal False Claims Act (FCA), a related law, prohibits submitting a fraudulent claim or making a false statement or representation in connection with a claim. It also encourages reporting suspected fraud and abuse against the government by protecting and rewarding people involved in *qui tam,* or whistle-blower, cases. Whistle-blowers are current or former employees of insurance companies or of medical facilities, program beneficiaries, and independent contractors.

- The Deficit Reduction Act (DRA) of 2005 gives states financial incentives for setting up their own false claims acts to prevent false claims under the Medicaid program. This act also requires training hospital staff and outside vendors to make sure they investigate and report fraud.

OIG Enforcement

The Office of the Inspector General enforces rules relating to fraud and abuse. The intent to commit fraud does not have to be proved by the accuser for the provider to be found guilty. Actions that might be viewed as errors or occasional slips might also be seen as establishing a pattern of violations, which constitutes the knowledge meant by "providers knew or should have known."

OIG has the authority to investigate suspected fraud cases and to *audit* the records of providers and payers. In an audit (a methodical examination), investigators review selected medical records to see whether the documentation supports the coding. The accounting records are often reviewed as well. When problems are found, the investigation proceeds and may result in charges of fraud or abuse against the provider.

Investigators look for patterns like these:

- Intentionally coding services that were not performed or documented

  EXAMPLES:
  A lab bills Medicare for two tests when only one was done.

  A physician asks a coder to report a telephone conversation with a patient as a physical examination.

- Coding services at a higher level than was carried out

  EXAMPLE: After a visit for a flu shot, the provider bills the encounter as a comprehensive physical examination plus a vaccination.

- Performing and billing for procedures that are not related to the patient's condition and therefore are not medically necessary

  EXAMPLE: After reading an article about Lyme disease, a patient is worried about having worked in her garden over the summer, and she requests a Lyme disease diagnostic test. Although no symptoms or signs have been reported, the physician orders and bills for the *Borrelia burgdorferi* (Lyme disease) confirmatory immunoblot test.

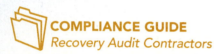

$ $ Billing Tip $ $

Avoid Double Billing
IPPS Services

Services that are paid under the IPPS should not also be reported for OPPS payment. For example, radiology services that are provided as part of an inpatient stay may not also be billed as an outpatient service.

COMPLIANCE GUIDE
Recovery Audit Contractors

The Tax Relief and Health Care Act of 2006 mandates the use of recovery audit contractors (RACs) in all states for all Part A and Part B claim types by 2010. RACs are a new contracting authority hired by CMS to identify and collect Medicare overpayments. Overpayments are identified through a careful review of individual Medicare claims to determine if the claims are medically necessary, correctly coded, and conform to Medicare payment policy.

Compliance Plans

Given all the concerns about HIPAA, fraud, and abuse violations, how does a hospital protect itself? A wise slogan is "the best defense is a good offense." For this reason, providers and other health care entities write and implement **compliance plans** to uncover and correct compliance problems. A compliance plan is a process for finding, correcting, and preventing illegal practices. It is a written document prepared by a compliance officer and committee that sets up the steps needed to (1) audit and monitor compliance with government regulations, (2) have policies and procedures that are consistent, (3) provide for ongoing staff training and communication, and (4) respond to and correct errors. The goal of the plan is to promote ethical conduct and establish a culture of compliance in the organization.

The goals of the compliance plan are to:

- Prevent fraud and abuse through a formal process to identify, investigate, fix, and prevent repeat violations relating to reimbursement for health care services
- Ensure compliance with applicable federal, state, and local laws, including employment and environmental laws as well as antifraud laws
- Help defend the entity if it is investigated or prosecuted for fraud by substantiating the desire to behave compliantly and thus to reduce any fines or criminal prosecution

Compliance plans cover all areas of government regulation beyond HIPAA, fraud, and abuse, such as Equal Employment Opportunity (EEO) regulations (for example, hiring and promotion policies) and Occupational Safety and Health Administration (OSHA) regulations (for example, fire safety and handling of hazardous materials such as blood-borne pathogens).

Guidance on Compliance Plans

Compliance plans vary according to the type of covered entity and its range of services, its location, and its business structure. The OIG has issued a **compliance program guidance** for the following entities:

OIG Compliance Program Guidance for Recipients of PHS Research Awards (Draft)	11/28/2005
Supplemental Compliance Program Guidance for Hospitals PDF [Original Compliance Program Guidance for Hospitals PDF (February 23, 1998)]	1/27/2005
Final Compliance Program Guidance for Pharmaceutical Manufacturers	4/28/2003
Final Compliance Program Guidance for Ambulance Suppliers PDF	3/24/2003
Final Compliance Program Guidance for Individual and Small Group Physician Practices	9/25/2000
Final Compliance Program Guidance for Nursing Facilities	3/16/2000
Final Compliance Program Guidance for Medicare+Choice Organizations	11/16/1999
Compliance Program Guidance for Hospices	9/30/1999
Compliance Program Guidance for the Durable Medical Equipment Prosthetics, Orthotics, and Supply Industry	6/22/1999
Compliance Program Guidance for Third-Party Medical Billing Companies	11/30/1998
Compliance Program Guidance for Home Health Agencies	8/7/1998
Compliance Program Guidance for Clinical Laboratories	8/24/1998

The content of each compliance program guidance is not a model plan, because good plans vary for each type of organization, but rather a description of what should be covered in a plan.

Parts of a Compliance Plan

Generally, according to the OIG, voluntary plans should contain seven elements:

1. Written policies and procedures
2. Appointment of a compliance officer and committee
3. Training
4. Communication
5. Auditing and monitoring
6. Disciplinary systems
7. Responding to and correcting errors

Written Policies and Procedures

The first component of a compliance plan is the organization's written policies and procedures. This material must cover a code of conduct, compliance policies and procedures, retention of patient medical records and of information systems, and how the policies and procedures are part of employee performance evaluation.

Compliance Officer and Committee

To establish the plan and follow up on its provisions, most organizations appoint a compliance officer who is in charge of the ongoing work. The compliance officer may also be the HIPAA-mandated privacy and/or security officer. A compliance committee is also usually established to oversee the program. The compliance officer and the committee analyze all areas that present a risk for out-of-compliance behavior by reviewing:

- Federal and state statutes
- Government-sponsored program regulations (Medicare and Medicaid)
- *Medicare Carrier Manual* and *Coverage Issues Manual*
- Other health plans' regulations
- Current and past years' OIG Work Plans
- OIG Fraud Alerts and audit reports

Ongoing Training

Compliance plans require a training program to keep professional and administrative staff up to date in pertinent regulatory matters. These training requirements affect managers, supervisors, employees, and business associates. Ongoing training also requires having the current annual updates, such as for HIPAA-mandated code sets, and researching changed regulations. Documentation improvement programs may be part of this training effort.

Effective Lines of Communication

The compliance plan describes how employees and business associates can report suspected noncompliant actions. The communications may be by telephone, by e-mail, face-to-face, or written. A separate method, such as a toll-free hotline, is required so that anonymous reporting of noncompliance is possible.

Ongoing Auditing and Monitoring

Another major aspect of the compliance plan is auditing and monitoring areas of concern, especially the coding and billing process. The person who is responsible for auditing and monitoring establishes a routine system for internal monitoring and regular compliance checks to ensure adherence to established policies and procedures.

To reduce the chance of an investigation by an enforcing agency and to reduce potential liability when one occurs, most compliance plans require **internal audits** to be conducted regularly. These audits are routine and are performed periodically without a reason to think that a compliance problem exists. They help determine whether financially related activities such as coding and billing are being done appropriately. The goal is to uncover problems so that they can be corrected. Internal audits often **benchmark** these activities (compare them against a standard). For example, statistics from the billing department of a hospital may be compared with statistics from comparable hospitals regarding the average length of stay for certain conditions or surgeries. Another method is to set up **triggered reviews,** in which certain events or certain repeated actions cause an audit of noncompliance. These types of events and actions are documented in the compliance plan.

In an **external audit,** an enforcing agency such as the OIG reviews selected records for compliance. Coding linkage, completeness of documentation, and adherence to documentation standards, such as the signing and dating of entries by the responsible health care professional, may all be studied. The accounting records are often reviewed as well.

Disciplinary Guidelines and Policies

A compliance plan must include written policies covering appropriate disciplinary actions if employees fail to comply with the organization's rules. Disciplinary actions are usually progressive, meaning that people are given opportunities to correct behavior before being fired. However, the disciplinary guidelines should also list offenses for which an employee can be fired without progressive discipline. Employees are responsible not only for compliance, but also for detecting noncompliance when routine observation would have provided adequate clues that a problem existed.

The compliance plan should also describe the organization's policies and procedures on requiring background checks to be sure that prospective employees and business associates have not previously been convicted of a crime or excluded from participation in a federal program.

Corrective Action

In the corrective action section of the compliance plan, the organization describes the steps to be taken when a report of noncompliance is received. These guidelines state how internal investigations should be conducted, options for corrective action, when to have an outside investigator brought in to conduct an investigation, and when noncompliant actions need to be reported to authorities, such as CMS, the OIG, or law enforcement personnel.

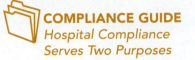

COMPLIANCE GUIDE
Hospital Compliance Serves Two Purposes

Hospital compliance with HIPAA privacy and security regulations helps the facility meet the Joint Commission's standards for privacy and security as well. These two sets of standards are fairly consistent, with HIPAA's being considerably more detailed.

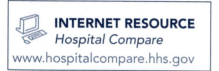

INTERNET RESOURCE
Hospital Compare
www.hospitalcompare.hhs.gov

Since 2002, CMS has launched a series of quality initiatives, including the Nursing Home Quality Initiative, the Hospital Quality Initiative, and the Physician Quality Reporting Initiative (PQRI), to encourage improved quality of care for patients in different health care settings. **Pay-for-performance programs** are growing rapidly as part of these initiatives. These programs consist of differential payments to hospitals and other providers based on the performance of a specified set of **quality measures,** including quality of patient care, clinical outcomes, patient satisfaction, and the implementation of information technology. The programs align financial incentives with the delivery of high-quality care.

As part of the Hospital Quality Initiative, the Hospital Quality Alliance (HQA) is a public-private collaboration to improve the quality of hospital care and to provide quality information to consumers and others. The HQA measures and publicly reports the quality of care in hospitals using a base set of quality measures. Each year new measures are added. Currently, a total of thirty-six measures report on how well hospitals follow various recommended treatments for heart attack, heart failure, and pneumonia; how well they follow various recommended procedures for surgical care improvement and surgical infection prevention; and how well they rate on a set of criteria that reflects patients' perspectives on hospital care. CMS links voluntary reporting of these measures to payment. Currently, 98 percent of eligible hospitals participate in the program.

❶ Medicare pays for inpatient services under its Inpatient Prospective Payment System (IPPS). This system is called *prospective* because rather than paying for each service based on what the hospital charges, the rate has been set in advance. The IPPS uses diagnosis-related groups (DRGs) to classify patients into similar treatment and length-of-hospital-stay units and sets prices for each classification group. A hospital's geographical location and labor and supply costs also affect the DRG pay rate it negotiates with CMS. Hospitals receive the predetermined DRG amount regardless of the actual cost of care, although adjustments may be made in some cases.

❷ In 2008, Medicare replaced the former CMS DRG system with the current Medicare-Severity DRGs (MS-DRGs) system to account for the different severities of illness among patients with the same diagnosis. Under the MS-DRG system, there are twenty-five major diagnostic categories and 745 DRGs. Each diagnosis code in ICD-9-CM is covered in one of the DRGs. To account for different severities of illness, every diagnosis code was assigned to one of three levels of CCs. CCs are secondary conditions—either comorbidities or complications—that affect the level of care.

The three levels of CCs are (a) major CCs (MCCs), which reflect a higher level of severity and require double the additional resources of a normal CC; (b) CCs, which involve regular or normal severity of illness and resource use; and (c) non-CCs, chronic conditions that do not require staff members to expend additional resources. Possible combinations of a principal diagnosis code and secondary codes are then grouped into DRG clusters to arrive at the appropriate DRG. A DRG cluster is a group of DRGs with the same principal diagnosis but varying degrees of severity in secondary condition codes.

❸ The Deficit Reduction Act (DRA) requires CMS to reduce payment in cases where patients develop hospital-acquired conditions that would move them from lower-paying to higher-paying DRGs. Unless any of the following eight conditions are present on admission, CMS does not assign higher paying DRGs to patients who, during their hospital stay, have or suffer from (a) a serious preventable event—object left in surgery; (b) a serious preventable event—air embolism; (c) a serious preventable event—blood incompatibility; (d) catheter-associated urinary tract infections; (e) pressure ulcers (decubitus ulcers); (f) vascular catheter-associated infection; (g) surgical site infection—mediastinitis after coronary artery bypass graft (CABG) surgery; or (h) falls.

❹ The Medicare Code Editor (MCE) is a software program used to detect and report errors in coding while processing inpatient hospital claims. The MCE software detects the following kinds of errors: (a) the code is not in the ICD-9-CM code set; (b) the code is not shown with its required fourth or fifth digit; (c) an E code is listed as the principal diagnosis; (d) entries are duplicated; (e) the age or gender of patient does not match the coding; (f) the code is not an acceptable principal diagnosis; (g) the discharge status code is not valid; (h) the operating room procedure is nonspecific or noncovered by Medicare; (i) the coded services have limited Medicare coverage.

5 The Medicare Outpatient Prospective Payment System (OPPS) is used to pay hospitals for services to Medicare patients that are provided on an outpatient basis. These services include most Medicare Part B services. Mirroring the DRGs for the IPPS, the OPPS is based on a prospective payment system that uses a pricing unit called the ambulatory payment classification (APC). APCs, which have predetermined payment amounts, are assigned for each outpatient procedure, service, or item. The total payment the hospital receives for the visit is computed as the sum of the individual APC payments for each service.

Similar to the DRG system, the APC system establishes groups of covered services so that the services within each group are comparable clinically and with respect to the use of resources. Payment rates are assigned to each group based on Medicare's analysis of the national median cost for outpatient procedures. Geographical differences are factored into the DRG payment rate and into the patient's copayment amount to account for differences in inflation across the country.

6 The Medicare Outpatient Code Editor (OCE) is a software program that is used to detect and report errors in coding while processing outpatient hospital claims. The OCE also assigns an APC number for each service that is covered under OPPS and returns information to be used as input to a pricer program. In addition to the Medicare edits built into the OCE, the OCE contains three types of National Correct Coding Initiative edits: (a) the column 1/column 2 code pair edits; (b) the mutually exclusive edits; and (c) the medically unlikely edits. The first two types are based on tables of code combinations used by Medicare to edit out those that do not match Medicare's payment rules. The third type involves unit-of-service edits that are used to determine the maximum allowed number of services for certain CPT/HCPCS codes.

7 The Health Care Fraud and Abuse Control Program, part of HIPAA, was enacted to prevent fraud and abuse in health care billing. This law, as well as the Federal False Claims Act and other related laws, are enforced by the Office of Inspector General (OIG).

8 A hospital compliance plan includes (a) consistent written policies and procedures; (b) appointment of a compliance officer and committee; (c) ongoing training; (d) effective lines of communication; (e) ongoing auditing and monitoring; (f) disciplinary guidelines and policies; and (g) corrective action.

9 CMS has launched various initiatives, such as the Physician Quality Reporting Initiative (PQRI), to encourage improved quality of care for patients in different health care settings. Pay-for-performance programs are rapidly expanding as part of these initiatives. Pay-for-performance programs consist of differential payment to hospitals and other providers based on the performance of a set of specified measures, including quality of patient care, clinical outcomes, patient satisfaction, and the implementation of information technology. These programs align financial incentives with the delivery of high-quality care.

✔ CHECK YOUR UNDERSTANDING

Write *T* or *F* to indicate whether you think the statement is true or false.

_____ **1.** Diagnosis-related groups (DRGs) are categories of inpatients.

_____ **2.** The predetermined rates for inpatient visits under the Medicare Inpatient Prospective Payment System (IPPS) are based on Medicare's analysis of how long people are hospitalized, on average, for similar conditions, and the average cost incurred.

_____ **3.** The Inpatient Prospective Payment System is called prospective because it pays for each service based on what the hospital charges rather than on a projected average cost.

_____ **4.** The greater the weight assigned to a DRG, the less resource-intensive it is.

_____ **5.** Medicare and hospitals use the MS Grouper software program to assign a patient's DRG.

_____ **6.** The new Medicare-Severity DRGs (MS-DRGs) differ from CMS DRGs in that they account for geographical differences in the inpatient population.

_____ **7.** CMS will not assign a higher paying DRG to patients who suffer from hospital-acquired conditions such as pressure ulcers.

_____ **8.** The Medicare Outpatient Prospective Payment System (OPPS) uses a pricing unit called a CMI (case mix index).

_____ **9.** Addendum B to the OPPS Final Rule contains a master list of CPT/HCPCS procedure codes with corresponding APC codes and payment rates.

_____ **10.** An inpatient-only procedure can be performed in an inpatient or outpatient setting; however, the hospital will be reimbursed only if it is performed in an inpatient setting.

_____ **11.** To bill when a procedure was not done is abuse; to bill when a procedure was not necessary is fraud.

_____ **12.** Pay-for-performance programs offer financial incentives for voluntary reporting of quality measures such as patient satisfaction and clinical outcomes.

Choose the best answer.

13. The system of analyzing conditions and treatments for similar groups of patients used to establish Medicare fees for hospital inpatient services is called the
    a. APC system
    b. *Federal Register*
    c. Correct Coding Initiative
    d. DRG system

14. In inpatient coding, the initials CC mean
    a. chief complaint
    b. comorbidities and complications
    c. cubic centimeters
    d. correct coding

15. Under the OPPS system, all CPC/HCPCS codes are linked to a _____ code that determines the hospital's payment.
    a. APC
    b. DRG
    c. MCC
    d. OCE

16. The _____ performs edits on claim data to identify errors and assigns an APC number for each service that is covered under OPPS.
    a. MS-Grouper
    b. Medicare pricer
    c. OCE
    d. MCE

17. Edits that represent the procedure and service combinations that cannot be billed together for the same patient on the same day of service because the codes could not have both reasonably been done are known as the
    a. CCI mutually exclusive edits
    b. medically unlikely edits
    c. CCI column 1/column 2 code pair edits
    d. non-CCI edits

18. Under appropriate circumstances, a _____ may be appended to a component code of a mutually exclusive code to bypass a CCI edit.
    a. relative weight
    b. status indicator
    c. APC code
    d. modifier

19. The Health Care Fraud and Abuse Control Program and the federal False Claims Act are enforced by
   a. CMS
   b. OIG
   c. HIPAA
   d. DRA

20. Most compliance plans require regular _____; these are performed periodically without a reason to think that a compliance problem exits.
   a. HIPAA training sessions
   b. internal audits
   c. triggered reviews
   d. external audits

COMPUTER EXPLORATION

Internet Application

1. The Centers for Medicare and Medicaid website contains a designated area for hospital information. To view this information, go to the CMS hospital website at www.cms.hhs.gov/center/hospital.asp. To view the range of topics available at the site, review the Important Links list. To learn more about the Acute Inpatient Prospective Payment System (PPS), click this subtopic (listed under the Payment heading), and then read the Overview. What did you learn about the role of DRGs in this payment system?

2. Visit the CMS website for the Medicare OPPS at www.cms.hhs.gov/HospitalOutpatientPPS/HORD/list.asp#TopOfPage. Click the link for the title "Final Changes to the Hospital Outpatient PPS and CY 2008 Payment Rates." In the list of files, select Addendum D-1 to view definitions of the current payment status indicators. How many status indicators are listed? List and describe three status indicators not mentioned in this chapter.

3. Visit the following website to obtain background information on the Outpatient Code Editor: www.cms.hhs.gov/OutpatientCodeEdit/. List one code edit that applies to hospital claims.

4. Visit the CMS website for the National Correct Coding Initiative at www.cms.hhs.gov/NationalCorrectCodInitEd/. Download the file "NCCI Policy Manual for Part B Medicare Claims" (a Microsoft Word document). In Chapter 1, locate any information on modifier −59. Find examples that describe the appropriate and inappropriate use of modifier −59.

5. Visit the Office of the Inspector General (OIG) website at http://oig.hhs. gov. Locate any cases of HIPAA violations, fraud, or abuse in the last year. Identify the type of violation, source of violation, and penalty.

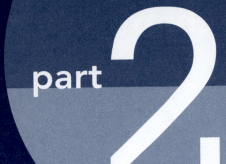

The UB-04 Claim Form

part **2**

Overview of the UB-04 Claim Form

LEARNING OUTCOMES

After completing this chapter, you will be able to define the key terms and:

1 Discuss the history of the UB-04 claim form in the medical health billing environment.

2 Discuss UB-04 claim creation and methods of transmittal to payers.

3 Describe the importance of preparing clean claims.

4 Describe the data elements and the general formats that are used for the form locators on the UB-04.

5 Explain the purpose of the seven form locators designated as unlabeled fields on the UB-04.

6 Explain the organization of the remaining chapters in Part 2 of this text.

KEY TERMS

- claim denial
- claim rejection
- clean claim
- CMS-1500
- CMS-1450
- delimiter
- detail-level code
- 837I
- 837P
- form locator (FL)
- HIPAA claim
- paper claim
- UB-04

Every payer—whether a government health plan such as Medicare or Medicaid or a commercial insurer such as Blue Cross and Blue Shield or CIGNA—has specific requirements for billing. Hospitals and other providers are responsible for gathering and recording the information about each patient's treatment that is required by the payer. A provider that fails to meet these requirements may be only partially paid, paid late, or not paid at all. The claim form used by institutional providers for gathering a patient's treatment information is known as the Uniform Bill (UB) and was developed by the National Uniform Billing Committee (NUBC).

Evolution of the Uniform Bill

The first attempt by the National Uniform Billing Committee to develop a single claim form with a standard data set that could be used for institutional health care claims nationwide was the Uniform Bill known as the UB-82. This bill, first introduced in 1982, aimed to balance the needs of payer organizations and providers. In 1992, after an eight-year moratorium on changes to the structure of the UB-82 data set design and several more years of evaluating its use, the UB-92 was developed and approved for use.

The UB-92 included improvements to the design and data set of the original form. The carefully designed, multipurpose billing form was used by hospitals, skilled nursing facilities (SNFs), and other providers to process inpatient and outpatient paper claims nationwide. Other facilities that used the form included psychiatric, drug, and alcohol treatment facilities; stand-alone clinics; ambulatory surgery centers (ASCs); subacute facilities; home health care agencies; and hospice organizations.

In 2003, as required by the HIPAA Electronic Health Care Transactions and Code Sets legislation, the electronic counterpart to the UB-92, known as the **HIPAA claim** or the **837I**, was introduced. It was designed to transmit the information contained in the UB-92 data set as a standard electronic file rather than on paper. CMS announced that, by HIPAA mandate, all but the smallest providers—those with fewer than twenty full-time or equivalent employees—had to begin using the 837I electronic format to submit Medicare Part A claims. Since most hospitals did not qualify as small providers, electronic claim submission soon became the norm in hospital billing. Today, according to the NUBC, more than 98 percent of Medicare hospital claims and more than 80 percent of all institutional claims are submitted electronically.

While the 837I format incorporated the same data as the paper claim, it also contained several new fields, such as the National Provider Identifier (NPI), that were or would be required in the future. Since the UB-92 claim form did not contain these new fields, the NUBC decided to update the paper form in 2004 to allow for better alignment with the electronic format, as well as to allow for more clinical data. The updated form, now called the **UB-04,** included a field for the NPI, expanded diagnosis and procedure code fields to accommodate larger ICD-10 codes, and space for more diagnosis codes and up to four modifiers for procedure codes—features already incorporated into the electronic form. The UB-04 officially replaced the UB-92 on March 1, 2007.

Because of HIPAA regulations, very few institutions use the paper UB-04 form to submit claims. The structure of the paper form, however, provides the best means of introducing the data fields on a hospital claim and for explaining the necessary connections between them. In the 837I, the information is broken down into loops, segments, and data elements. Both the terminology used to locate data and the sequencing of the data in the electronic file are designed to produce the most efficient electronic transmission; as a result, the logic inherent in the paper claim format is often lost. For this reason, CMS

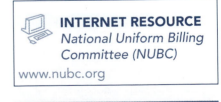

billing guidelines are based on the numbered fields on the paper claim, and the UB-04 is the basis of the chapter organization and the explanation of the preparation of hospital claims in this text as well.

For the most part, the information reported in the UB-04 and the 837I is the same. In instances where the 837I data requirements or format differ from that of the UB-04—for example, when the UB-04 contains a field, such as form locator 43 (Revenue Description), that is not in the 837I—an 837I Alert margin note is provided to notify you about the difference. (On the 837I, unlike the UB-04, the revenue code is reported without the use of a text description.)

Use of the UB-04 Claim Form

The UB-04 or its electronic HIPAA equivalent is used in hospitals everywhere because it is the only claim form accepted by Medicare fiscal intermediaries (FIs) and Medicare Administrative Contractors (MACs) for submitting claims for Medicare Part A reimbursement. Because of the flexibility of the UB-04 and the number of data variations it is designed to accept, it has been substantially adopted by most other payers as well. In an effort to promote the uniform use of the claim, the NUBC designed the form to accommodate the billing procedures and requirements of many types of provider facilities and of all major insurance carriers, including the various federal health programs. The UB-04 is also set up to accommodate the special billing requirements of certain illnesses, such as end-stage renal disease (ESRD), that follow a unique course of care and reimbursement. In addition, the claim form is designed to be easy to edit. Editing helps identify errors that would otherwise cause a claim to be denied or rejected.

Although the UB-04 is used to report hospital charges, it is not used to report the charges of physicians in the hospital. Physician charges, referred to as the professional component, are billed on the **CMS-1500** (formerly HCFA-1500) claim form. For example, if a patient receives a series of X rays during a hospital stay, the X-ray services are billed on the UB-04, while the radiologist's component is billed on the CMS-1500. With the exception of the professional component, the UB-04 represents a summary of all charges and data gathered from the various departments of the hospital during a patient's inpatient stay or for outpatient services.

Claim Creation and Transmission

The claim data on the UB-04 can be transmitted on paper by small providers and as electronic files by all others. The UB-04 **paper claim** can be designed as an optical character recognition (OCR) claim to be read by a scanner, or it can be converted to electronic format by Medicare. It is printed in red ink for scanning purposes and is designed to be typed or computer printed.

The electronic form, the 837I, is referred to as an electronic data interchange (EDI) transaction. EDI is the computer-to-computer exchange of routine business information using publicly available standards. In this case, the standard is the 837I format mandated by HIPAA for Medicare Part A claims.

The 837I is created and transmitted without the use of paper. The hospital's computer system stores required information about the services received by each patient in its database. When a claim is created, the computer system pulls together the information and transmits it from the hospital's computer to the computer of the payer or clearinghouse.

EDI claim transmittal has several advantages over sending paper. In general, electronic claims are more efficient and less expensive to process than paper claims. In addition, chances of error or omission are reduced with electronic filing because data are entered only once and do not have to be reentered or scanned on the receiving side. Another advantage is that Medicare reimburses EDI claims faster than paper claims. EDI claims are held by Medicare for thirteen days before they are released for payment, whereas paper claims are held for twenty-six days. Medicare offers faster reimbursement as an incentive for providers to file electronically. Because of these advantages, most claims, whether Medicare or non-Medicare, are submitted electronically.

Whether the provider uses paper or the EDI transmission, a software program is almost always used to create the claim. After the necessary claim data are obtained, the patient account specialist reviews the claim data, on paper or on-screen, to check for completeness, accuracy, and overall logic. When the information is complete and the claim is ready to be sent, the hospital's computer system transmits the data to the payer in the required 837I format. Alternatively, the hospital transmits the data to a clearinghouse, and the clearinghouse formats the data in 837I format and then transmits it to the payer.

Clean Claims

In insurance terminology, a claim that meets all the necessary specifications and passes all the predetermined data edits is a **clean claim.** For Medicare purposes, a clean claim is one that the FI does not need to investigate before paying because it has passed all FI-specific and common working file (CWF) edits. When an FI does not have all the data necessary to process a Medicare claim, the FI queries the provider. As long as the FI receives a definitive response to the query within seven days, the claim is considered clean. According to Medicare billing rules, a clean claim must be paid or denied by the thirtieth day after the date of receipt; otherwise, CMS must pay interest on it.

Following are some of the most common problems that keep a claim from passing the clean-claim requirements:

- Incorrect patient ID number
- Patient name and address that do not match the insurer's records
- Insufficient or no information about primary or secondary insurance coverage
- Incorrect dates of service
- Dates that lack the correct number of digits
- Revenue codes that are not listed in ascending order
- Missing data, such as a missing sex code in form locator 11
- Fee column that is blank or not itemized and totaled
- Invalid CPT and ICD-9-CM codes, or diagnosis codes that are not linked to the correct services or procedures

When a provider transmits a claim that does not meet the necessary specifications, the provider receives one of two responses from the payer—a claim denial or a claim rejection. A **claim denial** is received when the whole claim has been denied. In this case, the provider cannot resubmit the claim but can appeal the denial. A **claim rejection** is received when the whole claim has been rejected. In this case, the reverse is true—the provider may correct and resubmit a rejected claim but cannot appeal it.

Keeping Up with Changes

CMS and the NUBC revise information requirements for the data fields as well as the codes used in the UB-04 on a regular basis, and Medicare, Medicaid, and other major payers send periodic updates to providers. Keeping up with these changes is an important part of the job of a patient account specialist. In particular, update bulletins received within the last year should be carefully studied.

Sources of information on Medicare changes that affect billing and the UB-04 form can be located through the CMS Online Manual System, which contains links for the following items:

- The Internet-only manuals (IOMs)
- Future updates to the IOMs
- CMS transmittals
- Crosswalks (to assist in locating materials in the IOMs based on given locations in a paper manual)
- Paper-based manuals
- Program memoranda

The IOMs include important Medicare sources, such as the *Medicare Benefit Policy Manual*, the *Medicare Claims Processing Manual*, and the *Medicare National Coverage Determinations Manual*. Transmittals are used to communicate new or changed policies and procedures that will be incorporated into a CMS program manual. An important transmittal with regard to the UB-04 is Transmittal 1104. Issued November 3, 2006, Transmittal 1104 contains information on the implementation of the UB-04. More than a hundred pages long, it includes field-by-field instructions on completing a UB-04 claim for a Medicare beneficiary—information that will eventually be incorporated as Chapter 25 of the *Medicare Claims Processing Manual*.

Program memoranda (more recently referred to as "one-time notifications") clarify or give guidance on topics but do not contain information that will change the program manuals. Ongoing changes to the various billing and coding systems, including the Medicare Inpatient Prospective Payment System (PPS), outpatient fee schedules, ICD-9-CM and HCPCS coding systems, and billing and reimbursement policies, can be obtained from these sources.

Other sources of information on Medicare changes are the *MLN Matters* articles available through the Medicare Learning Network (MLN) and CMS mailing lists. *MLN Matters* (formerly known as *Medlearns Matters*) articles are national articles designed to inform physicians, other providers, and suppliers of the latest changes to the Medicare program. Located on the CMS website, they are user-friendly, and the content and language are tailored to the specific type of provider affected by a particular change. *MLN Matters* articles are efficient sources of information because of their brief format; they present the most pertinent information about complex material in an easy-to-understand style.

The CMS website also contains a list of more than eighty electronic mailing lists (listservs) that provide current Medicare information in the form of e-mail messages. Medicare listservs are available on a wide range of topics

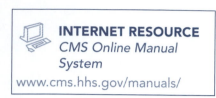

INTERNET RESOURCE
CMS Online Manual System
www.cms.hhs.gov/manuals/

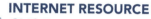

INTERNET RESOURCE
CMS Program Transmittals
www.cms.hhs.gov/transmittals

INTERNET RESOURCE
CMS Program Transmittal 1104:
UB-04 Implementation
www.cms.hhs.gov/transmittals/downloads/R1104CP.pdf

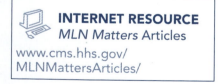

INTERNET RESOURCE
MLN Matters Articles
www.cms.hhs.gov/MLNMattersArticles/

and are easy to subscribe to. Listservs relevant to Medicare billing and the UB-04 include the following:

- HOSPITALS-ACUTE-L, which provides current Medicare information on acute inpatient hospitals
- OP-PPS-L, which provides current Medicare information for hospital outpatient billing
- HOSPITALODF-L, which provides information on monthly hospital Open Door Forum conference calls, including dial-in information for joining the next conference call

Because Medicare billing rules change regularly, learning how to make use of the vast amount of information available through the CMS website and the websites of local FIs is an important and ongoing job for the patient account specialist.

Form Locators

The UB-04 has eighty-one data elements contained in eighty-one different fields called form locators. A **form locator (FL)** is a numeric indicator that directs the reader to a specific box on a data collection form. Figures 6.1 and 6.2 on pages 134–135 show the front and back of a UB-04 claim form. Notice that there are eighty-one numbered boxes on the front of the claim.

Each form locator on the UB-04 is designed to record a specific type of billing data as determined by Medicare's billing rules. In most cases, other payers have the same or similar rules. Depending on the payer and the circumstances of the bill, completion of certain fields can be required, optional, or desirable. This is because some payers require information that others do not. Most of the UB-04 form locators are required fields for Medicare billing.

The billing rules for each form locator specify:

- The type of data that must be entered in the field—for example, an admission date or service charge
- The format of the data—for example, alphabetic or numeric
- The number of characters (letters, numbers, symbols, or spaces) allowed

The back of the UB-04 contains various certifications and authorizations connected with the processing of the claim. By submitting a claim, the submitter certifies that all the information contained on the front of the form is true, accurate, and complete; that the appropriate signature of the patient authorizing release of information and the assignment of benefits, if applicable, is on file; and that the physician's certifications, if required by contract, are on file; among other things. Verifications specific to particular payers are also contained on the back of the form: numbered paragraph 7 contains certifications that pertain to Medicare claims, paragraph 8 to Medicaid claims, and paragraphs 9(a) through 9(h) to TRICARE claims.

Form Locator Groupings

With the exception of eleven unlabeled form locators, each form locator on the UB-04 has a label indicating the type of data to be supplied in that particular field. Examples of labels are "Type of Bill," "Birthdate," "Condition Codes," "HCPCS/Rate/HIPPS Code," "Non-covered Charges," "Employer

Figure 6.1

UB-04 Claim Form—Front

1		2		3a PAT. CNTL #		4 TYPE OF BILL
				b. MED. REC. #		
				5 FED. TAX NO.	6 STATEMENT COVERS PERIOD FROM THROUGH	7

8 PATIENT NAME	a		9 PATIENT ADDRESS	a				
b				b		c	d	e

| 10 BIRTHDATE | 11 SEX | 12 DATE | ADMISSION 13 HR | 14 TYPE | 15 SRC | 16 DHR | 17 STAT | 18 | 19 | 20 | 21 | CONDITION CODES 22 23 24 25 26 27 28 | 29 ACDT STATE | 30 |

31 OCCURRENCE CODE DATE	32 OCCURRENCE CODE DATE	33 OCCURRENCE CODE DATE	34 OCCURRENCE CODE DATE	35 CODE	OCCURRENCE SPAN FROM THROUGH	36 CODE	OCCURRENCE SPAN FROM THROUGH	37
a								a
b								b

38		39 CODE	VALUE CODES AMOUNT	40 CODE	VALUE CODES AMOUNT	41 CODE	VALUE CODES AMOUNT
	a						
	b						
	c						
	d						

42 REV. CD.	43 DESCRIPTION	44 HCPCS / RATE / HIPPS CODE	45 SERV. DATE	46 SERV. UNITS	47 TOTAL CHARGES	48 NON-COVERED CHARGES	49
1							1
2							2
3							3
4							4
5							5
6							6
7							7
8							8
9							9
10							10
11							11
12							12
13							13
14							14
15							15
16							16
17							17
18							18
19							19
20							20
21							21
22							22
23	*PAGE ___ OF ___*	*CREATION DATE*		*TOTALS* ➡			23

50 PAYER NAME	51 HEALTH PLAN ID	52 REL INFO	53 ASG. BEN.	54 PRIOR PAYMENTS	55 EST. AMOUNT DUE	56 NPI
A						57 OTHER PRV ID
B						
C						

58 INSURED'S NAME	59 P. REL	60 INSURED'S UNIQUE ID	61 GROUP NAME	62 INSURANCE GROUP NO.
A				
B				
C				

63 TREATMENT AUTHORIZATION CODES	64 DOCUMENT CONTROL NUMBER	65 EMPLOYER NAME
A		
B		
C		

66 DX	67 A B C D E F G H I J K L M N O P Q	68

69 ADMIT DX	70 PATIENT REASON DX a b c	71 PPS CODE	72 ECI a b c	73

74 PRINCIPAL PROCEDURE CODE DATE	a. OTHER PROCEDURE CODE DATE	b. OTHER PROCEDURE CODE DATE	75	76 ATTENDING	NPI		QUAL
				LAST		FIRST	
c. OTHER PROCEDURE CODE DATE	d. OTHER PROCEDURE CODE DATE	e. OTHER PROCEDURE CODE DATE		77 OPERATING	NPI		QUAL
				LAST		FIRST	

80 REMARKS	81CC a	78 OTHER	NPI		QUAL
	b	LAST		FIRST	
	c	79 OTHER	NPI		QUAL
	d	LAST		FIRST	

UB-04 CMS-1450   APPROVED OMB NO. 0938-0997

NUBC National Uniform Billing Committee

THE CERTIFICATIONS ON THE REVERSE APPLY TO THIS BILL AND ARE MADE A PART HEREOF.

Figure 6.2

UB-04 Claim Form—Back

UB-04 NOTICE: THE SUBMITTER OF THIS FORM UNDERSTANDS THAT MISREPRESENTATION OR FALSIFICATION OF ESSENTIAL INFORMATION AS REQUESTED BY THIS FORM, MAY SERVE AS THE BASIS FOR CIVIL MONETARTY PENALTIES AND ASSESSMENTS AND MAY UPON CONVICTION INCLUDE FINES AND/OR IMPRISONMENT UNDER FEDERAL AND/OR STATE LAW(S).

Submission of this claim constitutes certification that the billing information as shown on the face hereof is true, accurate and complete. That the submitter did not knowingly or recklessly disregard or misrepresent or conceal material facts. The following certifications or verifications apply where pertinent to this Bill:

1. If third party benefits are indicated, the appropriate assignments by the insured /beneficiary and signature of the patient or parent or a legal guardian covering authorization to release information are on file. Determinations as to the release of medical and financial information should be guided by the patient or the patient's legal representative.

2. If patient occupied a private room or required private nursing for medical necessity, any required certifications are on file.

3. Physician's certifications and re-certifications, if required by contract or Federal regulations, are on file.

4. For Religious Non-Medical facilities, verifications and if necessary re-certifications of the patient's need for services are on file.

5. Signature of patient or his representative on certifications, authorization to release information, and payment request, as required by Federal Law and Regulations (42 USC 1935f, 42 CFR 424.36, 10 USC 1071 through 1086, 32 CFR 199) and any other applicable contract regulations, is on file.

6. The provider of care submitter acknowledges that the bill is in conformance with the Civil Rights Act of 1964 as amended. Records adequately describing services will be maintained and necessary information will be furnished to such governmental agencies as required by applicable law.

7. For Medicare Purposes: If the patient has indicated that other health insurance or a state medical assistance agency will pay part of his/her medical expenses and he/she wants information about his/her claim released to them upon request, necessary authorization is on file. The patient's signature on the provider's request to bill Medicare medical and non-medical information, including employment status, and whether the person has employer group health insurance which is responsible to pay for the services for which this Medicare claim is made.

8. For Medicaid purposes: The submitter understands that because payment and satisfaction of this claim will be from Federal and State funds, any false statements, documents, or concealment of a material fact are subject to prosecution under applicable Federal or State Laws.

9. For TRICARE Purposes:

   (a) The information on the face of this claim is true, accurate and complete to the best of the submitter's knowledge and belief, and services were medically necessary and appropriate for the health of the patient;

   (b) The patient has represented that by a reported residential address outside a military medical treatment facility catchment area he or she does not live within the catchment area of a U.S. military medical treatment facility, or if the patient resides within a catchment area of such a facility, a copy of Non-Availability Statement (DD Form 1251) is on file, or the physician has certified to a medical emergency in any instance where a copy of a Non-Availability Statement is not on file;

   (c) The patient or the patient's parent or guardian has responded directly to the provider's request to identify all health insurance coverage, and that all such coverage is identified on the face of the claim except that coverage which is exclusively supplemental payments to TRICARE-determined benefits;

   (d) The amount billed to TRICARE has been billed after all such coverage have been billed and paid excluding Medicaid, and the amount billed to TRICARE is that remaining claimed against TRICARE benefits;

   (e) The beneficiary's cost share has not been waived by consent or failure to exercise generally accepted billing and collection efforts; and,

   (f) Any hospital-based physician under contract, the cost of whose services are allocated in the charges included in this bill, is not an employee or member of the Uniformed Services. For purposes of this certification, an employee of the Uniformed Services is an employee, appointed in civil service (refer to 5 USC 2105), including part-time or intermittent employees, but excluding contract surgeons or other personal service contracts. Similarly, member of the Uniformed Services does not apply to reserve members of the Uniformed Services not on active duty.

   (g) Based on 42 United States Code 1395cc(a)(1)(j) all providers participating in Medicare must also participate in TRICARE for inpatient hospital services provided pursuant to admissions to hospitals occurring on or after January 1, 1987; and

   (h) If TRICARE benefits are to be paid in a participating status, the submitter of this claim agrees to submit this claim to the appropriate TRICARE claims processor. The provider of care submitter also agrees to accept the TRICARE determined reasonable charge as the total charge for the medical services or supplies listed on the claim form. The provider of care will accept the TRICARE-determined reasonable charge even if it is less than the billed amount, and also agrees to accept the amount paid by TRICARE combined with the cost-share amount and deductible amount, if any, paid by or on behalf of the patient as full payment for the listed medical services or supplies. The provider of care submitter will not attempt to collect from the patient (or his or her parent or guardian) amounts over the TRICARE determined reasonable charge. TRICARE will make any benefits payable directly to the provider of care, if the provider of care is a participating provider.

SEE http://www.nubc.org/ FOR MORE INFORMATION ON UB-04 DATA ELEMENT AND PRINTING SPECIFICATIONS

Name," and "Remarks." At first glance, the labels do not seem to be grouped in any particular order. On studying the form more carefully, however, a structure becomes apparent. Generally, the eighty-one data elements on the UB-04 are grouped into the following sections:

FLs 1–7	Provider information
FLs 8–17	Patient information
FLs 18–30	Condition codes
FLs 31–38	Occurrence codes and dates
FLs 39–41	Value codes and amounts
FLs 42–49	Revenue codes, descriptions, and charges
FLs 50–65	Payer, insured, and employer information
FLs 66–75	Diagnosis and procedure codes
FLs 76–79	Physician information
FLs 80–81	Remarks section and Code-Code field

The amount of detail and the compactness of the form are less overwhelming when the form is viewed as ten different sections, each containing a similar type of data, than when it is viewed as eighty-one different blocks of data. Because patient account specialists work with UB-04 claims regularly, they quickly become familiar with the different form locator groupings.

Required Formats

Each form locator on the UB-04 has a required format. Although detailed information on the format for each form locator is presented in subsequent chapters of Part 2, it is useful to know the range of formats that are acceptable on the UB-04 and some of the form's important formatting elements.

Numeric, alphabetic, alphanumeric, and text-based formats are used on the UB-04. Numeric formats are used in many form locators and include specialized codes particular to the UB-04, date formats, dollar amounts, certain units of measure, identification numbers, and a full range of diagnosis and procedure codes. The following are examples of numeric formats. Locate each example in Figure 6.3.

Numeric Entry	Meaning	Location on Form
12	12:00 (noon–12:59 p.m.)	FL 13, Admission Hour
7	Emergency room	FL 15, Source of Admission
1080.00	$1,080.00 per night	FL 44, HCPCS/Accommodation Rates/HIPPS Rate Codes
030410	March 4, 2010	FL 6, Statement Covers Period From
5	Number of nights	FL 46, Service Units
1288561733	National Provider Identifier	FL 56, NPI
2761	Hyposmolality	FL 67, Principal Diagnosis Code

Figure 6.3
Sample Completed UB-04 Form

1 HANOVER REGIONAL HOSPITAL	2			3a PAT. CNTL # 53820705		4 TYPE OF BILL
2600 RECORD STREET				b. MED. REC. # 3496815		0111
HANOVER, CT 06783				5 FED. TAX NO.	6 STATEMENT COVERS PERIOD FROM / THROUGH	7
860-376-2000				07-1282340	030410 / 030910	

8 PATIENT NAME	a		9 PATIENT ADDRESS	a 8 RIVER ROAD			
b ASTORE, GAIL			b HARTFORD		c CT	d 06516	e

10 BIRTHDATE	11 SEX	12 DATE	ADMISSION 13 HR 14 TYPE 15 SRC	16 DHR	17 STAT	18 19 20 21 CONDITION CODES 22 23 24 25 26 27 28	29 ACDT STATE	30
08051936	F	030410	12 1 7	16	06	C5		

31 OCCURRENCE CODE / DATE	32 OCCURRENCE CODE / DATE	33 OCCURRENCE CODE / DATE	34 OCCURRENCE CODE / DATE	35 OCCURRENCE SPAN CODE FROM THROUGH	36 OCCURRENCE SPAN CODE FROM THROUGH	37
a 05 030310	19 060103					
b						

38		39 CODE VALUE CODES AMOUNT	40 CODE VALUE CODES AMOUNT	41 CODE VALUE CODES AMOUNT
	a	45 23 00	80 5 00	
	b			
	c			
	d			

42 REV. CD.	43 DESCRIPTION	44 HCPCS / RATE / HIPPS CODE	45 SERV. DATE	46 SERV. UNITS	47 TOTAL CHARGES	48 NON-COVERED CHARGES	49
1	0121	MED-SURG-GY/SEMI	1080 00		5	5,400 00	
2	0250	PHARMACY				102 85	
3	0260	IV THERAPY				101 90	
4	0272	STERILE SUPPLY				42 39	
5	0301	CHEMISTRY TESTS				1,858 01	
6	0305	HEMATOLOGY TESTS				184 82	
7	0306	BACT & MICRO TESTS				44 18	
8	0320	DX X-RAY			1	809 25	
9	0351	CT SCAN/HEAD			1	485 66	
10	0420	PHYSICAL THERP				177 74	
11	0424	PHYS THERP/EVAL				154 21	
12	0450	EMERG ROOM			2	481 50	
13	0730	EKG/ECG				47 32	
23	0001	PAGE _1_ OF _1_	CREATION DATE 031210	TOTALS ➤		9,889 83	

50 PAYER NAME	51 HEALTH PLAN ID	52 REL INFO	53 ASG BEN	54 PRIOR PAYMENTS	55 EST. AMOUNT DUE	56 NPI 1288561733
A MEDICARE	00308	Y	Y			57 OTHER PRV ID 070089
B						
C						

58 INSURED'S NAME	59 P.REL	60 INSURED'S UNIQUE ID	61 GROUP NAME	62 INSURANCE GROUP NO.
A ASTORE, GAIL	18	102123712B		

63 TREATMENT AUTHORIZATION CODES	64 DOCUMENT CONTROL NUMBER	65 EMPLOYER NAME
A 01916931		

66 DX 2761	2920	72889	4019	30000	311	E8888		68

69 ADMIT DX 78079	70 PATIENT REASON DX	71 PPS CODE	72 ECI	73

74 PRINCIPAL PROCEDURE CODE DATE	a. OTHER PROCEDURE CODE DATE	b. OTHER PROCEDURE CODE DATE	75	76 ATTENDING NPI 1233281192 QUAL IG B18642
				LAST WOOD FIRST JOHN
c. OTHER PROCEDURE CODE DATE	d. OTHER PROCEDURE CODE DATE	e. OTHER PROCEDURE CODE DATE		77 OPERATING NPI QUAL
				LAST FIRST

80 REMARKS	81CC a B3 282N00000X	78 OTHER NPI QUAL
ACCIDENTAL FALL IN HOME,	b	LAST FIRST
NO LIABILITY	c	79 OTHER NPI QUAL
	d	LAST FIRST

UB-04 CMS-1450   APPROVED OMB NO. 0938-0997   **NUBC** National Uniform Billing Committee   THE CERTIFICATIONS ON THE REVERSE APPLY TO THIS BILL AND ARE MADE A PART HEREOF.

Alphabetic formats used on the UB-04 include names (provider, patient, payer, employer) and specialized codes particular to the UB-04, such as:

Alphabetic Entry	Meaning	Location on Form
Astore, Gail	Last name, first name	FL 8b, Patient Name
F	Female	FL 11, Sex
Medicare	Name of insurance	FL 50, Payer Name
Y	Yes	FL 53, Assignment of Benefits Certification Indicator

Alphanumeric formats contain both numbers and letters and are used on the UB-04 in addresses, ID numbers, and special codes particular to the UB-04, as well as in certain diagnosis and procedure codes:

Alphanumeric Entry	Meaning	Location on Form
C5	Postpayment review applicable	FLs 18–28, Condition Codes
E8888	E code (accidental fall)	FL 67 F, Other Diagnosis

A text-based format is used in FL 43 (Revenue Description) and FL 80 (Remarks). The revenue description is a narrative description—for example, "Pharmacy"—of the service charges associated with the revenue code in FL 42. The revenue description may also be a standard abbreviation, such as "PEDS/PVT," which stands for pediatric/private, the description used with revenue code 0113 (Routine service charges for accommodations in a private room, pediatric). The provider uses the Remarks field (FL 80) to enter information he or she deems necessary to substantiate the medical treatment and that is not shown elsewhere on the claim form. If Medicare is not the primary payer because of a workers' compensation or other liability plan, the provider may enter notes specific to the situation in this field.

Some form locators on the UB-04 contain a formatting element known as a delimiter. A **delimiter** is a character or symbol used in printed material to visually separate one group of words or values from another. A common delimiter is the vertical column of dots used to separate dollars and cents in a list of charges in form locators 39–41 (Value Codes and Amounts), 47 (Total Charges), 48 (Noncovered Charges), 54 (Prior Payments), and 55 (Estimated Amount Due). The delimiter makes the amount easier to read and compute on the UB-04.

Another important formatting element on the UB-04 is the use of a **detail-level code** in FL 42 (Revenue Code). A revenue code stands for a specific type of charge that is being billed. It identifies the hospital department that provided the service. In every revenue code, the first three digits stand for the type of service, and the fourth digit is used to define the detailed level of the code. The numbers 1 through 9 represent different details for different revenue codes, and 0 (zero) indicates the general classification. Following is an example of detail-level codes used with revenue code 044X, Speech therapy-language pathology. Note that the X in code 044X is a placeholder for the fourth-digit code; for billing purposes, the X must be replaced with a number from the subcategory list.

Fourth Digit	*Subcategory*	*Standard Abbreviation*
0	General classification	SPEECH THERAPY
1	Visit charge	SPEECH THERP/VISIT
2	Hourly charge	SPEECH THERP/HOUR
3	Group rate	SPEECH THERP/GROUP
4	Evaluation or reevaluation	SPEECH THERP/EVAL
5–8	Reserved	
9	Other speech therapy	OTHER SPEECH THERP

Based on this list of detail-level codes, a hospital billing for an evaluation session for speech therapy would show code 0444 in FL 42 (Revenue Code) on the UB-04.

The use of the fourth-digit detail-level code in the revenue coding system maximizes the options in the classification system but also retains the simplicity of the base three-digit code set. In most cases, a general revenue code (a code ending in 0) is all that is required for Medicare claims. In other cases, a detailed revenue code (a code ending in 1–9) is required so that the hospital can keep better track of the services rendered and to help determine the proper reimbursement.

Unlabeled Form Locators

Eleven UB-04 form locators are not labeled. Seven of these fields (FLs 7, 30, 37, 49, 68, 73, and 75) are reserved for national use in accordance with procedures and guidelines established by the NUBC. Unlike the other form locators, they are not intended for provider reporting. In this text, these seven form locators are referred to as unlabeled fields. They are included in the detailed description of each form locator in the subsequent chapters of Part 2, but no instructions on their use are given.

The remaining four unlabeled form locators are numbered 1, 2, 38, and 67. Despite being unlabeled on the UB-04, they are assigned fields intended for provider use. These form locators have the following names:

FL 1	Provider Name, Address, and Telephone Number
FL 2	Pay-to Name and Address
FL 38	Responsible Party Name and Address
FL 67	Principal Diagnosis Code and Present on Admission Indicator

Instructions on the use of FLs 1, 2, 38, and 67 appear in later chapters.

Similarly, there are unassigned codes in the various lists of codes used with certain form locators. In general, unassigned codes are designed to meet the future reporting needs of CMS and other regulatory agencies, such as for public health data reporting, and to accommodate future payer-specific requirements for hospital billing.

Chapter Organization and Coverage in Part 2

Each of the nine subsequent chapters in Part 2 provides a detailed description of a group of form locators on the UB-04:

Chapter 7	FLs 1–7	Provider information
Chapter 8	FLs 8–17	Patient information
Chapter 9	FLs 18–30	Condition codes
Chapter 10	FLs 31–38	Occurrence codes and dates
Chapter 11	FLs 39–41	Value codes and amounts
Chapter 12	FLs 42–49	Revenue codes, descriptions, and charges
Chapter 13	FLs 50–65	Payer, insured, and employer information
Chapter 14	FLs 66–75	Diagnosis and procedure codes
Chapter 15	FLs 76–81	Physician information, remarks section, and Code-Code field

Within each grouping, the chapter provides a general description of the information required in each form locator. The form locators are listed in numeric order with appropriate guidelines, formatting examples, billing tips, and compliance guides, including:

- The number of characters allowed in the field
- The type of formatting required
- Codes used to complete the field, if applicable
- Important connections to other information on the claim

Most of the guidelines and billing and coding tips apply to Medicare claims, and the varying guidelines for payers such as Medicaid, Blue Cross, and commercial insurers are mentioned only briefly. In addition, the main focus of the text is correct processing of hospital inpatient and outpatient claims, so codes for other billing entities, such as skilled nursing facilities (SNFs) and home health care agencies, are not discussed in detail.

FYI

Understanding the Codes

In explaining the coding system used for two of the form locators on the UB-04 (FL 4, Type of Bill, and FL 42, Revenue Code), an *X* is sometimes used as a temporary placeholder for one or two of the numbers that should be used in billing. For actual billing purposes, the appropriate subcategory number should replace the *X* in the code.

CHAPTER SUMMARY

1 The original Uniform Bill known as the UB-82 was introduced in 1982 by the National Uniform Billing Committee (NUBC) as its first attempt to devise a single hospital billing form that could be used nationally by most providers and payers. In 1992, after ten years of use, the UB-82 was updated and renamed the UB-92. The electronic HIPAA version of the Uniform Bill, known as the 837I, was introduced in 2003. It included the same data as the UB-92 and also several new fields and format changes required under HIPAA. In 2004, to better align the Uniform Bill with its new HIPAA equivalent, the NUBC introduced the UB-04, which officially replaced the UB-92 on March 1, 2007.

The UB-04 is also known as the CMS-1450 claim form. A wide range of facilities use the UB-04 or its electronic HIPAA equivalent. They include acute care facilities; SNFs; psychiatric, drug, and alcohol treatment facilities; stand-alone clinics; ambulatory surgery centers; subacute facilities; home health care agencies; and hospice organizations. The form is primarily designed for submitting claims for Medicare Part A reimbursement of both inpatient and outpatient services to Medicare FIs and MACs. Because of its flexibility, however, the UB-04 has also been adopted by most other payers as well. It is not used to report the charges of physicians, which are billed on the CMS-1500 claim form, also known as the 837P in its electronic HIPAA format.

2 The UB-04 claim form can be transmitted on paper or electronically. The electronic version is an EDI (electronic data interchange) transaction. In both formats, claims are usually created with a software program. The paper claim is transmitted to the payer on paper, however, and the EDI claim is transmitted from computer to computer. The advantages of EDI transmission include speed, economy, less possibility of data entry error, and faster turnaround. With HIPAA's mandate in 2003 that all but the smallest providers transmit data for Medicare claims electronically using the HIPAA claim, electronic claim transmission has become the predominant form.

3 When a claim meets all necessary specifications and passes all predetermined data edits, it is known as a clean claim. The patient account specialist aims to achieve clean-claim billing on all UB-04s. A claim that does not meet all the specifications of a clean claim is either denied or rejected by the payer. A provider cannot resubmit a denied claim but can appeal it. The reverse is true of a rejected claim: the provider can correct a rejected claim and resubmit it but cannot appeal it.

4 The UB-04 has eighty-one data elements contained in eighty-one different fields called form locators (FLs). The form locators on the UB-04 can be sequentially grouped into ten different sections based on similar types of data. The data included in each form locator are determined by Medicare's billing rules. In most cases, other payers have the same or similar rules. Most of the form locators are required fields for Medicare billing, and other payers' requirements may differ somewhat. The billing rules for each form locator specify (a) the type of data that must be entered in the field, (b) the format of the data, and (c) the number of characters—letters, numbers, symbols, or spaces—allowed. Specific formats for each form locator can be numeric, alphabetic, alphanumeric, or text-based.

5 Eleven form locators on the UB-04 are unlabeled. Seven of these fields (FLs 7, 30, 37, 49, 68, 73, and 75) are reserved for assignment by the NUBC and are not intended for provider use. The remaining four (FLs 1, 2, 38, and 67) are not labeled on the UB-04 but do have names in the documentation and are intended for provider use.

6 Each of the nine chapters that follow in Part 2 of this text provides a detailed walk-through of a group of form locators on the UB-04. Form locators are described and listed in numeric order, and guidelines, formatting examples, and billing and coding tips are provided. The detailed instructions apply mainly to Medicare claims. The billing entities are primarily acute care facilities, as the main focus of this text is the correct processing of inpatient and outpatient hospital claims.

✔ CHECK YOUR UNDERSTANDING

1. Define the following terms.
  a. form locator _____
  b. UB-04 _____
  c. EDI _____

2. Which of the following groups is responsible for deciding what data elements to include on the UB-04 claim form?
  a. CMS
  b. AHA
  c. NUBC
  d. ASC X12N Task Group on Health

3. True or False: The UB-04 can be used for preparing Medicare and Medicaid claims but not TRICARE claims. _____

4. What is the difference between the CMS-1500 and the CMS-1450? _____
  What is the name of the electronic HIPAA equivalent for each? _____

5. How many form locators are there on the UB-04? _____ How many of them are unlabeled?
  _____ Explain the use of the unlabeled form locators that are not intended for provider use.
  _____

6. A data entry of "A3 050611" in FL 31 (Occurrence Code and Date) is an example of what type of format?
  a. alphanumeric   **c.** numeric
  b. text-based   **d.** alphabetic

7. Following are the subcategories for revenue code category 021X (Coronary Care Unit). What revenue code would you enter in FL 42 (Revenue Code) if you were billing for the routine service charges for a heart transplant patient?

Fourth Digit	Subcategory	Standard Abbreviation
0	General classification	CORONARY CARE or CCU
1	Myocardial infarction	CCU/MYO INFARC
2	Pulmonary care	CCU/PULMONARY
3	Heart transplant	CCU/TRANSPLANT
4	Intermediate CCU	CCU/INTERMEDIATE
9	Other coronary care	CCU/OTHER

8. True or False: The difference between paper claims and electronic claims is that paper claims are not created on a computer. _____

9. Match the term on the left with its description on the right.

_____ clean claim   **a.** May be corrected and resubmitted by the provider

_____ claim rejection   **b.** Must be paid by the thirtieth day after the date of receipt

_____ claim denial   **c.** Can be appealed by the provider

10. List three reasons a claim may be returned to the provider without being paid.

_____

_____

_____

11. Which of the following items is not updated on a regular basis each year?

    a. Medicare Inpatient Prospective Payment System (PPS)

    b. ICD-9-CM and HCPCS

    c. outpatient fee schedules

    d. UB-04 form locators

12. True or False: The guidelines and coding tips presented in Part 2 of this text apply mainly to Medicare inpatient and outpatient hospital claims. _____

COMPUTER EXPLORATION

UB-04 Activity: Claim Analysis

The claim analysis activities at the end of each chapter in Part 2 are designed to increase your familiarity with the UB-04 by giving you the opportunity to analyze several sample claims. In each activity, a hospital claim is viewed onscreen using the Adobe Reader program. The activities present a series of questions about the claim to reinforce the concepts learned during that chapter.

Before you begin the claim analysis exercises, you will need to copy the pdf files of the sample claims to your computer. Refer to Chapter 16, for instructions on downloading the files from the text's Online Learning Center to your computer. Chapter 16 also provides brief instructions on how to open a pdf file in Adobe Reader and how to navigate through a form.

NOTE ON ADOBE READER: When you are finished viewing the file, simply exit Adobe Reader. You will not be asked about saving any changes you may have made to the form, since Adobe Reader does not allow you to save data entry on forms. The Print option on the File menu can be used at any time to print a copy of the data as it appears on screen; however, any changes to the original data will be lost automatically on exiting.

Viewing a Sample Claim

Open the file **Sample01.pdf** in Adobe Reader, and answer the following questions:

1. Roll the cursor over line 1 of form locator 1 (FL 1) and pause to display the rollover text. What rollover text appears?

2. Do the same for lines 2 through 4 of FL 1 to learn what type of information is reported in each line. For this claim, what is the billing provider's name and phone number?

3. Click inside FL 1 to orient the cursor, and then TAB over to FL 5. Notice the sequence the cursor makes as you TAB. The TAB stops move through every line of each FL in numeric order. SHIFT-TAB moves the cursor backwards through the same sequence. What rollover text is displayed in FL 5? Based on the data in FL 5, how many numbers are required in a federal tax ID?

4. As a means of analyzing the UB-04 form, the eighty-one numbered fields on the form are generally grouped into the sections listed below. Click once in each section and look over the fields contained in it. Use the rollover text as necessary to learn the content of each field. Notice the various formats used.

FLs 1–7	Provider information
FLs 8–17	Patient information
FLs 18–30	Condition codes
FLs 31–38	Occurrence codes and dates
FLs 39–41	Value codes and amounts
FLs 42–49	Revenue codes, descriptions, and charges
FLs 50–65	Payer, insured, and employer information
FLs 66–75	Diagnosis and procedure codes
FLs 76–79	Physician information
FLs 80–81	Remarks section and Code-Code field

5. Now that you are familiar with the various fields, locate the field for revenue codes. What is the number of the first revenue code on the claim?

6. What is the name of the beneficiary? How old is the beneficiary at the time of admission?

7. What is the principal diagnosis code?

8. What is the name of the attending provider? Is there an operating physician?

9. What type of insurance does the beneficiary have?

10. What is the charge for the anesthesia?

When finished viewing the claim, click Exit on the File menu.

Provider Information

LEARNING OUTCOMES

After completing this chapter, you will be able to define the key terms and:

1 Identify the types of provider information that belong in the first seven fields (FLs 1–7) of the UB-04 claim form.

2 Understand the different formats that are required for specific form locators.

3 Explain the difference between the patient control number (FL 3a) and the patient's medical record number (FL 3b).

4 Discuss the appropriate use of four-digit codes in FL 4 to indicate the type of bill (TOB) being generated.

5 Recognize which form locators contain data that necessitate data entry in other fields or data that must be coordinated with the data supplied in other fields.

6 Understand the importance of the from and through dates in FL 6 (Statement Covers Period), and know how to report the correct dates for different types of claims.

KEY TERMS

- comprehensive outpatient rehabilitation facility (CORF)
- continuing claim
- critical access hospital (CAH)
- interim bill
- medical/health record number
- patient control number
- statement covers period
- swing bed hospital
- type of bill (TOB)

This chapter provides instructions for filling in the first seven fields on the UB-04 claim form (see Figure 7.1). These fields contain information about the institutional provider of the services that are being billed. Medicare and other payers require this information to process payments correctly and efficiently. For example, the first field contains the provider's name, address, and telephone number, and the second field is used to report the pay-to address if the provider has a separate mailing address for receiving payments. Based on the information in the first two fields, the payer knows where to send a payment.

The provider information section of the UB-04 also supplies the basic information needed to identify the type of claim being billed. This information includes the type of facility at which the service was received, whether the bill is for inpatient or outpatient services, and whether the bill represents the beginning, middle, or end of an episode of care. Payers must have this information to determine which benefits are currently due, as well as to anticipate benefits due in the future.

Finally, the provider information on the UB-04 includes the from and through dates—the dates of service for the charges being billed. This information is especially important to payers in determining benefits for inpatient care.

FL 1 Provider Name, Address, and Telephone Number

FL 1 contains the name and service location of the provider submitting the bill. This information is needed for mailing payments. The payer will also use it to contact the provider if more information is needed. Up to four lines of text are allowed.

Line 1	Name of the provider
Line 2	Street address
Line 3	City, state (abbreviation), ZIP code (five- or nine-digit)
Line 4	Telephone and fax number (ten digits each), country code

Guidelines

Completion of this field is required for Medicare billing and for all other payers. The minimum entry for Medicare claims is the provider's name, city, state, and ZIP code (lines 1 and 3). The country code is required only when the address is outside the United States. Punctuation can be used in this field.

EXAMPLE:
ST REGIS HOSPITAL
2001 ULSTER AVENUE
FINEVIEW, NY 13640
315-425-9000

Figure 7.1

UB-04 Form—FLs 1–7

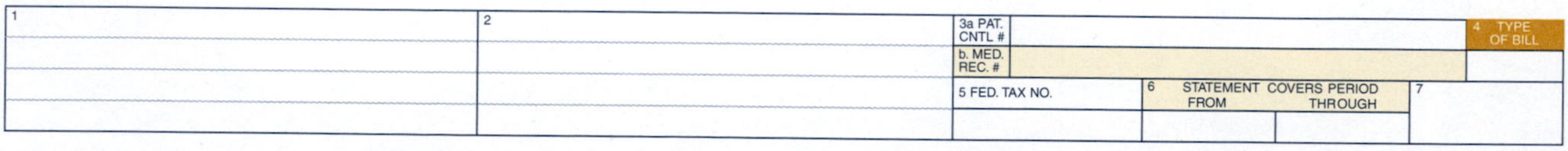

1	2	3a PAT. CNTL #		4 TYPE OF BILL
		b. MED. REC. #		
		5 FED. TAX NO.	6 STATEMENT COVERS PERIOD FROM THROUGH	7

FL 2 Pay-to Name and Address

FL 2 is used only if the address that payment is to be mailed to is different from the address reported in FL 1. For example, if payments to a hospital are to be mailed to a post office box number, the PO box address is reported in FL 2. Up to three lines of text are allowed:

Line 1	Pay-to name
Line 2	Street address or PO box number
Line 3	City, state (abbreviation), ZIP code (five-digit)

Guidelines

Line 4 of this field is reserved for assignment by the NUBC and therefore should be left blank.

EXAMPLE:
ST REGIS HOSPITAL
PO BOX 2990
FINEVIEW, NY 13640

FL 3a Patient Control Number

FL 3a contains a **patient control number,** a unique alphanumeric identifier assigned by the provider to each patient. The main purpose of the patient control number is to identify payments from third-party payers, who must use this number on payment checks, vouchers, or remittance advices such as the Medicare 835 remittance advice. The patient control number is usually associated with a single episode of care and is used to retrieve the patient's financial records and to post payments to the patient's account.

Guidelines

Completion of this field is required for Medicare billing and all other payers. Although there is space for twenty-four characters, HIPAA limits the patient control number to twenty alphanumeric characters. No spaces or special characters should be used.

EXAMPLE: AA201356098945

FL 3b Medical Record Number

FL 3b contains the number assigned by the provider to the patient's medical/health record. The **medical/health record number** provides a means of tracking a patient's medical history and treatment across multiple episodes of care. This number is different from the patient control number in FL 3a, which is used to locate an individual financial record for accounting purposes and is usually associated with a single episode of care. Although FL 3b is listed as a situational rather than a required field for Medicare claims, in practice most payers use it, since it enables the provider to identify the patient's medical record for future inquiries.

> **HIPAA TIP**
>
> *Medical Record Number and PHI*
> The HIPAA Privacy Rule covers the use and disclosure of patients' protected health information (PHI). A person's medical record number as reported on the UB-04 is considered a part of PHI.

Guidelines

The medical/health record number is a unique alphanumeric identifier and can contain up to twenty-four characters. Unlike the patient control number, the medical record number can span more than one episode of care.

EXAMPLE: RN3444J2X189000

FL 4 Type of Bill

837I alert✚

Type of Bill

On the electronic 837I claim, the leading zero in the TOB code is not reported. The leading zero is a new element in TOB reporting beginning with the UB-04.

HIPAA TIP

UB-04 Mapping to 837 Claim Transaction

The National Uniform Billing Committee publishes a manual on UB-04 claim completion called the *Official UB-04 Data Specifications Manual*. A table entitled "UB-04 Mapping to 837 Claim Transaction" in the appendix lists each UB-04 form locator with its corresponding mapping on the HIPAA equivalent form, the 837I. Each UB-04 form locator is mapped to a loop ID, reference designator, X12 data element number, and other data. Formatting notes such as "leading zero in FL 04 is not reported on 837," are also included. UB-04 form locators that do not map to any location on the 837I are noted as "No map" fields, indicating that the 837I does not contain that field.

The **type of bill (TOB)** is a four-digit code made up of a leading zero followed by three digits that relay three specific pieces of information for billing purposes: (1) the second digit in a TOB identifies the type of facility, (2) the third digit classifies the type of care being billed, and (3) the fourth digit, the frequency code, indicates the sequence of the bill within a given episode of care. Appendix A provides a listing of TOB codes for quick reference.

Guidelines

Completion of this field is required for Medicare billing and for all other payers. On a paper UB-04 claim, a four-digit code must always be used.

The TOB code, since it is made of up to three different types of information, has the most complicated structure of all the codes on the UB-04 claim. For simplification, the TOB is usually described as having two components rather than three. The second-digit code (type of facility) and the third-digit code (type of service received) together make up the first component, known as the *bill type*. For example, bill type 011X identifies charges for a hospital inpatient. The fourth-digit code makes up the second component, known as the *frequency code*. Frequency code 1, for example, identifies an admit-through-discharge claim, which means that the claim is expected to be the only bill submitted for the patient. The coding structure for each code in the TOB is described in more detail below.

Thinking of TOB codes in terms of two components rather than three helps in sorting out the various combinations of codes possible. Table 7.1 presents

Table 7.1

Medicare Bill Type Codes

Code	Bill Type	Code	Bill Type
011X	Hospital inpatient (Part A)	072X	Clinic ESRD (renal dialysis facility)
012X	Hospital inpatient Part B		
013X	Hospital outpatient	073X	Federally qualified health center
014X	Hospital other Part B		
018X	Hospital swing bed	074X	Clinic OPT (outpatient rehabilitation facility)
021X	SNF inpatient		
022X	SNF inpatient Part B	075X	Clinic CORF (comprehensive outpatient rehabilitation facility)
023X	SNF outpatient		
028X	SNF swing bed	076X	Community mental health center
032X	Home health		
033X	Home health	081X	Non-hospital-based hospice
034X	Home health (Part B only)	082X	Hospital-based hospice
041X	Religious nonmedical health care institution	083X	Hospital outpatient (ambulatory surgery center)
071X	Clinical rural health	085X	Critical access hospital

the list of bill type codes provided in the CMS Medicare Claims manual. Because the bill type codes in this table group patients by the type of facility they are in, the table is a good organizational tool for billing purposes.

EXAMPLE: TOB code 0134

In this example, the first component, bill type 013X, indicates a hospital outpatient. The second component, frequency code 4 (Interim—last claim), indicates that this is the final bill in a series of bills that have been submitted for this episode of care.

Coding Structure: Second Digit—Type of Facility

The following numbers, when used as second digits in a TOB, indicate the place of service. Each number represents a different type of facility.

1	Hospital
2	Skilled nursing facility (SNF)
3	Home health facility
4	Religious nonmedical health care institution—hospital
5	Reserved for national assignment by the NUBC
6	Intermediate care facility
7	Clinic or hospital-based renal dialysis facility (Use of this digit means that a special set of codes must be used for the third digit. These choices are covered below in the section "Third Digit—Classification for Clinics Only.")
8	Special facility or hospital ambulatory surgery center (Use of this digit means that a special set of codes must be used for the third digit. These choices are covered below in the section "Third Digit—Classification for Special Facilities Only.")
9	Reserved for national assignment by the NUBC

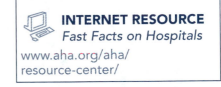

INTERNET RESOURCE
Fast Facts on Hospitals
www.aha.org/aha/
resource-center/

Coding Structure: Third Digit—Bill Classification

The following numbers, when used as third digits in the TOB, indicate the type of service received. There are three groups of services:

1. Bill classification—except clinics and special facilities
2. Classification for clinics only
3. Classification for special facilities only

The first group contains the major bill classifications based on the type of care received, such as inpatient care, outpatient care, or clinic care. If the second digit of the TOB is 7 or 8, however, the other two types of classification are used. Each contains a special set of codes—one for clinics and the other for special facilities—to further clarify the type of care received. The list of codes for each classification follows.

Third-Digit Bill Classification—Except Clinics and Special Facilities

1	Inpatient (including Medicare Part A)
2	Inpatient (Medicare Part B only), which includes home health agency visits under a Part B plan of treatment
3	Outpatient, which includes home health agency visits under a Part A plan of treatment and use of home health agency durable medical equipment under a Part A plan of treatment
4	Other (Medicare Part B), which includes home health agency medical and other health services that are not under a plan of treatment, hospital and skilled nursing facility diagnostic clinical laboratory services to nonpatients, and referred diagnostic services
5	Intermediate care—level I
6	Intermediate care—level II
7	Reserved for national assignment by the NUBC
8	Swing bed (Used to indicate billing for SNF level of care in a hospital with an approved swing bed agreement.)
9	Reserved for national assignment

Third-Digit Bill Classification—Classification for Clinics Only

1	Rural health clinic (RHC)
2	Hospital-based or independent renal dialysis facility
3	Freestanding provider-based federally qualified health center (FQHC)
4	Outpatient rehabilitation facility (ORF)
5	Comprehensive outpatient rehabilitation facility (CORF)
6	Community mental health center (CMHC)
7–8	Reserved for national assignment
9	Other

Third-Digit Bill Classification—Classification for Special Facilities Only

1	Hospice (non-hospital-based)
2	Hospice (hospital-based)
3	Ambulatory surgical center services to hospital outpatients
4	Freestanding birthing center
5	Critical access hospital (CAH)
6	Residential facility (Not used for Medicare.)
7–8	Reserved for national assignment
9	Other

Relating the Third-Digit Bill Classification to the Revenue Code

The third-digit bill classification codes in the TOB are often the main indicators of the type of revenue codes required in FL 42 (Revenue Code). For instance, in TOB 011X, the third-digit code 1 (Inpatient) means that a revenue code for some type of room charge is required in FL 42 because the patient stayed overnight. Conversely, in TOB 013X, the third-digit code 3 (Outpatient) means that a room charge cannot appear in FL 42 because the patient did not stay more than twenty-four hours.

One step in producing a clean claim is to verify that the third-digit code in a TOB logically matches the type of revenue code reported in FL 42. The coordination of data in the TOB and the Revenue Code fields is explained again in Chapter 12, "Revenue Codes, Descriptions, and Charges."

Coding Structure: Fourth Digit— Frequency of the Bill

Several fourth-digit codes in the TOB identify the frequency of the bill.

0   Nonpayment/Zero Claim

Frequency code 0 is used when the provider does not expect a payment as a result of submitting the bill; the information is instead being supplied to meet a specific reporting requirement. For example, if a patient has used up the benefits under a primary insurance plan and the secondary insurance plan should receive the claim, the claim first goes to the primary payer with frequency code 0 for a denial, and then goes to the secondary payer.

1   Admit Through Discharge Claim

Frequency code 1 reports an entire inpatient admission or the course of treatment of an outpatient. It is used when the claim is expected to be the only bill submitted for the patient.

2   Interim—First Claim

Frequency code 2 reports the first bill in an expected series of bills. A bill that does not cover a complete hospital stay is referred to as an **interim bill.** Frequency code 2 (Interim—first claim) is used for the first such interim claim. Additional bills are expected to be submitted for the same confinement or course of treatment either on a monthly basis (every thirty days) or every sixty days by Prospective Payment System (PPS) hospitals.

3   Interim—Continuing Claim (Not Valid for Inpatient Hospital PPS Bills)

Frequency code 3 is used for a **continuing claim**—a claim that is submitted after an initial bill has been sent for the same confinement or course of treatment and before the final bill. A TOB with frequency code 3 can be used only once every thirty days.

4   Interim—Last Claim (Not Valid for Inpatient Hospital PPS Bills)

Frequency code 4 is used for an interim bill that is the last in a series for a course of treatment. Further billing is not expected.

5   Late Charge(s) Only Claim

Frequency code 5 is used to report charges that are being billed late because the provider did not receive them in time to include them in the original claim. This code is used for billing outpatient services only. Late charge bills are not accepted for Medicare inpatient, home health, or ambulatory surgery center (ASC) claims.

6   Unassigned

This code is reserved for assignment by the NUBC.

7   Replacement of Prior Claim

This fourth-digit TOB code is used when a previously sent claim needs to be entirely changed except for the basic information that identifies the original claim. When frequency code 7 is used on a claim, the payer understands that the charges on the original claim are to be voided and that the revised claim is a complete replacement.

Condition codes that are used with frequency code 7 fall in the D0–D9 range (see Chapter 9, "Condition Codes") and include codes for making changes to service dates, charges, revenue codes/HCPCS/HIPPS rate codes, the sequence in an interim PPS bill, and ICD-9-CM codes, or changes to make Medicare the primary or secondary payer.

8   Void/Cancel of a Prior Claim

Frequency code 8 tells the payer that this bill is an exact duplicate of an incorrect bill that was previously submitted and paid. When this bill is submitted, the payer takes back the entire payment it made for the prior claim. Once the payer receives that payment, a separate claim with the corrected or replacement information, using frequency code 7, is usually submitted.

A void/cancel frequency code is usually used in the following cases only:

- To change the provider identification number in FL 51 (Health Plan ID)
- To change the beneficiary's health insurance identification number in FL 60 (Insured's Unique ID)
- To refund a duplicate payment

The appropriate condition code should also be reported in FLs 18–28 (see Chapter 9): either D5 (Cancel to correct insured's ID or provider ID) or D6 (Cancel only to repay a duplicate or OIG overpayment).

9   Final Claim for a Home Health PPS Episode

Frequency code 9 is used for home health billing only. It indicates that the bill should be processed as an adjustment to the request for anticipated payment (RAP)—the initial home health PPS bill.

FL 5 Federal Tax Number

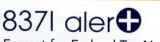

8371 alert

Format for Federal Tax Number

On the electronic claim, the hyphen in the federal tax number is not reported. The format is XXXXXXXXX.

The federal tax number is also known as the TIN (tax identification number) or the EIN (employer identification number). It is the number assigned to the provider by the federal government for tax-reporting purposes. On the UB-04, the federal tax number is reported on the bottom line of FL 5.

The top line of FL 5 may be used to report an affiliated subsidiary of the provider, such as a hospital psychiatric pavilion. If the provider has assigned the subsidiary a separate federal tax sub-ID, this number is reported on the top line.

Guidelines

Completion of this field is required for Medicare billing and by most other payers. The ten-character alphanumeric field allows for nine digits and a hyphen. The format is XX–XXXXXXX or XXXXXXXXX.

EXAMPLE: 92–3760176

FL 6 Statement Covers Period (From–Through)

FL 6 is used for reporting the dates of service for the full period included on the bill. **Statement covers period** refers to the from and through dates shown in FL 6 that represent the beginning and ending dates of service charged on the bill.

Guidelines

Completion of this field is required by all payers. Medicare and other payers use the from date to determine whether the claim has been filed within the payer's time limits.

Both from and through dates must be reported in six-digit MMDDYY numeric format. No hyphens or slashes (/) are used.

EXAMPLE: January 8, 2011, is entered as 010811.

The patient's admission date (FL 12) should not be confused with the from date in the Statement Covers Period field. These dates may or may not be the same. On an interim—continuing claim, for example, the admission date may be several months earlier. The from date represents the first day in that billing period, for example, the first day of the month if the claim's billing period is thirty days.

For same-day services (services provided on a single day), the from and through dates must be identical.

For an inpatient interim bill that has no discharge date (first claim or continuing claim, as indicated in FL 4, TOB), the through date in FL 6 is calculated as part of the total number of days (covered and noncovered) for the claim's billing period. In this case, the dates May 27 through May 31 will be calculated as five days.

On a final bill, the date of discharge or death must be entered in the through field; that date is not calculated in the total number of covered and noncovered days. For example, the dates May 27 through May 31 are calculated as four days in cases of discharge or death.

Dates of service before the patient's entitlement to Medicare are not shown. Reporting those days will lead to a Medicare rejection.

> ## 837I aler➕
> ### Date Format
> On the electronic HIPAA claim, dates, including the from and through dates in FL 6, are entered in the following eight-character format: CCYYMMDD
>
> EXAMPLE: January 8, 2011, is entered as 20110108.

> ## $ $ Billing Tip $ $
> ### FL 6: Covered Days + Noncovered Days
> For inpatient bills, the total number of days represented in FL 6 (Statement Covers Period) must be equal to the sum of covered days and noncovered days in the claim's billing period. On the UB-04, covered and noncovered days are reported in FLs 39–41 (Value Codes and Amounts) using value codes 80 and 81. Value codes and amounts are explained in Chapter 11.

FL 7 Unlabeled Field

On the UB-04, FL 7 is an unlabeled field that is reserved for national assignment by the NUBC. Previously, FLs 7–10 were used on the UB-92 claim form to report covered days, noncovered days, coinsurance days, and lifetime reserve days, respectively—all of which are closely connected to the dates in FL 6 (Statement Covers Period). To create space for other information, however, these field types were eliminated on the UB-04, and this information is now reported in FLs 39–41 (Value Codes and Amounts) using new value codes 80–83 (see Chapter 11). Appendix B, available at the text's Online Learning Center, contains a table comparing the UB-92 and the UB-04 claim forms.

> ## $ $ Billing Tip $ $
> ### Recurring Outpatient Bill
> A recurring outpatient bill often contains several nonconsecutive days during a billing period. For example, a patient may be treated on April 3, 10, 14, and 26. For such a bill, the from and through dates in FL 6 should reflect the first and last dates of service, in this case April 3 and April 26.

CHAPTER SUMMARY

1 FLs 1–7 on the UB-04 contain information about the provider of the services being billed. This includes provider identifying information, the patient account number and medical/health record number assigned by the provider, information identifying the type of claim being billed, a federal tax number, and the dates of service covered by the claim.

2 2. Each field on the UB-04 requires the use of a particular format for entering data. Important formatting requirements in the Provider section (FLs 1–7) include these: punctuation is acceptable, and up to four lines of text are allowed in FL 1 (Provider Name, Address, and Telephone Number); no spaces should be used between digits in FL 3a (Patient Control Number); FL 4 (TOB) must always contain a leading zero followed by three other digits; and the dates in FL 6 (Statement Covers Period) should be reported in the MMDDYY format. The formatting rules for some of these form locators are different on the corresponding electronic HIPAA claim.

3 The type of bill (TOB) code in FL 4 is a four-digit code comprised of a leading zero followed by three digits that relay three specific pieces of information about the services being billed. The second digit identifies the type of facility in which the services were received, for example, a clinic. The third digit classifies the type of care being billed, such as intermediate care. The last digit indicates the sequence of the bill within a given episode of care, for example, an admit through discharge claim. The TOB can be thought of as having two components: the second and third digits combined make up the bill type component, and the last digit makes up the frequency code.

4 Many fields on the UB-04 contain data that need to be coordinated with data in other fields. For example, certain TOB codes in FL 4 necessitate data entry in the Revenue Code field (FL 42) and/or in the Condition Codes fields (FLs 18–28).

5 An important field on the UB-04 is the Statement Covers Period field (FL 6). The dates of service reported here are key in determining a patient's benefits. For inpatient bills, the total number of days represented in this field must be equal to the sum of covered days and noncovered days recorded in FLs 39–41 (Value Codes and Amounts) on the UB-04 using value codes 80 and 81.

✔ CHECK YOUR UNDERSTANDING

1. Define the following terms, and specify which form locator on the UB-04 each occupies:

 a. patient control number _____

_____

 b. type of bill (TOB) _____

_____

c. medical/health record number _____

_____

d. statement covers period _____

_____

2. Practice assigning TOB (Type of Bill) codes to the following data. The information for each digit is listed in a separate column. After assigning a second-, third-, and fourth-digit code, add the leading zero and construct the four-digit TOB code in the column labeled FL 4.

2nd-digit	code	3rd-digit	code	4th-digit	code	FL 4
SNF	_____	Inpatient	_____	Interim—first claim	_____	_____
SNF	_____	Inpatient	_____	Interim—continuing claim	_____	_____
SNF	_____	Inpatient	_____	Replacement of prior claim	_____	_____
Clinic	_____	CORF	_____	Admit through discharge	_____	_____
Clinic	_____	Hospital-based	_____	Interim—last claim	_____	_____
Hospital	_____	Outpatient	_____	Admit through discharge	_____	_____
Hospital	_____	Inpatient	_____	Nonpayment claim	_____	_____
Hospital	_____	Inpatient	_____	Late charge claim	_____	_____
Special facility	_____	Critical access hospital	_____	Admit through discharge	_____	_____

3. Using the following provider information, complete FLs 1–7 below.

Provider of Service:	Wayne Memorial Hospital	TIN: 05-3557211
	Park Street	
	Honesdale, PA 18431-1498	
	phone: (570) 344-1001	
Service Dates:	Admitted: June 12, 2009	8:30 A.M.
	Discharged: June 12, 2009	11:30 A.M.
Patient Control No.:	0000H77654	
Med. Rec. No.:	TT813YS002C	

The patient was admitted to the hospital for a routine colonoscopy. This was the patient's only visit during the month of June. The June 2009 claim is being prepared.

UB-04 Form—FLs 1–7

1		2	3a PAT. CNTL #		4 TYPE OF BILL
			b. MED. REC. #		
			5 FED. TAX NO.	6 STATEMENT COVERS PERIOD FROM THROUGH	7

4. True or False: The second-digit code (type of facility) in the TOB is often the main indicator for whether some type of room charge code should appear in FL 42 (Revenue Code). _____

5. For each example, supply the correct TOB code for FL 4.

a. The second billing for a SNF patient admitted sixty days ago. The patient is expected to remain in the facility indefinitely. TOB _____

b. A non-hospital-based hospice billing for same-day outpatient services. TOB _____

c. A hospital billing for a patient receiving inpatient rehabilitation services for the second and final month. TOB _____

d. A community mental health center billing for a one-day service. TOB _____

6. A Medicare beneficiary elected to start using his lifetime reserve days after having used up the sixty covered hospital days and thirty coinsurance days allowed for this benefit period. He was admitted as an inpatient on March 15 and remains a patient. The June 2009 billing is being prepared. On what date did the beneficiary use his last coinsurance day? _____ How many lifetime reserve days did he use in June? _____

7. True or False: If a provider wants to determine how long a patient has been treated for a condition, the Medical Record Number rather than the Patient Control Number on the UB-04 should be used to help locate the information. _____

8. Using the following provider information, complete FLs 1–7 below.

Provider of Service:	Gateway General Hospital	TIN: 01-2999981
	2004 Fifth Ave.
	New Kennsington, PA 15068
	phone: (724) 335-8000
Service Dates:	Admitted: September 2, 2010	2:15 P.M.
	Discharged: September 16, 2010	9:00 A.M.
Patient Control No.:	0000H62622
Med. Rec. No.:	TT9387YS002CE

This bill is being prepared as a void/cancel bill for an inpatient admission claim because the patient's health insurance ID number (FL 60, Insured's Unique ID) was incorrect on the prior claim.

UB-04 Form—FLs 1–7

1		2	3a PAT. CNTL #		4 TYPE OF BILL
			b. MED. REC. #		
			5 FED. TAX NO.	6 STATEMENT COVERS PERIOD FROM THROUGH	7

9. Using the following information, complete FL 6 below. A patient is admitted to the hospital on December 8, 2009. The patient's entitlement to Medicare begins on December 10. The patient is discharged on December 18. A Medicare bill is being prepared.

UB-04 Form—FL 6

6 STATEMENT COVERS PERIOD FROM   THROUGH

10. True or False: If the TOB code on a claim is 0741, an admission date must appear in FL 12 (Admission Date). _____

COMPUTER EXPLORATION

UB-04 Activity: Claim Analysis

Viewing FLs 1-7: Provider Information

Open the file **Sample01.pdf** in Adobe Reader, and answer the following questions:

1. Two important billing fields in the Provider section are FL 4 (TOB) and FL 6 (billing period). Based on the TOB in FL 4, is this claim for inpatient or outpatient services?

2. At what type of facility did the patient receive the services?

3. Can you determine if the patient completed the treatment, or is the treatment ongoing?

4. How do the service dates in FL 45 correlate with the dates reported in FL 6? Were all of the services received on the same day?

5. Are the dates in FL 6 the same as the Admission date in FL 12? Can you think of a circumstance when these would be different?

6. On what date was the bill prepared? How many days did it take for the hospital to prepare the bill after the services were received?

7. FL 43 lists "OR SERVICES," meaning operating room services. Refer to Table 7.1 on page 148. If this patient received the same surgery at an ambulatory surgery center, what TOB would you expect to see?

8. Does the billing provider have a separate billing address?

9. If the patient returns to this facility again for a different condition, will the information in FLs 3a and 3b change?

10. Does the information in FL 5 (Federal Tax Number) remain the same for all bills the facility prepares, or does it vary depending on the patient?

When finished viewing the claim, click Exit on the File menu.

Patient Information

LEARNING OUTCOMES

After completing this chapter, you will be able to define the key terms and:

1. Identify the types of patient information that belong in FLs 8–17 of the UB-04 claim form.

2. Understand the correct format for entering a patient's identifying information.

3. Understand how the patient's admission information is reported on the UB-04.

4. Explain which codes are available for reporting the various types of inpatient admission.

5. Explain which codes are available for indicating the patient's point of origin for the inpatient or outpatient service being billed.

6. Understand the range of codes that are used to report the patient's status at the end of the period of care reported on a claim.

KEY TERMS

- admission date
- discharge date
- elective admission
- emergency
- Medicare distinct part unit
- patient discharge status
- point of origin for admission or visit
- self-referral
- urgent

This chapter provides instructions for filling in patient information on the UB-04. Patient information is contained in form locators 8–17. The form includes basic identifying information—the patient's name, address, date of birth, and sex. It also includes the details of the patient's admission and discharge—the date, hour, type, and point of origin for the admission, as well as the hour of discharge and the patient's condition at the time of discharge.

Medicare and other payers use patient information for a variety of purposes in processing UB-04 claims. It may be used to make sure the right patient receives the right benefits or to verify a beneficiary's eligibility for Medicare benefits. Patient information is also used for statistical purposes such as for Medicare's Quality Improvement Organization (QIO) reviews, for obtaining basic patient demographic information, and to help determine final Prospective Payment System (PPS) payments for inpatient services.

Accurate patient information is also important from the point of view of coding compliance. A common edit in claim processing is to check that a patient's sex and age are coordinated correctly with an age- or sex-related diagnosis or surgical procedure. For example, for a pediatric diagnosis, the patient's age must be between zero and seventeen to pass the corresponding edit. If the surgical procedure listed on the claim is a maternity procedure, the patient's sex must be female to pass the edit.

Figure 8.1

UB-04 Form—FLs 8–17

FL 8 Patient Name/Identifier

FL 8 has two lines: FL 8a and FL 8b. The bottom line, FL 8b, contains twenty-nine positions and is used to report the patient's last name, first name, and middle initial, if any. Titles such as Mrs., Sir, and Dr. are not used in this field.

The top line, FL 8a, which contains only nineteen positions, is available for reporting a patient identifier—a number assigned to the patient by the patient's insurance carrier. The patient identifier is reported only if it is different from the insured's identifier reported in FL 60 (Insured's Unique ID). Therefore, if the patient and the insured are the same, FL 8a is left blank. If the patient and the insured are different (for example, if the insured is a parent and the patient is her child) and the patient has been assigned a separate identifier by the payer, the patient identifier should be reported in FL 8a.

Guidelines

Completion of FL 8b (patient name) is required for Medicare billing and by all other payers.

For Medicare patients, the patient's name in FL 8b must be exactly as shown on the Medicare health insurance card. For example, if the card shows "Steven," then "Steve" is not valid. If the name on the card contains a suffix, such as "Jr.," the suffix must be included. Many billing errors on Medicare claims stem from discrepancies between the name as recorded on the Medicare card, or in Medicare's records, and the name reported in this field.

> **HIPAA TIP**
>
> *Patient's Identifying Information and PHI*
>
> A person's identifying information as reported on a UB-04, including name, address, and birth date, is considered a part of PHI.

The name is reported in the order of last name, first name, and middle initial. A comma (or space) is used to separate each component of the name. If the last name contains a suffix such as "III," the suffix is displayed after the last name, with no additional comma.

EXAMPLES:
Applebaum III, George
Riccardo Sr, Richard, J

If a name contains an apostrophe, the apostrophe is generally removed. (Computer systems often remove apostrophes and other punctuation automatically when the claim is processed).

EXAMPLE: OConnor (for O'Connor)

A name with a prefix, such as Von, should be displayed without a space.

EXAMPLES:
VonSchneider
MacHugh

The hyphen in a hyphenated name is usually retained (although some computer systems may remove it later while processing the claim).

EXAMPLE: Sanchez-Jones

FL 9 Patient Address

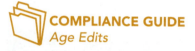
FL 9 is used to report the patient's full mailing address. It is divided into five subfields, labeled *a* through *e*. Each subfield is used to report a different part of the address.

a	Street address	40 positions
b	City	30 positions
c	State	2 positions
d	ZIP code	9 positions (5- or 9-digit codes allowed)
e	Country code	2 positions (used only if other than United States)

Guidelines

Completion of this field is required for Medicare billing and by all other payers. The full address, which is normally obtained and verified during the admission process, must be used. It is important to provide a correct address since Medicare uses the address to send Medicare notices, such as the beneficiary's Medicare Summary Notice (MSN).

FL 10 Patient Birth Date

FL 10 contains the patient's date of birth. The date of birth must contain eight characters and should be reported in the MMDDYYYY format.

EXAMPLE: July 12, 1957, is reported as 07121957.

Guidelines

Completion of this field is required for Medicare billing and by all other payers. The birth date may be used to verify eligibility for Medicare benefits. For hospitals reimbursed under the Medicare Prospective Payment System (PPS), the birth date is part of the diagnosis-related group (DRG) calculation.

On the paper UB-04, if the full correct date has not been obtained after reasonable efforts by the provider, the field should be filled with zeros, not left blank or partially filled.

FL 11 Patient Sex

FL 11 identifies the sex, or gender, of the patient as recorded at the time of admission, outpatient service, or start of care.

Guidelines

Completion of this field is required for Medicare billing and by all other payers. Only the characters *M* and *F* are valid in this field for Medicare claims. Other payers may accept *U* for "unknown."

The gender reported must be valid for male-only and female-only diagnosis and procedure codes. For example, if the diagnoses or surgical procedures reported in FLs 67–74 (see Chapter 14, "Diagnosis and Procedure Codes") contain gynecological and obstetrical codes, an *M* is not valid in this field.

COMPLIANCE GUIDE
Sex Edits

As with the patient's age, the software program used by Medicare FIs to analyze hospital outpatient claims also edits the patient's sex to ensure that it does not conflict with other fields on the form, such as the diagnosis (FL 67), principal procedure code (FL 74), or HCPCS procedure code (FL 44). If the claim does not pass the edit, it will be returned to the provider for correction.

FL 12 Admission, Start of Care Date

FL 12 contains the **admission date**—the date the patient was admitted to the health care facility for inpatient care or the start of care date for home health services. The date must be a valid month, day, and year recorded in the MMDDYY format.

EXAMPLE: February 24, 2009, is reported as 022409.

Guidelines

Completion of this field is required for Medicare billing for inpatient and home health care services. It is also required by most other payers. Although completion of this field is not required for most outpatient claims on the UB-04, an admission or start of care date is often reported on all claims.

FL 13 Admission Hour

The Admission Hour field contains the hour during which the patient was admitted for inpatient care. Completion of this field is not required for Medicare billing. However, it is required on inpatient claims by most other payers.

A set of hour codes, based on military time, is used for indicating the admission hour. Table 8.1, on page 162, lists each hour code and the period of time it represents. Each code has two numeric characters.

Table 8.1

Hour Codes

Code	A.M.	Code	P.M.
00	12:00 (midnight)–12:59	12	12:00 (noon)–12:59
01	1:00–1:59	13	1:00–1:59
02	2:00–2:59	14	2:00–2:59
03	3:00–3:59	15	3:00–3:59
04	4:00–4:59	16	4:00–4:59
05	5:00–5:59	17	5:00–5:59
06	6:00–6:59	18	6:00–6:59
07	7:00–7:59	19	7:00–7:59
08	8:00–8:59	20	8:00–8:59
09	9:00–9:59	21	9:00–9:59
10	10:00–10:59	22	10:00–10:59
11	11:00–11:59	23	11:00–11:59

EXAMPLES:

3:15 A.M. = 03
1:40 P.M. = 13
11:59 P.M. = 23

FL 14 Type of Admission or Visit

The Type of Admission or Visit field contains a code for establishing the priority or level of urgency of an inpatient admission.

Guidelines

Completion of this field is required for Medicare billing for inpatient claims only. It is also required for inpatient claims by most other payers. It is not required for outpatient claims; however, most outpatient claims report the admission type.

This field is used by carriers to determine benefit eligibility. It is also used for QIO review. The claim will be returned if the QIO determines that data are missing or incorrect.

The field contains single numeric codes as follows:

1   Emergency

An **emergency** is a type of admission in which the patient receives immediate medical care. The patient is usually, but not always, admitted through the emergency department. For Medicare purposes, an emergency admission indicates that the patient's condition is severe, life threatening, or potentially disabling if not treated.

2   Urgent

The **urgent** admission category indicates that the patient is suffering from a physical or mental disorder that requires immediate attention. The patient should be admitted to the first available suitable accommodation.

3 Elective

In an **elective admission,** the patient's condition permits adequate time to schedule the services, as the health of the patient is not in jeopardy. Admission to a suitable accommodation can be scheduled days or weeks in advance. An admission not classified as emergency or urgent is usually elective.

4 Newborn

The newborn admission type is used for a newborn baby, who may have been born inside the hospital submitting the claim or somewhere else. This code necessitates the use of a special set of codes pertaining to newborns in the next data field, FL 15 (Point of Origin for Admission or Visit). See the section "Coding Structure for Newborn Admissions" later in this chapter.

5 Trauma Center

Code 5 indicates a trauma center admission. Code 5 is most often used when the admission involves the activation of a trauma team, since some payers allow a separate activation fee to be billed with the code. Code 5 may also be used in the absence of trauma activation for statistical and follow-up purposes. The trauma center or trauma hospital visited by the patient must be properly designated or licensed by the state or local government authority or verified by the American College of Surgeons and capable of handling trauma activation.

6–8 Reserved for Assignment by the NUBC

9 Information Not Available

Code 9 is used when the hospital does not have information to classify the patient's admission. It is rarely used on the UB-04.

FL 15 Point of Origin for Admission or Visit

FL 15 contains a code that indicates the patient's point of origin for the inpatient admission or outpatient visit.

Guidelines

Completion of this field is required for Medicare billing for both inpatient and outpatient claims. Most other payers require the field to be completed on inpatient claims; outpatient requirements vary. It is not required for Medicaid billing.

There are two coding structures for indicating the patient's point of origin, each with its own set of single-digit codes. For all types of admission other than newborn, the first set of codes is used. For newborn admissions, a second set of codes that classifies the newborn's location at birth is used.

Coding Structure for All Admission Types Except Newborns

The following single-digit codes are used to indicate the point of origin for all admission types except newborns. Each number or letter represents the patient's place or point of origin that led to the inpatient or outpatient services that are being billed.

Point of Origin for Admission or Visit

The **point of origin for admission or visit** applies to the patient's point of origin for the emergency, elective, or other type of inpatient admission as indicated in FL 14 (Type of Admission or Visit) as well as the point of origin for outpatient services. The point of origin does not have to be a health care facility—for example, the patient may come from home, physician's office, or work—or the patient could have been transferred from another health care facility, such as a clinic or a skilled nursing facility (SNF), or from the emergency department. Another point of origin code is used when the patient is sent to the hospital under the direction of a court of law. For a newborn, the point of origin for admission is based on whether the baby was born in the billing hospital or somewhere else.

1   Non-Health Care Facility

For inpatients, code 1 indicates that the patient was admitted for inpatient care on the order of a physician. For outpatients, code 1 indicates that the patient came to the facility with an order from a physician for outpatient service or came for outpatient service that does not require an order, such as mammography. This includes nonemergency self-referrals. In a **self-referral,** the patient requests outpatient services on his or her own, independent of a physician. Code 1 includes patients coming from home, a physician's office, or a place of work.

2   Clinic

Code 2 indicates that the patient was either admitted for inpatient care or referred for outpatient or referenced diagnostic services as a transfer from a freestanding or non-freestanding clinic.

3   Reserved for Assignment by the NUBC

4   Transfer from a Hospital (Different Facility)

For an inpatient, code 4 indicates that the patient was admitted to the current facility for inpatient care after being transferred from a different acute care hospital at which he or she was an inpatient or an outpatient. For outpatients, code 4 indicates that the patient was referred to the current facility for outpatient or referenced diagnostic services after being transferred from a different acute care hospital at which he or she was an outpatient. (For transfer from the same facility, see code D below.)

5   Transfer from a Skilled Nursing Facility or Intermediate Care Facility

Code 5 indicates that the patient was either admitted for inpatient care or referred for outpatient or referenced diagnostic services after being transferred from a SNF or intermediate care facility (ICF) at which he or she was a resident.

6   Transfer from Another Health Care Facility

Code 6 indicates that the patient was transferred to the current facility for inpatient care or referred for outpatient or referenced diagnostic services from a type of health care facility not defined elsewhere in this code list at which he or she was an inpatient or outpatient.

7   Emergency Room

Code 7 is used when a patient is treated in the emergency department of the current health care facility and is then either admitted as an inpatient or discharged without an inpatient admission. This code includes emergency self-referrals that require immediate medical attention.

8   Court or Law Enforcement

Code 8 indicates that the patient was either admitted for inpatient care or referred for outpatient or referenced diagnostic services based on the direction of a court of law or at the request of a law enforcement agency representative.

9   Information Not Available

Code 9 indicates that the means by which the patient was either admitted to the hospital or referred to the hospital's outpatient department is not known.

A   Reserved for Assignment by the NUBC

B   Transfer from Another Home Health Agency

Code B indicates that the patient was admitted to the current home health agency (HHA) as a transfer from another HHA.

C   Readmission to Same Home Health Agency

Code C is used when a patient is readmitted to the same HHA within the same episode of home health care (based on a sixty-day payment period). This code is for use with Medicare bill type 032X, Home Health under PPS.

D   Transfer from One Distinct Unit of the Hospital to Another Distinct Unit of the Same Hospital Resulting in a Separate Claim to the Payer

For inpatients, code D indicates that the patient was admitted to the facility as a transfer from one distinct unit of the hospital at which he or she was an inpatient to another distinct unit of the same hospital, resulting in a separate claim to the payer. For example, the patient was in acute care and was transferred to a separate inpatient psychiatric facility in the same hospital. A **Medicare distinct part unit** or facility is a distinct unit or a unique level of care in a hospital that operates under its own payment system and therefore requires a separate claim to the payer.

For outpatients, code D indicates that the patient received outpatient services in one distinct unit of the hospital after being transferred from another distinct unit within the same hospital, resulting in a separate claim to the payer.

E   Transfer from Ambulatory Surgery Center

Code E indicates that the patient was either admitted for inpatient care or referred for outpatient or referenced diagnostic services as a transfer from an ambulatory surgery center.

F   Transfer from Hospice and Is Under a Hospice Plan of Care or Enrolled in a Hospice Program

Code F indicates that the patient was either admitted for inpatient care or referred for outpatient or referenced diagnostic services as a transfer from hospice. The patient is still under a hospice plan of care or is enrolled in a hospice program.

G–Z Reserved for Assignment by the NUBC

Coding Structure for Newborn Admissions

When the code in FL 14 (Type of Admission or Visit) is 4 (newborn), the Point of Origin for Admission or Visit field (FL 15) must contain a single-digit code from the following set of codes for newborn admissions.

1–4 Reserved for Assignment by the NUBC

5   Born Inside This Hospital

Code 5 is used to when the baby is delivered inside the hospital that is submitting the claim.

FYI

Medicare Distinct Part Units or Facilities

Examples of Medicare distinct part units include observation services, psychiatric and rehabilitation units, units in a critical access hospital, and swing beds located in an acute care hospital. They also include psychiatric, children's, and cancer hospitals. Such units are exempt from the inpatient PPS and must meet certain Medicare requirements.

6 Born Outside of This Hospital

Code 6 is used when the baby is delivered somewhere other than the hospital submitting the claim.

7–9 Reserved for Assignment by the NUBC

FL 16 Discharge Hour

FYI

Discharge Date

The date a patient is released from a hospital or a SNF is called the patient's **discharge date.** Discharged patients include people who are discharged to home or to another facility as well as patients who die during their stay.

FL 16 is used to report the hour during which an inpatient is discharged from inpatient care. Completion of this field is not required for Medicare billing; however, it is either required or considered desirable by other payers.

The same set of hour codes used for indicating the admission hour (FL 13) is used for reporting the discharge hour. Table 8.1 on page 162 lists each hour code and the period of time it represents. Each code contains two numeric characters.

EXAMPLES:

$$10:55 \text{ A.M.} = 10$$
$$1:01 \text{ P.M.} = 13$$

FL 17 Patient Discharge Status

$ $ Billing Tip $ $

Discharged Status

Codes 1–20 in this field are used to indicate a discharged status. The patient may be discharged to home or transferred to another facility, or in the case of code 20, the patient may have expired during the stay. On a UB-04, a discharged status in FL 17 indicates the end of a billing period and should therefore be reflected in the last digit of the Type of Bill field (FL 4, TOB). Valid TOBs for a claim with a discharge status in FL 17 include those that end with 1 (admit through discharge) or 4 (interim—last claim). The patient status and TOB codes are used by payers to determine whether additional bills are expected for the described services and from whom they are expected.

FL 17 contains a code for the patient discharge status. The **patient discharge status** is an indicator of the patient's disposition or status as of the through date of the billing period (reported in FL 6, Statement Covers Period). Although there are many patient discharge status codes, they fall into one of four basic categories: routine discharge, discharged to another facility, still a patient, or expired.

Guidelines

Completion of this field is required for Medicare billing for all Part A inpatient, SNF, hospice, home health, and outpatient hospital services. Patient discharge status information affects the final PPS payment for inpatient services. It is also used to determine Medicare eligibility. Most other payers also require this information on inpatient claims.

FL 17 (Patient Discharge Status) is a two-digit field. Following are the two-digit codes that can be used in this field. Each represents a type of discharge status (routine discharge, discharged to another facility, still a patient, or expired).

01	Discharged to home or self-care (routine discharge).
02	Discharged and transferred to a short-term general hospital for inpatient care.
03	Discharged and transferred to a SNF with Medicare certification in anticipation of covered skilled care. *Note:* For a hospital with an approved swing bed arrangement, use code 61 below. For reporting discharges and transfers to a noncertified SNF, see codes 04 and 64 below.
04	Discharged and transferred to an intermediate care facility.

05	Discharged and transferred to a designated cancer center or children's hospital. *Note:* Transfers to nondesignated cancer hospitals should use code 02.
06	Discharged and transferred to home under care of an organized home health service organization in anticipation of covered skilled care.
07	Left against medical advice or discontinued care.
08	Reserved for assignment by the NUBC.
09	Admitted as an inpatient to this hospital.
10–19	Reserved for assignment by the NUBC.
20	Expired. *Note:* When patient status code 20 is used on a claim, the through date in FL 6, Statement Covers Period, should reflect the date of the patient's death. Code 20 is not valid on a Medicare hospice claim; see codes 40–42 below, which are used for hospice claims only.
21–29	Reserved for assignment by the NUBC.
30	Still a patient or expected to return for outpatient services. *Note*: Code 30 is typically used when billing a subsequent, or interim, claim for a Medicare beneficiary who is still a patient. For example, when a patient stays in a health care facility for several months and each month is billed separately, code 30 is used on each subsequent bill to indicate that the person is still a patient—until the month the patient is discharged. On each subsequent claim, the original admission date should be used. Only the dates in the from and through fields are changed each month to reflect the current month's dates of service.
	Code 30 is also used when billing for leave of absence days—days when a patient is temporarily away from the hospital—to indicate that the person is still a patient.
31–39	Reserved for assignment by the NUBC.
40	Expired at home. *Note:* For use only for Medicare and TRICARE billing on hospice claims.
41	Expired in a medical facility, such as a hospital, SNF, ICF, or freestanding hospice. *Note:* For use only for Medicare and TRICARE billing on hospice claims.
42	Expired, place unknown. *Note:* For use only for Medicare and TRICARE billing on hospice claims.
43	Discharged and transferred to a federal health care facility. *Note:* Examples include transfers to a Department of Defense hospital, a Veteran's Administration hospital, or a Veteran's Administration nursing facility, whether the patient lives there or not.
44–49	Reserved for assignment by the NUBC.
50	Discharged and transferred to hospice—home.
51	Discharged and transferred to hospice—medical facility (certified) providing hospice level of care.
52–60	Reserved for assignment by the NUBC.

COMPLIANCE GUIDE
Outpatient Versus Inpatient Services

Code 09 is used on Medicare outpatient claims only. For example, a Medicare patient receives outpatient surgery at a facility. Observation services that follow the surgery result in the patient's admission to the facility. There is an additional rule that applies to the use of code 09 in this situation. The outpatient services must have occurred more than three days before the admission or else be unrelated to the reason for admission. Otherwise, the outpatient services are considered part of the patient's inpatient stay and will be processed as inpatient services.

(continued)

61	Discharged and transferred within this institution to a hospital-based Medicare-approved swing bed.
62	Discharged and transferred to an inpatient rehabilitation facility (IRF) including rehabilitation distinct part units of a hospital.
63	Discharged and transferred to a Medicare-certified long-term care hospital (LTCH).
64	Discharged and transferred to a nursing facility certified under Medicaid but not under Medicare.
65	Discharged and transferred to a psychiatric hospital or psychiatric distinct part unit of a hospital.
66	Discharged and transferred to a critical access hospital.
67–69	Reserved for assignment by the NUBC.
70	Discharged and transferred to another type of health care institution that is not defined elsewhere in this code list.
71–99	Reserved for assignment by the NUBC.

1 FLs 8–17 on the UB-04 contain various types of patient information. One type is the patient's identifying information, including the full name, address, date of birth, and sex. Patient admission information and patient discharge information are also reported in these form locators.

2 There are important formatting requirements for reporting the patient's identifying information (FL 8b). For example, the name is reported in the order of last name, first name, and middle initial, with a comma or space separating each part. For Medicare patients, the name must be exactly as shown on the Medicare health insurance card. A full and correct mailing address must be provided, including a valid ZIP code. The patient's date of birth must contain eight characters reported in the MMDDYYYY format.

3 The patient's admission information includes the date and hour of admission, as well as the type and point of origin for admission. This information is used by payers to determine patients' benefits. Type of admission data is also used for QIO review. The Admission, Start of Care Date field (FL 12) contains the date the patient was admitted for inpatient care or the start of care date for home health services. The Admission Hour field (FL 13) contains the hour during which the patient was admitted for inpatient care.

4 The Type of Admission or Visit field (FL 14) contains one of several single-digit codes that establish the level of urgency of an inpatient admission: emergency, urgent, elective, or newborn.

5 The Point of Origin for Admission or Visit field (FL 15) contains two sets of single-digit codes for reporting the point of origin for the admission or outpatient registration represented by the claim. The point of origin can be a non-health care facility such as home, work, or a physician's office; a transfer from a health care facility or emergency department; an order from a court of law or a law enforcement agency representative; or in the case of a newborn, birth inside the billing hospital or elsewhere. The first set of codes applies to all admission types except newborn admissions. The second set classifies newborn admissions.

6 The patient's discharge information includes the Discharge Hour field (FL 16) and the Patient Discharge Status field (FL 17). Patient discharge status is an indicator of the patient's disposition at the end of the billing period represented on the claim. There are numerous two-digit patient status codes that fall into one of four categories: routine discharge, discharged to another facility, still a patient, or expired. Payers require this information to determine whether to expect additional bills and from whom to expect them.

1. Define the following terms and specify which form locator each occupies on the UB-04.

a. admission date _____

_____

b. point of origin for admission or visit _____

_____

c. patient discharge status _____

_____

2. Using the following patient information, complete FLs 8–17 on the UB-04 claim form below.

Patient Name:	Irene R. Penn-Slozak	D.O.B. 12-22-27
Patient Address:	109 Fairview Avenue	
	Verona, NJ 07044	
Service Dates:	Admitted: September 9, 2010 4:15 A.M.	
	Discharged: September 11, 2010 8:30 A.M.	

The patient came to the emergency room during the middle of the night complaining of severe chest pains. She was not able to contact her doctor. She was admitted to the hospital for tests of heart function. The tests were negative, and it was determined that she was suffering from acute indigestion. She was sent home two days later. She is insured under her husband's plan, and her patient identifier, which is separate from his, is BC1079A.

UB-04 Form—FLs 8–17

8 PATIENT NAME	a				9 PATIENT ADDRESS	a									
b					b				c	d			e		

10 BIRTHDATE	11 SEX	12 DATE	ADMISSION 13 HR	14 TYPE	15 SRC	16 DHR	17 STAT	18	19	20	21	CONDITION CODES 22	23	24	25	26	27	28	29 ACDT STATE	30

3. True or False: Completion of FL 14 (Type of Admission or Visit) is required for Medicare billing for inpatient claims only. It is not necessary for outpatient claims. _____

4. Rewrite the following names in the format required for patient names on the UB-04.

a. Melanie Guidry _____

b. Paddy S. Trehorn III _____

c. Cheryl-Sue MacAllister _____

d. Gerald R. Brown, Esquire _____

e. Dr. Margaret B. Di Paola _____

f. Kara Von Essen _____

g. Juan Clemente, Sr. _____

h. Mei W. Sing-Chang _____

i. Sara T. O'Bryan _____

5. Use the required hour codes to report the following admission times as they would be reported on a UB-04.

a. midnight _____

b. 3:59 A.M. _____

c. 1:12 P.M. _____

d. 11:00 A.M. _____

e. noon _____

f. 5:00 P.M. _____

g. 9:22 A.M. _____

h. 11:00 P.M. _____

6. Which of the following are valid admission types for FL 14 on the UB-04?

   a. urgent

   b. emergency

   c. baby born in hospital

   d. newborn

   e. nonemergency self-referral

7. Indicate the correct code for FL 15 (Point of Origin for Admission or Visit) in each of the following situations.

   a. A patient is admitted to the current facility as an inpatient and is being transferred from an ICF at which she was a resident. _____

   b. A patient with severe burns is admitted directly from the ER to the burn unit of the same hospital. _____

   c. A baby was born in the emergency department of the billing hospital. _____

   d. A battered woman and child are brought to the hospital by two police officers. _____

   e. A patient is admitted to the facility as a transfer from hospice but is still under a hospice plan of care. _____

   f. A patient is admitted to the psychiatric distinct part unit of a hospital after having been discharged from the acute short-term care unit of the same hospital, resulting in a separate claim. _____

   g. A physician at a freestanding clinic refers a patient to the current facility for a series of outpatient diagnostic services. _____

8. Indicate the correct code for FL 17 (Patient Discharge Status) in each of the following situations.

   a. A patient is admitted on November 5 but leaves the hospital on November 8 against the medical advice of his doctor. _____

   b. A TRICARE patient is admitted to a hospital-based hospice on September 2 and passes away on September 5. _____

   c. A patient in an acute care hospital is discharged to a psychiatric distinct part unit of the hospital. _____

   d. A patient is transferred back to the Veteran's Administration hospital in which he lives. _____

   e. A patient undergoes same-day surgery and returns home at 4:00 P.M. _____

   f. A patient is admitted to the hospital on August 5 and passes away on August 7. _____

   g. A patient is admitted to the hospital on May 5 and remains a patient until June 17. May is being billed. _____

   h. A patient is discharged from acute care in a private hospital to a designated cancer center. _____

UB-04 Form—FLs 8–17

1 ST JOACHIM HOSPITAL	2		3a PAT. CNTL # 20000096A			4 TYPE OF BILL
8900 TENTH AVE			b. MED. REC. # XYZ3330			
OAKLAND, CA 94610			5 FED. TAX NO.	6 STATEMENT COVERS PERIOD FROM / THROUGH		7
510-834-2220			10-9879564	102809 / 103109		

8 PATIENT NAME	a AE62G		9 PATIENT ADDRESS	a 223 VERNON ST				
b MCFARLAND, BETH			b OAKLAND			c CA	d 94610	e

10 BIRTHDATE	11 SEX	12 DATE	ADMISSION 13 HR	14 TYPE	15 SRC	16 DHR	17 STAT	18	19	20	21	CONDITION CODES 22	23	24	25	26	27	28	29 ACDT STATE	30
01031949	F	102809	08	3	4	14	50													

9. Answer the following questions based on the top portion of the UB-04 form shown here.

   a. Given the data shown, do you think the TOB on the claim is 011X or 013X? _____

   b. Are the patient and the insured the same or different? _____

   c. In what month was the patient born? _____

d. Was the patient admitted as an emergency case, or did she choose the date of her admission? _____

e. Where did the patient come from before being admitted? _____

f. Was the patient discharged in the morning or afternoon? _____

g. What is the patient's discharge status? _____

10. True or False: If code 4 (Transfer from a hospital, different facility) is used on an inpatient claim in FL 14 (Point of Origin for Admission or Visit), it indicates that the patient was admitted to the current facility after being transferred from a distinct inpatient unit in the same hospital. _____

COMPUTER EXPLORATION

UB-04 Activity: Claim Analysis

Viewing FLs 8-17: Patient Information

Open the file **Sample02.pdf** in Adobe Reader, and answer the following questions:

1. Is the patient male or female?

2. What is the patient's age at the time of admission?

3. Is this an inpatient or outpatient claim?

4. What type of facility provided the services? Is this a final bill?

5. What is the admission type?

6. Compare the dates in FL 6 (Statement Covers Period) with the Admission Date in FL 12. How long was the patient in the facility?

7. What time did she arrive? Based on the data in FLs 14 and 15, suggest the likely point of origin for this admission. Note also the description of the services received in FL 43.

8. In the first sample claim, each service described in FL 42 (Revenue Code Description) had a corresponding service date in FL 45 (Service Date). Does this claim report service dates?

9. Do the service units reported in FL 45, line 1 reflect the dates in FL 06 accurately?

10. What is the date and time of the patient's discharge? What does the patient's discharge status in FL 17 indicate?

When finished viewing the claim, click Exit on the File menu.

Condition Codes

LEARNING OUTCOMES

After completing this chapter, you will be able to define the key terms and:

1. Discuss the codes that are used in FLs 18–28 of the UB-04 to report special conditions about a claim that may affect its processing and payment.

2. Become familiar with the major categories of condition codes.

3. Explain various billing situations that arise when particular condition codes are used.

4. Recognize the condition codes that must be coordinated with data supplied in other fields of the UB-04.

5. Discuss the use of FL 29 to report the state in which an accident occurred in a claim with services related to an auto accident.

KEY TERMS

- condition code
- focused medical review
- outlier
- 72-hour rule
- working aged person

This chapter provides the information needed for filling in FLs 18–28 of the UB-04. This group of fields is used to describe special conditions about a claim that may affect its processing and payment. The chapter also covers FL 29, Accident State, and unlabeled FL 30 (See Figure 9.1).

Some claims are straightforward, and payers easily understand what benefits are due. Other claims are more complex and may contain information that seems contradictory, incomplete, or illogical to a payer. Unless the payer understands the special circumstances surrounding the request for payment, the claim is either held up or denied. The codes reported in FLs 18–28 are used to explain such conditions so that claims can be processed efficiently and accurately.

For example, suppose the patient is a woman who kept her maiden name after she married. Although she has benefits under her husband's insurance plan, the insurance company will not recognize her as eligible for the benefits because she does not use the same last name as her husband. Reporting the appropriate condition code, in this case code 18 (Maiden name retained), in FL 18 explains the situation.

Many members of the hospital's team share responsibility for identifying and assigning condition codes with the patient account specialist. Coordination with the members of other departments, including utilization review, admissions, coding, and health information management staff members, is essential for gathering correct data for billing.

FL 29 (Accident State) in this section of the UB-04 is used to report the state in which an accident occurred when the claim involves an auto accident. The last field in this section, FL 30, is an unlabeled field.

Figure 9.1

UB-04 Form—FLs 18–30

18	19	20	21	CONDITION CODES 22	23	24	25	26	27	28	29 ACDT STATE	30

FLs 18–28 Condition Codes

FLs 18–28 are used for reporting condition codes on the UB-04. A **condition code** is a two-digit numeric or alphanumeric code that identifies a special condition or unique circumstance about a claim. Most condition codes are designed to help the payer determine a patient's eligibility and benefits. For example, condition codes show whether the patient is covered by more than one type of insurance, whether medical necessity affects room assignment, and whether an injury or illness is related to employment. Condition codes are not associated with dates.

Condition codes cover a wide range of circumstances, including claim changes. For example, when a change in the amount charged for a service necessitates an adjustment to a claim that was already processed, condition code D1 (Changes to charges) is reported on the adjustment claim to explain the reason. Condition codes range from 01 to 99 and A0 to ZZ. Many codes are reserved for national assignment and payer assignment. In this chapter, each condition code is described briefly. Billing tips on how and when to use certain codes are provided in the margins.

Guidelines

If a condition code is applicable on a claim, the field must be filled in for Medicare claims and for all other payers.

Eleven condition codes may be listed on a single claim—one each in FLs 18–28. The codes should be listed in ascending order, beginning with numbers and followed by letters.

EXAMPLE:

FL 18	FL 19	FL 20	FL 21	FL 22	FL 23	FL 24	FL 25	FL 26	FL 27	FL 28
02	38	C5								

In the example, code 02 indicates that the condition is employment related, code 38 that a semiprivate room is not available, and code C5 that a postpayment review of the claim may apply.

If more than eleven codes are required for a claim, FL 81 (Code-Code field) is used to report the overflow. Chapter 15, "Physician Information, Remarks, and Code-Code Field," explains how to use FL 81 to report additional condition codes.

Insurance Codes

The condition codes related primarily to insurance issues are described below.

01   Military Service Related

Code 01 indicates that the patient's treatment is related to a condition that occurred during active military service. Because of this, coverage will need to be coordinated with the Department of Veterans Affairs. This code is not required for Medicare claims, but it is used when it applies to other payers.

02   Condition Is Employment Related

Code 02 is used when a patient alleges that the injury or illness represented on the claim is due to the environment or events resulting from his or her employment; for example, it is used for workers' compensation claims. If it applies, this code is required for Medicare claims as well as for commercial payers and TRICARE.

The use of this code flags a possible MSP (Medicare Secondary Payer) situation (see Chapter 3, "Hospital Insurance"). Coverage may need to be coordinated with the beneficiary's workers' compensation insurance.

03   Patient Covered by Insurance Not Reflected Here

Code 03 indicates that the patient stated during the admission process that other insurance coverage may be in effect that is not reflected on the claim. This code is not needed for Medicare claims. It is required for commercial and TRICARE billing if applicable.

04   Information Only Bill

Code 04 is used when the bill is being submitted for informational purposes only. For example, it may be used on a claim that is being submitted as a utilization report. It may also be used on a claim for a beneficiary enrolled in a risk-based managed care plan, such as a Medicare Advantage plan, where the hospital expects to receive payment from the plan. If it applies, code 04 is required for Medicare claims.

05   Lien Has Been Filed

Code 05 indicates that the provider has filed a legal claim for recovery of funds from a patient in response to a legal action initiated by the patient.

HIPAA TIP

HIPAA 837I Not Required with Workers' Compensation Claims

The HIPAA mandate to file claims electronically for all but the smallest providers does not cover workers' compensation plans.

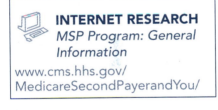
INTERNET RESEARCH
MSP Program: General Information
www.cms.hhs.gov/
MedicareSecondPayerandYou/

$ $ Billing Tip $ $

Understanding Hospice Benefits

Without condition code 07, the Medicare-covered service being billed will not be paid because patients who choose hospice benefits waive their rights to other benefits for services related to the terminal diagnosis. Code 07 indicates to the payer that the services are not related to the terminal diagnosis and therefore should be covered as regular Medicare services. For the same reasons, the Type of Bill (TOB) code in FL 4 must not be 082X (Special facility, Hospice, X) when condition code 07 is used.

The provider's action is intended to collect the funds potentially due to the patient as a result of the legal action. If it applies, this code must appear on Medicare claims. An MSP situation may exist because of a pending liability case.

06   ESRD Patient in the First Thirty Months of Entitlement Covered by Employer Group Health Insurance

If the patient also is covered by employer group health insurance during the first thirty months of ESRD (end-stage renal disease) benefits, code 06 indicates a possible MSP situation. If it applies, this code is required for all claims.

07   Treatment of Nonterminal Condition for Hospice Patient

Code 07 indicates that the patient has chosen Medicare hospice benefits for treating a terminal condition, but that the reporting provider is treating the patient for another condition and is asking for regular Medicare payment. This code is required for Medicare billing if it applies.

08   Beneficiary Would Not Provide Information Concerning Other Insurance Coverage

Code 08 is used when the patient refuses to supply information about other insurance coverage. This code is required for Medicare and TRICARE claims. The patient account specialist should be prepared to prove that the beneficiary would not provide this information. The fiscal intermediary (FI) will contact the beneficiary to settle the question.

09   Neither Patient Nor Spouse Is Employed

Code 09 indicates to Medicare that both the patient and his or her spouse have responded to MSP development questions by stating that they are not employed (and therefore do not have other insurance through an employer). If it applies, this code is required for Medicare claims. It notifies Medicare that neither the patient nor the patient's spouse is a working aged person, so no further MSP development is necessary.

10   Patient and/or Spouse Is Employed but No EGHP Coverage Exists

Code 10 indicates that the patient and spouse have responded to MSP development questions by stating that they have no group health insurance under an EGHP (employer group health plan) even though one or both are employed. This code is required for Medicare billing when applicable. It notifies Medicare that neither the patient nor the patient's spouse have group health insurance as a working aged person, so no further MSP development is necessary.

11   Disabled Beneficiary, but No Large Group Health Plan Coverage

Code 11 indicates that, during MSP development questioning, a disabled beneficiary and/or his or her family members stated that although one or more family members are employed, no one is covered by group health insurance from a large group health plan (LGHP) or other employer-sponsored or employer-provided health insurance that would cover the patient. Medicare requires this code, if it applies, to recognize that no further MSP development along these lines is necessary.

12–16 Reserved for Payer Use Only

Providers do not report these codes.

Patient Condition Codes

Condition codes connected to a variety of special circumstances and student status are listed below.

17 Patient Is Homeless

This code is used to communicate that the patient is homeless.

18 Maiden Name Retained

Code 18 is used when a dependent spouse is entitled to benefits but does not use her husband's last name. The code is not needed for Medicare claims, but it is used for commercial payers and TRICARE.

19 Child Retains Mother's Name

Code 19 is used when the patient is a dependent child entitled to benefits who does not have his or her father's last name. The code is not needed for Medicare claims, but it is used for commercial payers and TRICARE.

20 Beneficiary Requested Billing

Code 20 indicates that the provider knows that the services on the claim are not covered but the beneficiary has asked for a written notice of determination from the payer anyway. This is known as a demand bill. The claim will be suspended for medical review of the noncovered charges; depending on the circumstances, a disputed charge could be covered. When it applies, this code is required for Medicare home health and inpatient SNF claims.

21 Billing for Denial Notice

Code 21 is used on a no-pay claim, meaning that it indicates that the provider knows that the services are not covered but is requesting a written notice of the denial from Medicare in order to bill the claim to another payer, such as Medicaid, a supplementary payer, or the patient. The code is required for Medicare billing when applicable.

22 Patient on Multiple Drug Regimen

Code 22 is used to describe situations in which a patient is receiving multiple IV drugs while on home IV therapy. When it applies, the code is required for Medicare claims.

23 Home Caregiver Available

Code 23 is used when a caregiver is available at home to assist the patient with self-administration of IV drugs. When it applies, the code is required for Medicare claims.

$ $ Billing Tip $ $

Medicare Noncovered Services and Advance Beneficiary Notices

When an outpatient service is denied to a beneficiary because Medicare does not consider it medically necessary under the circumstances or because the service is one of a number of screening services (for example, a screening mammography or prostate cancer screening) that was performed more frequently than Medicare covers, Medicare participating providers must notify the beneficiary in writing before providing the service. An Advance Beneficiary Notice of Noncoverage (ABN) stating that the charge for the service will not be paid by Medicare is given to the patient. If the provider does not issue an ABN, the patient could potentially hold the hospital liable for the cost of the service.

When outpatient services are denied to a beneficiary based on categorical or technical denials (for services not considered to be Medicare benefits, such as cosmetic surgery, routine foot care, or most self-administered drugs), Medicare participating providers, although encouraged to issue ABNs, are not legally required to do so. When a service is noncovered because it is excluded from the list of Medicare benefits, regardless of whether the patient receives an ABN for such services, the beneficiary may be held liable for the cost of the service.

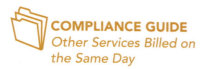
When using condition codes 20 and 21, special care should be taken regarding the billing of other covered services on the same day. Each code follows a different rule. When using condition code 20 (for a demand bill), covered and noncovered charges should be recorded on two separate bills. (Claims using condition code 20 are exempt from the usual same-day billing rules that require a single bill.) When using condition code 21 (for a no-pay bill), however, covered and noncovered charges should be included on the same bill; a split bill is not allowed. To distinguish the noncovered charges, modifier −GY is used to trigger beneficiary liability for the noncovered services.

FYI

Sole Community Hospital

A sole community hospital is the only source of inpatient services in a given geographical area. A hospital is eligible to be classified as a sole community hospital if it is located more than thirty-five miles from other like hospitals. In a rural area, a hospital may be classified as a sole community hospital when the distance to similar hospitals is less than thirty-five miles provided it meets certain other criteria. Sole community hospitals are paid under Medicare's PPS; however, because of their importance to the community, they receive certain financial advantages.

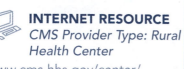

INTERNET RESOURCE
CMS Provider Type: Rural Health Center
www.cms.hhs.gov/center/rural.asp

24 Home IV Patient Also Receiving Home Health Agency Services

Code 24 is used when a patient is under the care of a home health agency while receiving home IV therapy services. When it applies, the code is required for Medicare claims.

25 Patient Is a Non-U.S. Resident

Code 25 is used to indicate that the patient is not a resident of the United States.

26 Veterans Affairs-Eligible Patient Chooses to Receive Services in Medicare-Certified Facility

Code 26 is used to report that a patient is eligible for VA benefits at a VA facility but chooses to receive services in a Medicare-certified facility. When it applies, the code is required for Medicare claims.

27 Patient Referred to a Sole Community Hospital for a Diagnostic Laboratory Test

Code 27 can be reported by sole community hospitals only. It should not be used when a specimen is sent only for testing. It is used to indicate that the laboratory service is paid at 62 percent of the fee schedule amount rather than at 60 percent. When it applies, the code is required for Medicare claims.

28 Patient and/or Spouse's Employer Group Health Plan Is Secondary to Medicare

Code 28 reports the following situation: In response to MSP development questions, the patient and/or spouse indicates that one or both are employed and have group health insurance from an EGHP. However, their EGHP is secondary to Medicare either because it is a single employer plan and the employer has fewer than twenty full- and part-time employees, or because it is a multiple employer plan that elects to pay secondary to Medicare for employees and spouses aged sixty-five and older for those participating employers with fewer than twenty employees. When it applies, the code is required for Medicare claims.

29 Disabled Beneficiary and/or Family Member's Large Group Health Plan Is Secondary to Medicare

Code 29 reports the following situation: In response to MSP development questions, the patient and/or family members indicate that one or more are employed and have group health insurance from a LGHP. However, the LGHP is secondary to Medicare either because it is a single employer plan and the employer has fewer than one hundred full- and part-time employees, or because it is a multiple employer plan and all participating employers have fewer than one hundred full- and part-time employees. This code is required for Medicare claims when applicable.

30 Qualifying Clinical Trials

Code 30 is used to indicate nonresearch services being provided to all patients, including managed care plan members, who are part of a qualified clinical trial.

31–34 Student Status Codes

Student status condition codes are required when the patient is over eighteen years old and is covered by an insurance plan as a dependent child. Only one of the codes should be used on a claim. The codes are not required for Medicare billing, but they are required for commercial payers and for TRICARE billing.

31	Patient is a student (full-time day)
32	Patient is a student (cooperative/work study program)
33	Patient is a student (full-time night)
34	Patient is a student (part-time)

35   Reserved for National Assignment

Room Codes

The following condition codes describe special situations relating to accommodations.

36   General Care Patient in a Special Unit

Code 36 indicates that the patient was temporarily placed in a special care unit because no general care beds were available. When it applies, this code should be reported for Medicare, commercial, and TRICARE claims. However, code 36 is not used for hospitals under the PPS.

37   Ward Accommodation at Patient's Request

Code 37 indicates that the patient was assigned to ward accommodations at his or her own request. This code is required for Medicare claims and commercial payers. It is not used by PPS hospitals.

38   Semiprivate Room Not Available

Code 38 indicates situations in which a patient was placed in a ward or private room because no semiprivate rooms were available. This code is required for Medicare, commercial, and TRICARE claims when applicable. Code 38 is not used by PPS hospitals.

39   Private Room Medically Necessary

Code 39 indicates that the patient was assigned a private room for medical reasons. This code is required for Medicare and all other payers, but is not used by PPS hospitals.

40   Same-Day Transfer

Code 40 indicates that the patient was transferred to another facility before midnight on the day of admission. It is required for Medicare billing when applicable.

41   Partial Hospitalization

Code 41 indicates that the claim is for partial hospitalization services. For outpatients, this includes a variety of psychiatric programs (such as for drug

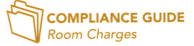

COMPLIANCE GUIDE
Room Charges

When condition code 36 is used, the accommodation room charges on the bill should be based on the hospital's typical semiprivate room rate, not on the rate for the special care unit.

$ $ Billing Tip $ $

Private Room Charges and Revenue Codes

Code 38 should be used with the appropriate accommodation revenue code for a private, private deluxe, or ward accommodation reported in FL 42 (Revenue Code; see Chapter 12). Code 39 should be used with the appropriate accommodation revenue code for a private room.

and alcohol abuse), and the code is used to distinguish partial hospitalization services from routine outpatient psychiatric services. This code is required for Medicare billing when applicable.

42 Continuing Care Not Related to Inpatient Admission

Code 42 is used if the patient's continuing care plan is not related to the condition or diagnosis that brought about the inpatient hospital admission. When used with patient discharge status 06 in FL 17 (Discharged/transferred to home under care of organized home health service organization in anticipation of covered skilled care), this code will generate the full payment for the diagnosis-related group (DRG), which is greater than the amount that would be received for a transferred patient.

43 Continuing Care Not Provided Within Prescribed Postdischarge Window

Code 43 is used if the patient's continuing care plan is related to the condition or diagnosis that brought on the inpatient hospital admission, but care did not start within the postdischarge window (usually a three-day window) after the date of discharge. As with code 42, when used with patient discharge status 06 (Discharged/transferred to home under care of organized home health service organization in anticipation of covered skilled care), this code will generate the full DRG payment, which is greater than the amount that would be received for a transferred patient.

44 Inpatient Admission Changed to Outpatient

Code 44 is used only on an outpatient claim when the physician ordered inpatient services, but the internal utilization review (UR) performed while the patient was still in the hospital (and before an inpatient claim was submitted) determined that the services received did not meet the UR inpatient criteria. Therefore, the claim is being billed as an outpatient claim. This change also requires the physician's concurrence, which must be documented in the patient's medical record.

45 Ambiguous Gender Category

This code is used to indicate that the patient's gender characteristics are ambiguous. This would refer to transgender patients, for example, or patients with one of a group of conditions known as DSDs (disorders of sex development).

TRICARE, Product Replacement, and SNF Information Codes

The following condition codes contain information that relates specifically to TRICARE, product replacement, and SNF claims.

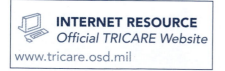

INTERNET RESOURCE
Official TRICARE Website
www.tricare.osd.mil

46 Nonavailability Statement on File

Code 46 indicates that a nonavailability statement is on file for the TRICARE claim being filed. This code is required for TRICARE claims when it applies. It is not required for Medicare billing.

47 Reserved for TRICARE

48 Psychiatric Residential Treatment Centers for Children and Adolescents

Code 48 identifies claims submitted by a psychiatric residential treatment center (RTC) for children and adolescents. The facility must be TRICARE-authorized. This code is required for TRICARE claims when applicable. It is not required for Medicare billing.

49 Product Replacement Within Product Life Cycle

Code 49 indicates that a product has been replaced earlier than its anticipated life cycle based on an indication that it is malfunctioning.

50 Product Replacement for Known Recall of a Product

Code 50 is used to indicate that either the manufacturer or the FDA has identified a product for recall and, therefore, replacement.

51–54 Reserved for National Assignment

55 SNF Bed Not Available

Code 55 indicates that the patient's SNF admission was delayed more than thirty days after hospital discharge because a SNF bed was not available. This code is required for Medicare and TRICARE billing when applicable.

56 Medical Appropriateness

Code 56 communicates that the patient's SNF admission was delayed more than thirty days after hospital discharge because the patient's condition made it inappropriate to begin active care within that period. This code is required for Medicare and TRICARE billing when applicable.

57 SNF Readmission

Code 57 indicates that, within thirty days of the current SNF readmission, the patient had received Medicare-covered SNF care.

Other Special Codes

58 Terminated Medicare Advantage Enrollee

Code 58 communicates that the patient is a terminated enrollee in a Medicare Advantage plan whose three-day inpatient hospital stay was waived.

59 Nonprimary ESRD Facility

Code 59 is used by a facility that is not the patient's primary dialysis facility to indicate that an ESRD beneficiary received unscheduled or emergency dialysis services. Code 59 is used along with the appropriate condition code that represents the renal dialysis setting (see codes 70–76 below).

60 Day Outlier

This code is used by fiscal intermediaries only.

Nonavailability Statement

Formerly, if a patient covered by TRICARE lived within a certain distance of a military hospital (usually within a forty-mile radius) and the hospital was unable to admit the patient, that hospital had to file a *nonavailability statement* with the DEERS database before the patient could be covered at a civilian hospital. A nonavailability statement was required for nonemergency inpatient care only. Currently, under the 2002 National Defense Authorization Act, this requirement is eliminated, except for nonemergency inpatient mental health care services. In addition, some military treatment facilities that are granted an exemption may still require the statement.

$ $ Billing Tip $ $

Condition Codes 56 and 57

When code 56 or 57 is used, occurrence span code 70 (Qualifying stay dates for SNF use only) should be reported in FL 35 or 36 (Occurrence Span Codes and Dates). The qualifying stay dates should be the same as those used for the initial admission fewer than thirty days earlier, and the qualifying stay must be at least a three-day inpatient hospital stay.

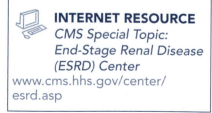
61   Cost Outlier

This code is used by fiscal intermediaries only.

62–65 Payer Only Codes

These codes are used only by payers for internal use.

66   Provider Does Not Wish Cost Outlier Payment

Code 66 indicates that a hospital paid under a PPS is not requesting additional payment for this stay as a cost outlier. It is required for Medicare billing when applicable.

67   Beneficiary Elects Not to Use Lifetime Reserve (LTR) Days

Code 67 is required for Medicare and TRICARE billing when applicable.

68   Beneficiary Elects to Use LTR Days

Code 68 indicates that the beneficiary has elected to use LTR days when charges are lower than LTR coinsurance amounts. This code is required for Medicare and TRICARE billing when applicable.

69   IME/DGME/N&A Payment Only

Code 69 indicates that a hospital is requesting a supplemental payment for IME (indirect medical education), DGME (direct graduate medical education), or N&A (nursing and allied health). Hospitals may use this code to request a supplemental payment for beneficiaries enrolled in a Medicare managed care plan, such as Medicare Advantage, for the IME portion of the DRG payment. To do so, condition code 04 (Information only bill) should be reported together with this code. Code 69 is required for Medicare billing if applicable.

Renal Dialysis Setting Codes

Seven condition codes that describe various renal dialysis settings for patients' treatments are described below. With the exception of condition code 75 (Home—100 percent reimbursement), which is not used for Medicare, all the codes in this category are required for Medicare billing when applicable.

70   Self-Administered Anemia Management Drug

Code 70 indicates that the bill is for a home dialysis patient who self-administers an anemia management drug such as erythropoetin alpha (EPO) or darbepoetin alpha. If code 70 is used, FL 42 (Revenue Code) should list the revenue code for EPO (0635). The appropriate value code (code 48, 49, or 68) and amount are also required in FLs 39–41 (see Chapter 12, "Revenue Codes, Descriptions, and Amounts," and Chapter 11, "Value Codes and Amounts").

71   Full Care in Unit

Code 71 indicates that the bill is for a patient who received staff-assisted dialysis services in a hospital or renal dialysis facility.

72 Self-Care in Unit

Code 72 indicates that the bill is for a patient who managed his or her own dialysis services without staff assistance in a hospital or renal dialysis facility.

73 Self-Care Training

Code 73 indicates that the bill is for special dialysis services in which the patient and a helper (if necessary) were learning to perform dialysis.

74 Home

Code 74 indicates that the bill is for a patient who received dialysis services at home and for whom code 75 does not apply.

75 Home—100 Percent Reimbursement

Code 75 indicates that the bill is for a patient who received dialysis services at home using a dialysis machine that was purchased by Medicare under the 100 percent program. This code is not used by Medicare. Other payers, however, may use it.

76 Backup In-Facility Dialysis

Code 76 indicates that the bill is for a home dialysis patient who received backup dialysis services in a facility. Emergency backup maintenance dialysis is only allowed due to medical necessity or because the patient is traveling. At all other times, treatment should be provided by the patient's home facility.

Miscellaneous Codes

A miscellaneous category containing four other condition codes follows. Each applicable code is required for Medicare billing. Code 77 is also required for Blue Cross, commercial, and TRICARE claims.

77 Provider Accepts or Is Obligated/Required, Due to a Contractual Arrangement or Law, to Accept Payment by a Primary Payer as Payment in Full

Code 77 indicates that the provider has accepted or is obligated or required to accept the primary insurer's payment as payment in full due to a contractual arrangement or law and, therefore, that no Medicare payment is due (no MSP will be made). For Medicare claims, when condition code 77 is used, FL 4 (Type of Bill) should contain the code for a no-payment bill (TOB code 0XX0). When code 77 is used, an MSP value code stating the amount received from the primary payer is required in FLs 39–41 (see value codes 12–16 and 41–43 in Chapter 11, "Value Codes and Amounts").

78 New Coverage Not Implemented by Managed Care Plan

Code 78 is used on a bill for a service that is newly covered by Medicare for which a managed care plan does not pay. (On outpatient bills, when code 78 is used, condition code 04 should be omitted.)

79 CORF Services Provided Offsite

Code 79 communicates that offsite physical therapy, occupational therapy, or speech pathology services were provided.

80 Home Dialysis-Nursing Facility

Code 80 indicates that the patient is receiving dialysis services at home and that the patient's home is a SNF or a nursing facility. Code 80 should be reported in conjunction with the condition code for a home renal dialysis setting (code 74—Home) to further clarify that home, in this case, is a nursing facility.

81–99 Reserved for National Assignment

Special Programs

The following condition codes cover a variety of special programs.

A0 TRICARE External Partnership Program

Code A0 is used to identify TRICARE claims submitted under the External Partnership Program.

A1 EPSDT/CHAP

Code A1 is used to identify services related to the EPSDT (Early and Periodic Screening, Diagnostic, and Treatment) program. This code is required for Medicaid billing if applicable.

A2 Physically Handicapped Children's Program

Services provided under this program receive special funding for the handicapped through Title VII of the Social Security Act or through TRICARE. Code A2 is used to indicate these services. It is required for Medicaid and TRICARE billing when applicable.

A3 Special Federal Funding

Code A3 is designed for uniform use by the state uniform billing committees (SUBCs). It is required for Medicare and Medicaid billing.

A4 Family Planning

Code A4 is designed for uniform use by the SUBCs. The code is required for Medicaid billing if applicable.

A5 Disability

Code A5 is designed for uniform use by the SUBCs. If applicable, this code is required for Medicare and Medicaid billing.

A6 Vaccines/Medicare 100 Percent Payment

Code A6 indicates that the pneumococcal pneumonia and influenza vaccine (PPV) services received are reimbursable under special Medicare program provisions. For these services, therefore, the Medicare deductible and coinsurance do not apply. This code is required for Medicare and Medicaid billing.

A7–A8 Reserved for National Assignment

A9 Second Opinion Surgery

Code A9 is used when the services were requested to support a second opinion on surgery. This code is required for Medicare and Medicaid claims if it applies. When code A9 is used, the Part B deductible and coinsurance do not apply to the claim.

AA Abortion Performed Due to Rape

AB Abortion Performed Due to Incest

AC Abortion Performed Due to Serious Fetal Genetic Defect, Deformity, or Abnormality

AD Abortion Performed Due to a Life-Endangering Physical Condition Caused by, Arising from, or Exacerbated by the Pregnancy Itself

AE Abortion Performed Due to Physical Health of Mother That Is Not Life Endangering

AF Abortion Performed Due to Emotional/ Psychological Health of the Mother

AG Abortion Performed Due to Social or Economic Reasons

AH Elective Abortion

AI Sterilization

AJ Payer Responsible for Copayment

AK Air Ambulance Required

Code AK is used on ambulance claims only. It indicates that an air ambulance was required because the time needed to transport the patient posed a threat.

AL Specialized Treatment/Bed Unavailable

Code AL is used on ambulance claims only. It indicates that a specialized treatment or bed was unavailable and that the patient was therefore transported to an alternate facility.

AM Nonemergency Medically Necessary Stretcher Transport Required

Code AM is used on ambulance claims only. It indicates that the patient required a nonemergency, medically necessary stretcher for transport.

> **INTERNET RESOURCE**
> *CMS Provider Type: Ambulance Services Center*
> www.cms.hhs.gov/center/ambulance.asp

AN   Preadmission Screening Not Required

Code AN is used when the person meets the criteria for an exemption from preadmission screening.

AO–AZ Reserved for National Assignment

B0   Medicare Coordinated Care Demonstration Claim

Code B0 is used to report that the patient is a participant in a Medicare coordinated care demonstration.

B1   Beneficiary Ineligible for Demonstration Program

The full definition of code B1 is pending.

B2   Critical Access Hospital Ambulance Attestation

Code B2 is used by a critical access hospital (CAH) to state that the facility meets the criteria for exemption from the ambulance fee schedule.

B3   Pregnancy Indicator

Code B3 communicates that the patient is pregnant. It is required when mandated by law. The determination of the pregnancy should be completed in compliance with the applicable law.

B4   Admission Unrelated to Discharge on Same Day

Code B4 is used in circumstances where a patient is discharged and then readmitted to the same acute care PPS hospital on the same day. It indicates that the patient's admission, as determined by the hospital, is unrelated to the patient's discharge that same day. The symptoms must be unrelated to the patient's earlier medical condition. The code is used so that two separate DRG payments, subject to QIO review, will be generated.

B5–BZ Reserved for National Assignment

QIO Approval Indicator Services

The following codes apply to quality improvement organization (QIO) approvals. For Medicare billing, the QIO approval indicator codes are no longer required except on Medicare inpatient claims that contain excluded diagnoses.

QIOs, as explained in Chapter 2, are groups hired by Medicare to assess the medical necessity of planned procedures. Utilization review (UR) companies that specialize in precertification perform a similar function for private payers. Medical reviews are conducted either before the patient's admission or planned procedure or after discharge. Payment may be made in whole or in part, or it may be denied, depending on the terms of the insurance plan. The reviewers consider the necessity, appropriateness, and quality of certain inpatient and outpatient surgical procedures. The URs and QIOs can assist in the assignment of codes C1, C3, and C4.

Claims containing codes C1, C3, and C4 are excluded from the billing timeliness and accuracy standard because of the additional time that may be required to obtain a medical review.

C0 Reserved for National Assignment

C1 Approved as Billed

Code C1 indicates that the claim was reviewed by the QIO/UR and was fully approved, including any outlier. This code is required for Medicare billing when applicable. It is also required by most other payers.

C2 Automatic Approval as Billed Based on Focused Review

Code C2 flags a case that is automatically approved based on the fact that it is part of a category of cases that the QIO/UR has determined need not be reviewed under a focused medical review program. This code is no longer used for Medicare billing. However, it is required by most other payers when applicable.

C3 Partial Approval

Code C3 indicates that the claim has been reviewed by the QIO/UR and that some portion (days or services) was denied. This code is required for Medicare billing and for all other payers when applicable.

C4 Admission/Services Denied

Code C4 indicates that the patient's need for inpatient services was reviewed by the QIO/UR and that all the services were denied because the stay was medically unnecessary. If it applies, this code is required by all payers.

C5 Postpayment Review Applicable

Code C5 indicates that the QIO medical review of the claim will be completed after the claim is paid. The bill may be a cost outlier, part of a review sample, or reviewed for other reasons, or it may not be reviewed. When applicable, this code is required by all payers.

C6 Admission Preauthorization

Code C6 is used to indicate that the QIO/UR has authorized this admission or procedure, although it has not reviewed the services provided. When applicable, this code is required by all payers.

C7 Extended Authorization

Code C7 indicates that the QIO has authorized the services for an extended length of time but has not reviewed them. When applicable, this code is required for all payers.

C8–CZ Reserved for National Assignment

Claim Change Reasons

The condition codes that are used to report claim changes are described below, along with several other miscellaneous codes. Only one of the claim change reason codes may be reported on the new claim. The single reason that best describes the change being made should be used.

If more than one claim change reason code applies to the adjustment, code D9 (Any other change) is reported. Code D9 is used when none of the usual

---

FYI

Focused Medical Review

The goal of a **focused medical review** is to identify abuse of the Medicare payment system by focusing medical review efforts on claims that represent the greatest risk of inappropriate payment. National data, such as internal billing, utilization, and payment data, are collected and analyzed, and the results are passed on to the Medicare fiscal intermediaries. Local medical review policies are then developed to identify such claims in an attempt to reduce the number of noncovered claims or unnecessary services.

$$ Billing Tip $$

Occurrence Codes and Condition Code C3

A claim containing condition code C3 includes some covered and some noncovered services. Both covered and noncovered levels of care must be listed on the claim. FLs 35–36 (Occurrence Span Codes and Dates) are used to report both the QIO/UR approved stay dates (occurrence span code M0) as well as the noncovered days or services (occurrence span code 77). Occurrence span codes and dates are discussed in Chapter 10.

$$ Billing Tip $$

Condition Code C6 and FL 63

When condition code C6 is used, the authorization number received from the payer should be reported in FL 63 (Treatment Authorization Codes) on the UB-04. FL 63 is described in Chapter 13, "Payer, Insured, and Employer Information."

claim change reasons in D0–D8 applies or when more than one change is required. Most of the codes that follow (except G0 and H0) are required for Medicare billing if applicable.

Adjustment bills use a type of bill (TOB) code that ends with frequency code 7 (0XX7) or 8 (0XX8) in FL 4. TOB code 0XX7 is used to replace a previously submitted bill, and TOB code 0XX8 is used to cancel a prior claim. Most adjustment claims use TOB 0XX7.

D0   Changes to Services Dates

Use claim change reason code D0 on adjustment claims to make changes in the service dates (FL 6, Statement Covers Period) reported on a previously submitted claim. When the dates of service are incorrect on the original claim, a replacement claim (TOB 0XX7) with this condition code is submitted to correct the error. The entire adjustment request is submitted as if it were an initial bill.

D1   Changes to Charges

Use claim change reason code D1 on an adjustment claim to make a change in a charge reported on a previously submitted claim. This code is used to adjust the total charges or the charges related to a specific line item reported in FL 47 (Total Charges). The entire revenue line to be changed must be entered on the replacement bill. TOB 0XX7 is reported.

D2   Changes in Revenue Codes/HCPCS/HIPPS Rate Code

Use claim change reason code D2 on an adjustment claim to make a change in the revenue codes or HCPCS/HIPPS rate codes reported on a previously submitted claim. This code is used to change data in FL 42 (Revenue Code) or FL 44 (HCPCS/Rates/HIPPS Rate Codes). TOB 0XX7 is reported.

D3   Second or Subsequent Interim PPS Bill

Use claim change reason code D3 on an adjustment claim to submit a second or subsequent interim PPS bill. TOB 0XX7 is reported. When condition code D3 is used, the through date in FL 6 (Statement Covers Period) is updated (PPS bills are generally issued every sixty days). The from date remains the same. In addition, the code in FL 17 (Patient Discharge Status) must be 30 (Still a patient).

D4   Change in ICD-9-CM Diagnosis and/or Procedure Codes

Use claim change reason code D4 on an adjustment claim to make a change in a diagnosis code (FL 67) or procedure code (FL 74) reported on a previously submitted claim (see Chapter 14, "Diagnosis and Procedure Codes"). When code D4 is used, a brief explanation of the change should be provided in the Remarks field (FL 80). TOB 0XX7 is reported.

D5   Cancel to Correct Insured's ID or Provider ID

Code D5 is used to indicate that a claim is being cancelled only to correct a health insurance claim number (HICN) or provider identification number. The health insurance claim number is located in FL 60, and the provider identification number is located in FL 51. A copy of the claim to be cancelled is first submitted with TOB 0XX8. Then a new claim containing the correct information and TOB 0XX7 is submitted.

D6 Cancel Only to Repay a Duplicate or OIG Overpayment

Code D6 indicates that a claim is being cancelled only to repay a duplicate payment or Office of Inspector General (OIG) overpayment, including the cancellation of an outpatient bill containing services that are required to be included on an inpatient bill. A copy of the claim to be cancelled is first submitted with TOB 0XX8. If applicable, a new claim containing the correct information is then submitted (with TOB 0XX7).

D7 Change to Make Medicare the Secondary Payer

Use claim change reason code D7 on an adjustment claim to make Medicare the secondary rather than primary payer. TOB 0XX7 is reported. The amount paid by the primary payer is indicated using the appropriate value code and amount (see Chapter 11). The MSP insurer's name, address, and employer information are also reported.

D8 Change to Make Medicare the Primary Payer

Use claim change reason code D8 on an adjustment claim to make Medicare the primary payer. TOB 0XX7 is reported. Provide a brief explanation of the reason for the change in FL 80 (Remarks Field).

D9 Any Other Change

Use claim change reason code D9 on an adjustment claim to make any other changes to a claim that was already submitted. This code should be used only when any of the above claim change reason codes do not apply or when the adjustment requires more than one change. For example, code D9 can be used to make a change to the units of service (FL 46) or to a value code that was incorrectly reported. Provide a brief explanation of the reason for the change in FL 80 (Remarks Field).

DA–DQ Reserved for National Assignment

DR Disaster Related

This code is used to identify claims that are or may be affected by specific payer or health plan policies related to a national or regional disaster.

DS–DZ Reserved for National Assignment

E0 Change in Patient Status

Use claim change reason code E0 on an adjustment claim to change the reported patient discharge status (FL 17) on a processed claim. Use TOB 0XX7.

E1–FZ Reserved for National Assignment

G0 Distinct Medical Visit

Use code G0 when the patient visited the same revenue center more than once during a day, but the visits were not related to each other. An example is a beneficiary who presented at the emergency department twice on the same day for two unrelated reasons, such as a broken arm in the morning and chest pain later in the day.

The Outpatient Code Editor will reject multiple medical visits on the same day with the same revenue code unless condition code G0 is used. When condition code G0 is used, the two visits should be reported on separate lines in FL 44 (HCPCS/Rates), rather than on one line with multiple service units, indicating that the second visit is a distinct medical visit.

G1–GZ Reserved for National Assignment

H0 Delayed Filing, Statement of Intent Submitted

Code H0 indicates that a statement of intent was submitted within the allowed qualifying period to specifically identify the existence of another third-party liability situation. Without code H0, the claim will be rejected due to untimely filing.

H1–LZ Reserved for National Assignment

M0–MZ Reserved for Payer Assignment

N0–0Z Reserved for National Assignment

P0–PZ Reserved for Public Health Data Reporting Only

Q0–ZZ Reserved for National Assignment

FL 29 Accident State

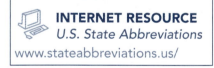

INTERNET RESOURCE
U.S. State Abbreviations
www.stateabbreviations.us/

837I No Map Field
The Accident State field is new on the UB-04. There is currently no field on the 837I electronic claim for reporting the accident state.

FL 29 is used to report the state in which an accident occurred on a claim containing services related to an automobile accident.

Guidelines

This field contains two positions for reporting the two-character state abbreviation of the state, for example, NY to indicate New York or FL for Florida. It is not used for Medicare billing. Other payers require it when applicable.

FL 30 Unlabeled Field

1 FLs 18–28 on the UB-04 are used for reporting condition codes—two-digit numeric or alphanumeric codes that identify special conditions or unique circumstances that affect the processing and payment of the claim. Condition codes are used to clarify a patient's eligibility and benefits. For example, they help the payer determine whether coverage exists under more than one type of insurance, whether primary or secondary insurance coverage is to be administered, whether medical necessity affects room assignment, whether an injury or illness is related to employment, and other details about a patient's circumstances so that the claim can be processed efficiently and accurately.

2 The UB-04 allows eleven condition codes to be listed at one time—one each in FLs 18–28. Condition codes can be grouped as follows: insurance codes, patient condition codes, room codes, TRICARE/product replacement/SNF information codes, and other special codes, including codes for renal dialysis settings, miscellaneous codes, and codes for special programs, QIO approval indicator services, and claim change reasons. Many condition codes are reserved for national or payer assignment or are currently payer-only codes.

3 When particular condition codes are used, various billing situations arise. For example, many of the insurance codes require MSP development—that is, verification of Medicare's responsibility for the claim; one TRICARE information code is used when a nonavailability statement is on file; and certain codes connected to QIO approvals are automatically excluded from the billing timeliness and accuracy standard.

4 Many condition codes must also be coordinated with data in other fields on the UB-04. For example, the room codes require particular accommodation revenue codes in FL 42; the renal dialysis setting codes require a revenue code for dialysis services in FL 42; the QIO approval code for admission preauthorization requires a treatment authorization code in FL 63; all the claim change reason codes require the document control number assigned to the previously submitted claim to be listed in FL 64, and many also require an explanation of the change in the Remarks field (FL 80) or a particular occurrence code and date (FLs 31–34) to justify the change.

5 FL 29 (Accident State) is new to the UB-04 and is used to report the state in which an accident occurred for claims containing services related to an auto accident. FL 30 is an unlabeled field reserved for future assignment by the NUBC.

✔ **CHECK YOUR UNDERSTANDING**

1. Define *condition code* and specify which form locator(s) on the UB-04 it occupies.

_____

_____

_____

2. Which of the following categories is not a grouping for condition codes?
   a. TRICARE information codes
   b. room codes
   c. occurrence codes and dates
   d. claim change reason codes
   e. product replacement information codes

3. Which of the following represents the correct order for listing condition codes on a claim?
   a. 09, 20, AJ, D1
   b. AJ, D1, 09, 20
   c. 09, 20, D1, AJ

4. True or False: Condition code 02 (Condition is employment related) indicates possible Medicare Secondary Payer development. _____

5. When claim change reason codes D0–D9 are used, which of the following types of data must always be reported?
   a. treatment authorization code
   b. TOB 0XX7
   c. brief explanation for change in Remarks field
   d. document control number

6. True or False: Medical necessity reviews are always conducted before the patient's admission or planned procedure. _____

7. Determine which condition code applies to each of the following circumstances.
   a. A provider is requesting regular Medicare payment for treating a patient who has otherwise elected Medicare hospice benefits. _____
   b. A patient was admitted to an acute care hospital in the morning and transferred to a different short-term facility in the afternoon of the same day. _____
   c. A patient requires a stretcher for transport in a nonemergency situation for medical reasons. _____
   d. A child is entitled to benefits under her father's insurance but doesn't have her father's last name. _____
   e. A patient is admitted at the end of the month to the same SNF he had been in for five days at the beginning of the month. _____
   f. A claim is submitted as a utilization report, rather than for payment. _____
   g. The UR has authorized this procedure but has not reviewed the services provided. _____
   h. An inpatient's second PPS bill is prepared after sixty days. _____

i. A patient residing in a nursing facility (SNF) is receiving dialysis services at the nursing facility. _____ and _____

j. The patient's discharge status code on the original bill was 01 (Discharged to home) but it should have been 06 (Discharged to home under care of organized home health service organization in anticipation of covered skill care). _____

k. The patient claims her fall was a result of the poor condition of her company's parking lot. _____

l. A patient has a stent replaced because of a recall by the manufacturer. _____

m. A duplicate payment is received. Payment for the same claim was received a week ago. _____

n. The QIO fully approves a claim containing a cost outlier. _____

o. A patient is discharged from an acute care PPS hospital at noon and is then readmitted to the same facility at 10:00 P.M. that night. The symptoms for the two admissions are unrelated. _____

8. A patient is involved in a car accident in Boston and is sent to the emergency room for treatment. What entry is reported in FL 29? _____

9. Answer the following questions based on the top portion of the UB-04 form shown here.

UB-04 Form—FLs 1–30

1 BELLAIRE HOSPITAL	2	3a PAT. CNTL # 9R33795	4 TYPE OF BILL
222 RTE 9		b. MED. REC. # R7770X9100	0117
LAKE KATRINE, NY 12449		5 FED. TAX NO.	6 STATEMENT COVERS PERIOD FROM / THROUGH	7
845-336-4000		23-7776669	040209 / 073009	

| 8 PATIENT NAME a | | 9 PATIENT ADDRESS a 629 ROUTE 28 | | |
| b OPPENHEIM, REGINA | | b SHOKAN | c NY d 12481 | e |

| 10 BIRTHDATE | 11 SEX | 12 DATE | ADMISSION 13 HR | 14 TYPE | 15 SRC | 16 DHR | 17 STAT | 18 | 19 | 20 | 21 | CONDITION CODES 22 23 24 25 26 27 28 | 29 ACDT STATE | 30 |
| 04181940 | F | 040209 | 10 | 2 | 1 | | 30 | 28 | D3 | | | | | |

a. On what date was the patient admitted? _____

b. What is the patient's discharge status? _____

c. What does the frequency code in the TOB code indicate? _____

d. How long has the patient been in the hospital? _____

e. What code is reported in FL 19, and what does it indicate? _____

f. Based on a sixty-day billing period, is this the first, second, or third bill that has been prepared for this patient's hospital visit? _____

g. How old is the patient? _____

h. Are either the patient or the patient's spouse employed? _____

i. Do either the patient or the patient's spouse have more than one health insurance plan? _____

j. Who is the primary payer on the claim? _____

10. A Medicare patient is admitted to an acute care hospital for outpatient diagnostic testing. When he returns home, a complication develops from the tests, and he is admitted as in inpatient the next day to treat the complication. He remains in the hospital for two days and is then discharged. How many claims should be filed?
    a. two claims, one for the outpatient services and one for the inpatient services
    b. one outpatient claim that combines both the outpatient and inpatient services
    c. one inpatient claim that combines both the inpatient and outpatient services
    d. either b or c

UB-04 Activity: Claim Analysis

Working with Condition Codes: FLs 18-28

Open the file **Sample01.pdf** in Adobe Reader, and answer the following questions:

1. What condition code is reported on the claim? What does it indicate?

2. Who is the payer on the claim?

3. Based on the patient's age at the time of admission, is the patient potentially a working aged person?

4. What questionnaire did the patient and/or the patient's spouse complete during registration in connection with the information reported in FL 18?

5. How many form locators are provided for condition codes?

6. Suppose the patient is participating in a qualified clinical trial in connection with the condition on this claim. What condition code would be added to indicate this?

7. Are condition codes sequenced based on chronology, seriousness of the condition, or numeric order?

8. Suppose condition code 38 is reported on this claim. Why would the claim be edited?

9. Assume that, after submitting the claim, the billing office is informed that the date of service on the claim is incorrect—it should be November 25. When submitting an adjustment claim, what condition code is used to indicate the change? What TOB should be used on the adjustment claim?

10. List the form locators where the new date needs to be recorded. Assume you have received the remittance advice for the first claim. What information from the remittance advice should also be reported on the adjustment claim?

When finished viewing the claim, click Exit on the File menu.

Occurrence Codes and Dates

LEARNING OUTCOMES

After completing this chapter, you will be able to define the key terms and:

1. Discuss the codes that are used in FLs 31–34 of the UB-04 to report significant events, or occurrences, connected with claims that affect how they are processed and paid.

2. Understand the four categories of occurrence codes.

3. Discuss the types of codes that are used in FLs 35–36 of the UB-04 to report occurrence spans and dates.

4. Explain various billing situations that arise when particular occurrence codes and occurrence span codes are used.

5. Recognize which occurrence codes and occurrence span codes contain data that must be coordinated with other fields on the UB-04.

6. Explain what information belongs in FL 38, Responsible Party Name and Address, of the UB-04 form.

KEY TERMS

- conditional payment
- guarantee of payment provision
- leave of absence (LOA) days
- Medicare Conditional Payment request
- occurrence code
- occurrence span code
- spell of illness

FLs 31–34 of the UB-04 are used to record significant occurrences connected with claims that affect how payers evaluate them. For example, the fact of an automobile accident or the dates on which speech therapy was provided affect payments for claims. The payer needs to know the details of the occurrence—in particular, the date it happened—to decide what benefits are due. The events may be related to such factors as liability decisions, patient coverage, the appropriateness of the services rendered, and Medicare Secondary Payer (MSP) development during the admissions process.

Two other fields of the UB-04, FLs 35 and 36, Occurrence Span Codes and Dates, are used to report similar information. In these two form locators, however, the significant event being reported is defined by a span of time rather than by a single date. For example, occurrence span code 76 (Patient liability) is used to report a period of noncovered care for which the patient is responsible. Another code, occurrence span code 70, is used to report a period of skilled nursing-level care that occurs during an inpatient acute care hospital stay. The period must be at least a three-day stay.

Chapter 10 also covers FLs 37 and 38. FL 37 is an unlabeled field reserved for national assignment. FL 38 (Responsible Party Name and Address) is not required for Medicare billing but is used on commercial claims to report the name and mailing address of the beneficiary or other person responsible for the bill. FL 38 is positioned on the UB-04 so that the address will show through the window of the envelope if the claim is mailed in an envelope with a window.

As is the case with the condition codes described in Chapter 9, many members of the hospital staff—not only the patient account specialist—must coordinate their work to identify and assign correct occurrence codes and occurrence span codes for timely filing. Chapter 10 describes each occurrence code and occurrence span code briefly and provides billing tips when appropriate. Appendix A also contains a list of occurrence codes for easy reference.

Figure 10.1

UB-04 Form—FLs 31–38, with Occurrence Code Fields Highlighted

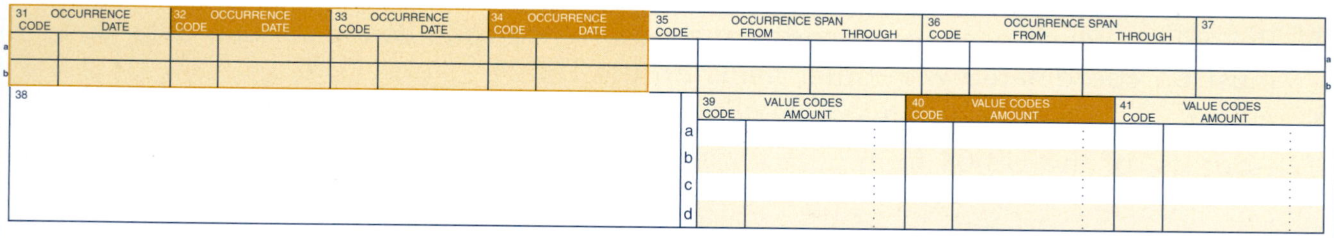

FLs 31–34 Occurrence Codes and Dates

FYI

Date Formats for Occurrence Codes

Every occurrence code must be accompanied by a date. The date should be recorded in the Date box to the right of the occurrence code using the MMDDYY format. (*Note:* The electronic version of the UB-04 requires dates to be reported in the CCYYMMDD format.)

FLs 31–34 are used to define occurrence codes and their associated dates. An **occurrence code** is a two-digit numeric or alphanumeric code that defines a significant event—an occurrence—that happened in connection with a claim and that affects payer processing of the claim. Occurrence codes and dates help payers decide liability issues, coordinate benefits, and determine what benefits are due. As with condition codes, occurrence codes cover a range of billing circumstances.

Guidelines

Completion of this field is required for Medicare billing and all other payers when applicable. Occurrence codes range from 01 to 69 and A0 to LZ. They are usually grouped into four categories for ease of reference:

1. Accident-related codes
2. Medical condition codes

3. Insurance-related codes

4. Service-related codes

The same occurrence code can appear only once on a claim, although as many as eight different codes and associated dates may be reported on a single claim. If more than one occurrence code is reported, enter the codes in alphanumeric sequence (with numbered codes preceding alphabetical codes) in the following order: FLs 31a–34a should be filled in first (line 1), then FLs 31b–34b (line 2). If more than eight codes are required, the next two fields (FLs 35–36, Occurrence Span Code and Date) can be modified to report the overflow. This is done by using the from date in FLs 35–36 and leaving the through date blank. If FLs 35–36 are not available, FL 81 (Code-Code field) may be used with the appropriate qualifier to report the additional occurrence codes and dates (FL 81 is covered in Chapter 15, "Physician Information, Remarks, and Code-Code Field").

Accident-Related Codes

The occurrence codes and dates related to accidents are described below.

01   Accident/Medical Coverage

Code 01 is used to report the date of an accident-related injury for which there is medical payment coverage. This code indicates that Medicare is not the primary payer for the claim and that MSP provisions apply. When the code applies, it is required for Medicare and most other payers' claims.

If the provider sends the claim to the liability insurer first and no payment is received after 120 days, the provider may issue a Medicare Conditional Payment request.

02   No-Fault Insurance Involved—Including Auto Accident/Other

Code 02 reports the date of an accident, auto or other, occurring in a state with no-fault liability laws. Under these laws, liability can be settled without admission or proof of guilt. Code 02 indicates that Medicare is not the primary payer for the claim and that MSP provisions apply. When applicable, this code is required for Medicare and most other payers' claims.

03   Accident/Tort Liability

Code 03 reports an accident (excluding an automobile accident) caused by another person's action that may require a lawsuit to obtain payment from that person. Unlike codes 01 and 02, which are used to report auto accidents, code 03 is used to report accidents that are not auto-related. The code applies when liability is involved other than no-fault liability. Code 03 indicates that Medicare is not the primary payer for the claim. This code is required for Medicare billing and by most other payers when applicable.

If the provider sends the claim to the liability insurer first and can show that no payment is expected to be received within 120 days, the provider may issue a Medicare Conditional Payment request.

04   Accident/Employment-Related

Accident code 04 is used to report an accident and corresponding date when the accident relates to the patient's employment. Code 04 is used for workers'

In general, the date associated with an occurrence code must fall within the from and through dates specified in FL 6 (Statement Covers Period). If the occurrence code date is not logical, the claim will be edited. For example, the date associated with code 41 (Date of first test for preadmission testing) must be on or before the admission date to avoid an edit on the claim, based on the logic that preadmission comes before admission.

FYI

Conditional Payments

When an accident claim is pending payment, the provider may issue a **Medicare Conditional Payment request,** a form requesting a **conditional payment**—a payment made while the provider is waiting for the actual claim to be paid. To do this, the provider must have reason to believe that the primary payer (the liability insurer) will not pay within 120 days due to the lengthy processing delay often associated with third-party liability. If so and if Medicare is the secondary payer on the claim, the provider may ask Medicare to make the conditional payment. Once the primary payer makes a payment, a refund or request for reconsideration must be sent to Medicare within 60 days.

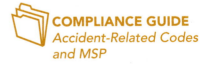

COMPLIANCE GUIDE
Accident-Related Codes and MSP

The six codes in the accident-related category require review for compliance with the Medicare Secondary Payer (MSP) program. With any type of MSP claim, the patient account specialist must check carefully to make sure the most accurate codes are used and that the event is clearly documented, when necessary, in the Remarks field (FL 80) in order for the claim to be processed smoothly.

compensation claims. This code is required for Medicare billing and by all other payers when applicable.

Medicare is not the primary payer for a workers' compensation claim. When a workers' compensation claim is pending payment, if the payment is not expected to be made within 120 days, the provider may issue a Medicare Conditional Payment request.

05 Accident/No Medical or Liability Coverage

Code 05 reports an accident, such as a burn received while cooking at home, that is not described by any of the previous accident-related codes 01–04. It is used for accidents where no liability is involved. This code is required for Medicare billing and by all other payers when applicable. The accident should be described in the UB-04 Remarks field (FL 80; see Chapter 15), noting where and how it occurred—for example, "patient received burn at home while cooking, no liability involved."

06 Crime Victim

Accident code 06 indicates that the patient was a crime victim on the date reported. Medicare does not require this code, but it is required for Medicaid, commercial, and TRICARE billing when applicable.

07–08 Reserved for National Assignment

Medical Condition Codes

Occurrence codes that relate primarily to medical conditions are described below.

09 Start of Infertility Treatment Cycle

Code 09 is used to report the start of an infertility treatment cycle. This code is not required for Medicare billing. It may be required by other payers.

10 Last Menstrual Period

Code 10 reports the last menstrual period. It is used only when a patient is being treated for a maternity-related condition. This code is not required for Medicare billing. It may be required by other payers.

11 Onset of Symptoms/Illness

Code 11 indicates the date the patient first became aware of the symptoms or illness that is being treated. It is used with an illness or injury that results in the need for outpatient therapy services, such as physical therapy. Code 11 is required for Medicare claims as well as by other payers when applicable.

12 Date of Onset for a Chronically Dependent Individual

Code 12 reports the date that the patient or beneficiary is declared a chronically dependent individual (CDI), as certified by a physician. This is the first month of the three-month period required immediately before a beneficiary can qualify for Medicare respite care. This code is required for Medicare home health agency (HHA) billing only when applicable.

13–15 Reserved for National Assignment

Insurance-Related Codes

Occurrence codes that relate primarily to insurance issues are as follows.

16 Date of Last Therapy

Code 16 indicates the last day of services for therapies such as physical therapy, occupational therapy, or speech therapy. It is required for Medicare billing if applicable.

17 Date Outpatient Occupational Therapy Plan Established or Last Reviewed

Code 17 is used to report the date a plan for occupational therapy was established or last reviewed. This code is required for Medicare outpatient billing when applicable.

18 Date of Retirement of Patient/Beneficiary

Code 18 indicates the date of retirement for the patient or beneficiary. This code is required for Medicare billing when applicable. It is used to notify Medicare that the patient or beneficiary is not a working aged person and, therefore, that Medicare is the primary payer.

19 Date of Retirement of Spouse

Code 19 indicates the date of retirement for the patient's spouse. This code is required for Medicare billing when applicable. It is used to notify Medicare that the patient's or beneficiary's spouse is not a working aged person and, therefore, that Medicare is the primary payer (FL 50A).

20 Guarantee of Payment Began

Code 20 indicates the date on which the provider began claiming Medicare payment under the guarantee of payment provision (see FYI on page 200). This code is required for Medicare Part A inpatient bills only when applicable (TOB codes 011X and 041X). Medicare payment under the guarantee of payment provision can go into effect only after the beneficiary's coinsurance days and lifetime reserve days are exhausted.

21 UR Notice Received

Code 21 reports the date the skilled nursing facility (SNF) or hospital received the finding by the utilization review (UR) committee, or Quality Improvement Organization (QIO), or other responsible group that an admission or continued inpatient stay was not medically necessary. This code is required for Medicare billing, as well as for TRICARE billing when applicable.

Value code 46 (Number of grace days) should also be reported in FLs 39–41 (Value Codes and Amounts) to report the number of grace days the UR committee or QIO determined were necessary to arrange for the patient's care after discharge.

22 Date Active Care Ended

Code 22 indicates the date on which a covered level of care in a SNF or general hospital ended. This date is defined as the last covered day preceding a noncovered day. It is required for Medicare billing, as well as for TRICARE billing when applicable. It is not required when code 21 (UR notice received) is used.

FYI

Workers' Compensation Plans

Each state administers its own workers' compensation program and has its own statutes that govern workers' compensation, so coverage varies from state to state. Employers or their insurance carriers must file proof of workers' compensation insurance with the state Workers' Compensation Board.

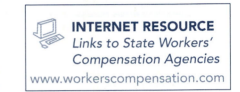

INTERNET RESOURCE
Links to State Workers' Compensation Agencies
www.workerscompensation.com

$ $ Billing Tip $ $

Relating Occurrence Code 11 and Other Occurrence Codes

Occurrence code 11 is often used with other occurrence codes, such as one of the following codes that show when treatment began for a particular type of therapy:

- Code 35, Date treatment started for physical therapy
- Code 44, Date treatment started for occupational therapy
- Code 45, Date treatment started for speech therapy
- Code 46, Date treatment started for cardiac rehabilitation

Note that the date treatment started changes for each subsequent billing period. However, the onset date associated with code 11 must remain the same until the current course of therapy is finished.

Code 22 is also used to indicate the date on which active care ended in a psychiatric or tuberculosis hospital, or the date on which a patient was released on a trial basis from a residential facility.

23   Date of Cancellation of Hospice Election Period

Code 23 is for fiscal intermediary use only. Providers do not report this code.

24   Date Insurance Denied

Occurrence code 24 reports the date a health care facility received an insurance denial from an insurer (other than Medicare). It is required for Medicare, Medicaid, and TRICARE billing when it applies.

25   Date Benefits Terminated by Primary Payer

Code 25 reports the date when insurance coverage (including workers' compensation benefits or no-fault coverage) is no longer available to the patient. This code is not required for Medicare billing. It is required, however, for Medicaid and TRICARE claims when it applies.

26   Date SNF Bed Became Available

Occurrence code 26 reports the date on which a SNF bed became available to a hospital inpatient who required only a SNF level of care. This code is required by Medicare when applicable. It is also required for commercial and TRICARE claims.

27   Date of Hospice Certification or Recertification

Code 27 reports the date of certification or recertification of the hospice benefit period, beginning with the first two initial benefit periods of ninety days each and the subsequent sixty-day benefit periods. This code is required for Medicare billing and by most other payers when applicable.

28   Date Comprehensive Outpatient Rehabilitation Facility Plan Established or Last Reviewed

Code 28 reports the date a comprehensive outpatient rehabilitation facility (CORF) plan of treatment was established or last reviewed. This code is required for Medicare and TRICARE billing when applicable. A hospital would not use this code for billing unless it owns the CORF.

29   Date Outpatient Physical Therapy Plan Established or Last Reviewed

Code 29 is used to report the date a plan of treatment was established or last reviewed for outpatient physical therapy. Code 29 is required for Medicare and TRICARE billing when applicable. When this code is used, the patient account specialist should verify that the claim contains a charge for physical therapy services (revenue code 042X in FL 42) and a corresponding diagnosis code (FL 67).

30   Date Outpatient Speech Pathology Plan Established or Last Reviewed

Code 30 is used to report the date a plan of treatment for outpatient speech pathology was established or last reviewed. This code is required for Medicare and TRICARE billing when applicable. When occurrence code 30 is reported, a charge for speech therapy services (revenue code 044X in FL 42) and at least one diagnosis code (FL 67) that reflects the need for speech therapy should also be present on the claim.

31 Date Beneficiary Notified of Intent to Bill (Accommodations)

Code 31 indicates the date the hospital provided notice to the patient that the patient no longer requires inpatient care and that coverage has therefore ended. This code is required for Medicare and TRICARE billing when applicable.

32 Date Beneficiary Notified of Intent to Bill (Procedures or Treatments)

Code 32 indicates the date of notice provided to the beneficiary by the hospital that the requested care (diagnostic procedures or treatments) may not be considered reasonable or necessary under Medicare. This code is required for Medicare and TRICARE billing when applicable. It indicates the date an advance beneficiary notice of noncoverage (ABN) was given to the beneficiary.

Only service for which an ABN was given should be reported on a claim with occurrence code 32. Services not pertaining to the ABN should be reported on a separate claim using different statement dates. However, if the statement dates are the same and a single claim containing both ABN and non-ABN services must be submitted, the modifier –GA should be appended to the HCPCS code (FL 44) for the line item associated with the ABN to set it apart.

33 First Day of the Medicare Coordination Period for ESRD Beneficiaries Covered by an EGHP

Code 33 indicates the first day of the coordination period during which Medicare or TRICARE benefits are secondary to benefits payable under an employer group health plan (EGHP). This code is required for end-stage renal disease (ESRD) beneficiaries only. It is required for Medicare ESRD and TRICARE billing when applicable.

34 Date of Election of Extended Care Services

Code 34 reports the date the patient chose to receive extended care services (used by religious nonmedical health care institutions only).

35 Date Treatment Started for Physical Therapy

Code 35 reports the date services were initiated for physical therapy. This code is required for Medicare billing when applicable. It is used for outpatient claims only.

Occurrence code 35 is used when physical therapy services are being billed on the claim (revenue code 042X in FL 42). It is used together with occurrence code 11 (Onset of symptoms/illness), occurrence code 29 (Date outpatient physical therapy plan established or last reviewed), and a relevant diagnosis code in FL 67. In FLs 39–41 (Value Codes and Amounts), value code 50 (Physical therapy visits) should be present with the total number of visits reported from the onset of treatment through this billing period.

Figure 10.2 on page 202 shows an outpatient claim for physical therapy that includes the required occurrence codes, value codes, and revenue codes.

Figure 10.2

Sample of Occurrence Codes, Value Codes, and Revenue Codes on a Physical Therapy Claim

31 OCCURRENCE CODE	DATE	32 OCCURRENCE CODE	DATE	33 OCCURRENCE CODE	DATE	34 OCCURRENCE CODE	DATE	35 CODE	OCCURRENCE SPAN FROM	THROUGH	36 CODE	OCCURRENCE SPAN FROM	THROUGH	37
a 11	021010	29	030110	35	030210									
b														

38					39 CODE	VALUE CODES AMOUNT	40 CODE	VALUE CODES AMOUNT	41 CODE	VALUE CODES AMOUNT
				a	50	5 00				
				b						
				c						
				d						

42 REV. CD.	43 DESCRIPTION	44 HCPCS / RATE / HIPPS CODE	45 SERV. DATE	46 SERV. UNITS	47 TOTAL CHARGES	48 NON-COVERED CHARGES	49
1 0421	PHYS THERP/VISIT	97110GP	030210	1	28 05		1
2 0421	PHYS THERP/VISIT	97110GP	030410	1	28 05		2
3 0421	PHYS THERP/VISIT	97140GP	030610	1	29 30		3
4 0421	PHYS THERP/VISIT	97140GP	030710	1	29 30		4
5 0421	PHYS THERP/VISIT	97140GP	031410	1	29 30		5
6 0424	PHYS THERP/EVAL	97001GP	030110	1	154 98		6
7							7
8							8
9							9
10							10
11							11
12							12
13							13
14							14
15							15
16							16
17							17
18							18
19							19
20							20
21							21
22							22
23 0001	**PAGE** 1 **OF** 1	**CREATION DATE** 033110	**TOTALS** ➡	298 98			23

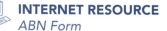

INTERNET RESOURCE

ABN Form

www.cms.hhs.gov/BNI/
Downloads/CMSR131G.pdf
Refer to Figure 3.2 for a draft of
the newly revised ABN.

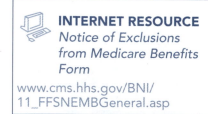

INTERNET RESOURCE

*Notice of Exclusions
from Medicare Benefits
Form*

www.cms.hhs.gov/BNI/
11_FFSNEMBGeneral.asp

Similar codes are used for billing occupational therapy, speech therapy, and cardiac rehabilitation.

36 Date of Inpatient Hospital Discharge for Covered Transplant Patient

Code 36 reports the date of discharge for an inpatient hospital stay during which the patient received a transplant procedure that is covered. It is required only when billing immunosuppressive drugs furnished to transplant patients. This code is required for Medicare billing when applicable.

37 Date of Inpatient Hospital Discharge for Noncovered Transplant Patient

Code 37 reports the discharge date for an inpatient hospital stay during which the patient received a noncovered transplant procedure. It is required only when billing immunosuppressive drugs furnished to transplant patients. This code is required for Medicare billing when applicable.

38 Date Treatment Started for Home IV Therapy

Code 38 is used to report the date the patient was first treated at home with IV therapy. It is required for Medicare billing when applicable and is used by home IV providers (TOB code 085X).

39 Date Discharged on a Continuous Course of IV Therapy

Code 39 reports the date the patient was discharged from the hospital on a continuous course of IV therapy. It is required for Medicare billing when applicable and is used by home IV providers (TOB code 085X).

Service-Related Codes

Occurrence codes that relate primarily to service issues are as follows.

40 Scheduled Date of Admission

Code 40 reports the date when a patient will be admitted to the hospital as an inpatient. This code may be used on an outpatient claim only. It is not required for Medicare billing, but it is required for commercial billing when applicable and must be used with code 41.

41 Date of First Test for Preadmission Testing

Code 41 indicates the date on which the first outpatient diagnostic test was performed as part of a preadmission testing program. This outpatient claim code is required for Medicare and commercial billing when applicable. It must be used with code 40, and the date of the first test must be the same day or before the admission date reported with code 40. It can be used only if the date of admission was scheduled prior to the administration of the tests.

42 Date of Discharge

Code 42 is used on hospice claims only. It indicates the date on which a beneficiary terminated his or her election to receive hospice benefits from the facility rendering the bill, or when hospice care ends due to decertification, revocation, or death. The frequency code in the TOB should be for a final bill (last digit 1 or 4). This code is required for Medicare and Medicaid billing whenever applicable.

43 Scheduled Date of Canceled Surgery

When an outpatient surgery is canceled, code 43 is used to indicate the date on which the surgery was scheduled.

44 Date Treatment Started for Occupational Therapy

Code 44 reports the date services were initiated for occupational therapy. This code is required for Medicare billing when applicable. It is used for outpatient claims only.

Occurrence code 44 is used when occupational therapy services are being billed on the claim (revenue code 043X in FL 42). It is used together with occurrence code 11 (Onset of symptoms/illness), occurrence code 17 (Date outpatient occupational therapy plan established or last reviewed), and a relevant diagnosis code in FL 67. In FLs 39–41 (Value Codes and Amounts), value code 51 (Occupational therapy visits) should be present with the total number of visits from the onset of treatment through this billing period reported.

45 Date Treatment Started for Speech Therapy

Code 45 reports the date services were initiated for speech therapy. This code is required for Medicare billing when applicable. It is used for outpatient claims only.

Occurrence code 45 is used when speech therapy services are being billed on the claim (revenue code 044X in FL 42). It is used together with occurrence code 11 (Onset of symptoms/illness), occurrence code 30 (Date outpatient speech therapy plan established or last reviewed), and a relevant diagnosis code in FL 67. In FLs 39–41 (Value Codes and Amounts), value code 52 (Speech therapy visits) should be present with the total number of visits from the onset of treatment through this billing period reported.

46 Date Treatment Started for Cardiac Rehabilitation

Code 46 reports the date services were initiated for cardiac rehabilitation. This code is required for Medicare billing when applicable. It is used for outpatient claims only.

Occurrence code 46 is used when cardiac rehabilitation services are being billed on the claim (revenue code 0943 in FL 42). It is used together with occurrence code 11 (Onset of symptoms/illness) and a relevant diagnosis code in FL 67. In FLs 39–41 (Value Codes and Amounts), value code 53 (Cardiac rehabilitation visits) should be present with the total number of visits from the onset of treatment through this billing period reported.

47 Date Cost Outlier Status Begins

Code 47 is used to report the first day of cost outlier status (the first day after the day the inpatient cost outlier threshold is reached). For Medicare purposes, a beneficiary must have regular coinsurance and/or lifetime reserve days available beginning on this date to allow coverage of additional daily charges for the purpose of making cost outlier payments. This code is required for Medicare billing when applicable.

48–49 Payer Codes

Providers do not report these codes.

50–69 Reserved for National Assignment

70–99 Reserved for Occurrence Span Codes

See occurrence span codes below.

A0 Reserved for National Assignment

A1 Birth Date—Insured A

Code A1 indicates the birth date of the person in whose name the insurance reported in FL 50 (Payer Name), line A, is carried.

A2 Effective Date—Insured A Policy

Code A2 indicates the first date the insurance listed in FL 50, line A, is in force.

A3 Benefits Exhausted

Code A3 indicates the last date for which benefits are available for the insurance listed in FL 50, line A, after which no payment can be made by payer A. This code is required for Medicare billing when applicable and is used to report the date on which the patient's Part A benefits have been exhausted.

A4   Split Bill Date

Code A4 reports the date the patient became eligible for Medicaid due to medically needy spenddown (sometimes referred to as the "split bill date").

A5–AZ Reserved for National Assignment

B0   Reserved for National Assignment

B1   Birth Date—Insured B

Code B1 indicates the birth date of the person in whose name the insurance reported in FL 50 (Payer Name), line B, is carried.

B2   Effective Date—Insured B Policy

Code B2 indicates the first date the insurance listed in FL 50, line B, is in force.

B3   Benefits Exhausted

Code B3 indicates the last date for which benefits are available for the insurance listed in FL 50, line B, after which no payment can be made by payer B. This code is required for Medicare billing when applicable.

B4–BZ Reserved for National Assignment

C0   Reserved for National Assignment

C1   Birth Date—Insured C

Code C1 indicates the birth date of the person in whose name the insurance reported in FL 50 (Payer Name), line C, is carried.

C2   Effective Date—Insured C Policy

Code C2 indicates the first date the insurance listed in FL 50, line C, is in force.

C3   Benefits Exhausted

Code C3 indicates the last date for which benefits are available for the insurance listed in FL 50, line C, after which no payment can be made by payer C. This code is required for Medicare billing when applicable.

C4–CZ Reserved for National Assignment

D0–DQ Reserved for National Assignment

DR   Reserved for Disaster-Related Code

DS–LZ   Reserved for National Assignment

Occurrence codes pertaining to Insured E, F, and G (codes E1–E3, F1–F3, and G1–G3) were discontinued on March 1, 2007.

M0–ZZ   Reserved for Occurrence Span Codes

See the following section on occurrence span codes.

Occurrence span codes and dates identify significant events that happened over a span of time and that affect claim processing and payment.

Figure 10.3

UB-04 Form—FLs 31–38, with Occurrence Span Code Fields Highlighted

31 OCCURRENCE CODE DATE	32 OCCURRENCE CODE DATE	33 OCCURRENCE CODE DATE	34 OCCURRENCE CODE DATE	35 OCCURRENCE SPAN CODE FROM THROUGH	36 OCCURRENCE SPAN CODE FROM THROUGH	37
a						a
b						b

38		39 VALUE CODES CODE AMOUNT	40 VALUE CODES CODE AMOUNT	41 VALUE CODES CODE AMOUNT
	a			
	b			
	c			
	d			

FYI

Occurrence Span Codes

An **occurrence span code** is a two-digit numeric or alphanumeric code describing an event that occurred over a period of time that relates to the current billing period. Every occurrence span code must be accompanied by a beginning (from) date and an ending (through) date. The dates should be recorded in the appropriate From and Through boxes to the right of each occurrence span code on the UB-04 using the MMDDYY format. (*Note:* The electronic version of the UB-04 requires the CCYYMMDD format when reporting dates.)

INTERNET RESOURCE
Provider Type: Skilled Nursing Facility
www.cms.hhs.gov/center/snf.asp

Guidelines

Occurrence span codes and dates must be completed for Medicare claims and for commercial and TRICARE claims when they apply. They may be required by Medicaid if applicable. For Blue Cross billing, they are required only when specified under a particular plan or contract.

If more than one code is reported, enter the codes in alphanumeric sequence (with numeric codes preceding alphanumeric codes) in the following order: FLs 35a and 36a should be filled in first (line 1), then FLs 35b and 36b (line 2). If more than four codes are required, FL 81 (Code-Code field) may be used with the appropriate qualifier (A3) to report the overflow (FL 81 is covered in Chapter 15, "Physician Information, Remarks, and Code-Code Field").

There are two ranges of occurrence span codes: 70–99 and M0–ZZ.

70   Qualifying Stay Dates for SNF Use Only

Code 70 indicates the from and through dates when the patient was hospitalized for at least a three-day inpatient stay (excluding the day of discharge). This is the required time period to qualify the patient for Medicare payment of the SNF services billed on this claim. The code is required for Medicare Part A SNF level of care billing only when applicable.

71   Prior Stay Dates

Code 71 indicates the from and through dates supplied by the patient for any hospitalization that ended within sixty days of the present hospital or SNF admission. This code is required for Medicare Part A billing only when applicable. It is also required for TRICARE billing. It is not valid for outpatient claims. Similar to occurrence span code 78 described below, code 71 is used to report a continued spell of illness (see FYI on page 207).

72   First/Last Visit Dates

Code 72 indicates the actual dates of the first and last outpatient visits occurring in this billing period when these dates differ from those in FL 6, Statement Covers Period. This code is required for Medicare and commercial billing when it applies. It is used for repetitive and related services that are submitted on one monthly bill. The dates should be the first and last times the patient visited during the statement period reported in FL 6.

73 Benefit Eligibility Period

Code 73, for TRICARE claims only, reports the inclusive dates during which TRICARE medical benefits are available to a sponsor's beneficiary as shown on the beneficiary's identification card.

74 Noncovered Level of Care/Leave of Absence Dates

Code 74 reports the from and through dates of a period that is at a noncovered level of care or that represents a leave of absence during an otherwise covered stay. The code excludes any period reported with occurrence span code 76 (Patient liability), 77 (Provider liability period), or 79 (Payer code only) described below. Note that most noncovered care is reported with codes 76 and 77. Code 74 is required for Medicare and TRICARE billing when applicable.

75 SNF Level of Care Dates

Code 75 indicates the from and through dates of a period of SNF level of care during an inpatient hospital stay. It does not apply to swing bed hospitals. This code is required for Medicare and TRICARE billing when applicable.

76 Patient Liability

Code 76 reports the from and through dates for a period of noncovered care for which the hospital is permitted to charge the Medicare beneficiary. Code 76 is used together with occurrence code 31 (Date beneficiary notified of intent to bill—accommodations) and/or code 32 (Date beneficiary notified of intent to bill—procedures or treatment) in FLs 31–34. Code 76 should be used only when the fiscal intermediary or QIO has approved the charges in advance and the patient has been notified in writing three days prior to the from date. This code is required for Medicare billing when applicable.

77 Provider Liability Period—Utilization Charged

Code 77 reports the from and through dates for a period of noncovered care (other than custodial care or care that lacks medical necessity) for which the provider is liable. The beneficiary's record is charged by the fiscal intermediary with Part A days used, Part A or Part B deductible, and Part B coinsurance. Only the Part A or Part B deductible and coinsurance may be collected from the beneficiary. This code is required for Medicare billing if applicable.

Code 77 is used either separately or with occurrence span code 76 (Patient liability) to indicate that the bill is for noncovered services. It may be used, for example, when the provider is responsible for part of the admission. The total of noncovered days is reported in FLs 39–41 with value code 81 (Noncovered days).

78 SNF Prior Stay Dates

Code 78 reports the from and through dates, as reported by the patient, for any SNF or nursing home stay that ended within sixty days of the present hospital or SNF admission. It is used to indicate a continued spell of illness. This code is for Part A claims only.

79 Payer Code

This code is not for provider reporting.

80–99 Reserved for National Assignment

> **FYI**
>
> **Spell of Illness**
> A **spell of illness** is a benefit period for hospitalization as defined by a health plan. For Medicare patients, a spell of illness begins with admission to a hospital or other facility and ends when the patient has not received inpatient care anywhere for sixty consecutive days. A Medicare beneficiary pays a deductible for each benefit period.
>
> For example, a Medicare patient is admitted on May 1 and discharged on May 5. Until sixty days after discharge (July 3), the same spell of illness is in effect. If the patient is readmitted within this sixty-day period, the beneficiary is not required to pay the Medicare deductible because he or she is in the same spell of illness, regardless of the reason for readmission.

> **FYI**
>
> **Leave of Absence Days**
> **Leave of absence (LOA) days** are days during which a patient is temporarily discharged from the hospital, with readmission expected for follow-up care or surgery. LOA situations occur, for example, when surgery cannot be scheduled right away or a specific surgical team is not available, and the patient does not require hospitalization during the interim period. The patient may also need further treatment that cannot be given immediately.

M0 QIO/UR Approved Stay Dates

Code M0 is used to report the from and through dates of the approved portion of a billing period if condition code C3 (Partial approval) is used in FLs 18–28. This code indicates that the total days or services provided in this billing period have been subject to medical review and partially denied and that the dates shown represent the approved portion. It is required for Medicare billing as well as by all other payers when applicable.

M1 Provider Liability—No Utilization

Code M1 indicates the from and through dates for a period of noncovered care that is denied as custodial care or due to a lack of medical necessity and for which the provider is liable. The beneficiary is not charged with utilization. The provider may not collect the Part A or Part B deductible or coinsurance from the beneficiary. This code is required for Medicare billing when applicable.

M2 Dates of Inpatient Respite Care

Code M2 indicates the from and through dates of a period of inpatient respite care for hospice patients (TOB 81X or 82X). It is required for Medicare billing if applicable.

M3 Intermediate Care Facility (ICF) Level of Care

Code M3 is used to report the from and through dates of a period of intermediate level of care during an inpatient hospital stay.

M4 Residential Level of Care

Code M4 is used to report the from and through dates of a period of residential level of care during an inpatient stay.

M5–MQ Reserved for National Assignment

MR Reserved for Disaster-Related Occurrence Span Code

MS–ZZ Reserved for National Assignment

FL 37 Unlabeled Field

FL 38 Responsible Party Name and Address

FL 38 is used for reporting the name and address of the party responsible for the bill (the beneficiary or someone handling the beneficiary's affairs). Completion of this field is not required by Medicare, Blue Cross, Medicaid, or TRICARE. For commercial claims, however, completion of the field is desirable. When a window envelope is used for mailing the bill, the name and mailing address of the responsible party will show through the window.

For Medicare claims, the five blank lines in FL 38 may be used to report the name and address of the other payer when a claim involves a payer that is primary to Medicare. FL 80, Remarks, may also be used to report this information.

1 FLs 31–34 on the UB-04 are used for reporting occurrence codes—two-digit numeric or alphanumeric codes that identify significant events connected with a claim that affect its processing and payment. Payers use occurrence code information and corresponding dates to determine liability issues, coordinate benefits, clarify patient eligibility, and make final decisions about the benefits due on a claim.

2 Occurrence codes are generally grouped into four categories for ease of reference: accident-related codes, medical condition codes, insurance-related codes, and service-related codes.

3 FLs 35–36 on the UB-04 are used to record occurrence span codes and dates. Like occurrence codes, occurrence span codes identify significant events—that occur over a period of time—that influence the payment process. For example, occurrence span code 76 (Patient liability) and its corresponding dates indicate the period of noncovered care for which the hospital is permitted to charge the Medicare beneficiary.

4 Various billing situations arise when particular occurrence codes and occurrence span codes are used. For example, the accident-related occurrence codes (01–06) indicate that Medicare is not the primary payer for the claim and that MSP provisions apply. If code 24 (Date insurance denied) is used to bill Medicare for a conditional payment, the claim must contain an explanation of the request for the conditional payment in the Remarks field (FL 80); without such an explanation, the payer will not be able to process the claim properly. When occurrence span code 74 (Noncovered level of care/leave of absence dates) is used, it excludes any period reported with the usual occurrence span codes that are used to report noncovered care (codes 76 and 77).

5 Most occurrence codes and occurrence span codes contain data that must be coordinated with data in several other fields on the UB-04. For example, when an accident code is used, the accident hour as well as the appropriate value code and amount paid by the primary payer must also be reported in FLs 39–41 (Value Codes and Amounts). Similarly, when occurrence span code 76 (Patient liability) is used to report a span of noncovered care for which the patient is responsible, FLs 39–41 should report the appropriate value code and amount the patient is responsible for, as well as the appropriate value code to report the total number of noncovered days and either occurrence code 31 (Date beneficiary notified of intent to bill—accommodations) or 32 (Date beneficiary notified of intent to bill—procedures or treatment).

6 FL 37 on the UB-04 is an unlabeled field that is reserved for national assignment. FL 38, Responsible Party Name and Address, is used mostly by commercial carriers. The name and address of the party responsible for the bill are recorded in this form locator and can show through when the bill is mailed in a window envelope. Although not required for Medicare claims, FL 38 may be used to report the name and address of a payer that is primary to Medicare when Medicare is not the primary payer on the claim.

✔ CHECK YOUR UNDERSTANDING

1. Define the following terms and specify the form locators they occupy on the UB-04.

   a. occurrence codes _____

   _____

   b. occurrence span codes _____

   _____

2. Which of the following categories are used for grouping occurrence codes?

   a. insurance-related codes

   b. special program indicator codes

   c. condition codes

   d. accident-related codes

3. Which of the following form locators should be used to report an occurrence span code and its corresponding dates when FLs 35a and 36a are full?

   a. FL 37

   b. FL 80

   c. FL 81

   d. FL 35b

4. True or False: Occurrence codes range from 01–99, and occurrence span codes range from A0–ZZ. _____

5. Occurrence code 44 (Date treatment started for occupational therapy) is used for which claims only?

   a. Medicare

   b. rehabilitation

   c. inpatient

   d. outpatient

6. True or False: Occurrence code 21 (UR notice received) is used with value code 46 (Number of grace days) to report the number of grace days required for arranging the patient's postdischarge care. _____

7. Determine which occurrence codes or occurrence span codes apply in the following situations. In several situations, more than one code may apply.

   a. The patient's medical condition resulted from an accident at work on this day. _____

   b. One week after the onset of symptoms, a speech pathology plan was established; the speech therapy treatment began on the following day. _____

   c. The patient reported the dates of a prior hospital stay, and these dates were a month ago, indicating the same spell of illness benefit period for the current hospital admission. _____

   d. The patient is being held liable for two days of noncovered care in a hospital after being notified in writing six days ago that a continued stay was noncovered. _____

   e. On this day, a patient was discharged from the hospital and placed on a continuous course of home IV therapy. _____

   f. A Medicare beneficiary has spent down her money as of this date and has become eligible for Medicaid. _____

   g. This three-day stay in the hospital qualified the patient for Medicare Part A SNF benefits billed on the claim. _____

   h. A patient was scheduled for admission on this date. The first preadmission testing began one day before. _____

i. During this period of an inpatient hospital stay, the beneficiary was at an intermediate level of care. _____

j. The patient's medical condition is the result of an alleged criminal action on the date reported. _____

k. The provider has reason to believe that the liability insurer will not pay promptly because the claim, which involves an auto accident, is being held up in a lengthy litigation process. The provider is therefore billing Medicare for a conditional payment. _____

8. When occurrence code 31 (Date beneficiary notified of intent to bill—accommodations) is reported on a claim, which of the following items should also be reported on the UB-04?

a. time span of the patient liability (occurrence span code)

b. number of noncovered days (value code)

c. Medicare rate code (value code)

d. amount of patient liability (value code)

9. Answer the following questions based on the top portion of the UB-04 form shown here. Appendix A contains a table of occurrence codes for quick reference.

UB-04 Form—FLs 1–49

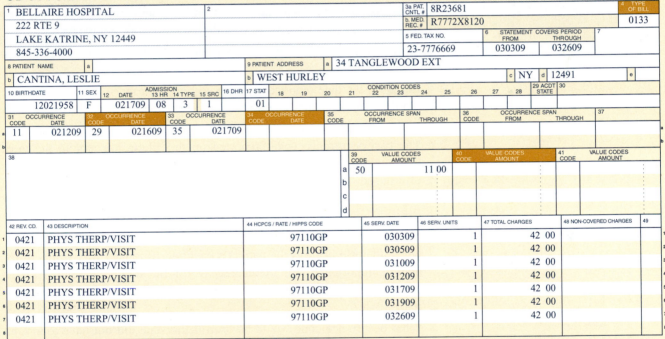

a. Based on the TOB (0133), is this the first physical therapy claim for the patient for this condition? _____

b. Has the patient finished treatment? _____ Explain. _____

c. Do the dates of service in FL 45, lines 1–7, correspond with the dates reported in FL 6 (Statement Covers Period)? _____

d. Based on the data in FLs 31–33, when was the patient evaluated for physical therapy treatment? _____

e. When did the patient begin receiving treatment? _____

f. How many treatments are being reported on this claim? _____

g. Value code 50 in FL 39 is used to report the number of physical therapy visits from the onset of treatment through this billing period. How many treatments did the patient receive in February? _____

h. When did the patient first become aware of the symptoms that are being treated? _____

UB-04 Activity: Claim Analysis

Working with Occurrence Codes: FLs 31–34

Open the file **Sample01.pdf** in Adobe Reader, and answer the following questions:

1. What is the first occurrence code reported on the claim? What does it indicate?

2. Before using the ICD-9-CM codebook to look up the principle diagnosis code (FL 67), make an educated guess at what type of treatment the patient received based on the description of services in FL 43? The description OR SERVICES in FL 43 indicates surgery. What type of surgery do you think the patient had?

3. Locate a copy of the ICD-9-CM codebook, and look up the diagnosis code reported in FL 67 to determine the patient's principal diagnosis. Refer to Chapter 4 if necessary for information on using the ICD-9-CM. What diagnosis does the code indicate? Based on the date reported in FL 31, how long has the patient been aware of this illness or its symptoms?

4. What is the second occurrence code reported on the claim? What does it indicate?

5. Based on the date reported with the second occurrence code, at what age did the patient retire? Given that Medicare is the payer on the claim, why is the patient's retirement information reported?

6. The two occurrence codes reported on this claim are among the most often used codes. In addition, accident-related occurrence codes are often used. Suppose a separate claim for this patient is being prepared and the patient has been in an auto accident in a state that has no-fault liability laws. What occurrence code would be used to report the date of the accident?

7. Given that Medicare is the patient's primary insurance, why is this information important? Will Medicare pay for the treatment related to the auto accident? What is the main purpose of an accident-related occurrence code?

8. What occurrence code would be used if the state did not have a no-fault policy for auto accidents?

9. What other form locator is filled in when the claim involves an auto accident in particular?

10. If the patient tripped over his pet at home and broke his arm, what accident-related occurrence code would be used to report the date of the accident?

When finished viewing the claim, click Exit on the File menu.

Value Codes and Amounts

LEARNING OUTCOMES

After completing this chapter, you will be able to define the key terms and:

1 Describe the types of value codes that are used in FLs 39–41 on the UB-04 to report monetary data that affect the way the claim is processed and paid.

2 Explain the relationship between value codes and the dollar amounts, units, or number of visits that are reported with them.

3 Recognize various billing patterns that arise in connection with value codes.

4 Understand which value codes contain data that must be coordinated with data supplied in other fields on the UB-04.

KEY TERMS

- Medicare blood deductible
- MSP value code
- noncovered days
- value code

Hospital bills routinely include information about monetary amounts. Examples include the amount of a no-fault insurance payment made on behalf of a Medicare beneficiary and the amount to be applied to the patient's deductible by the provider. These financial data elements are grouped together under a set of codes called value codes. Depending on the billing circumstances, the appropriate value codes and related amounts are recorded in FLs 39–41 on the UB-04. Several lines are provided in each field because more than one value code is often required on a single claim.

The payer needs to know the information conveyed by the value code and amount in order to pay the claim accurately and in a timely manner. This chapter provides instructions on what value codes are available, how related dollar amounts (units or number of visits) are reported for each code, and which codes are required in various billing situations. The codes relate to a wide range of billing circumstances.

In this chapter, each numerical value code is briefly described, and important details and billing tips are explained. General value codes are listed first, followed by a group of codes that are mostly specific to home health services or are payer-only codes. At the end of the chapter, the relevant alphanumeric codes (A0–ZZ) are described. Appendix A provides a list of value codes for quick reference.

Figure 11.1

UB-04 Form—FLs 39–41

	39 CODE	VALUE CODES AMOUNT	40 CODE	VALUE CODES AMOUNT	41 CODE	VALUE CODES AMOUNT
a						
b						
c						
d						

FLs 39–41 Value Codes and Amounts

FYI

Value Codes

A **value code** is a two-digit numeric or alphanumeric code used to identify a dollar amount, unit amount, or number of visits associated with a claim. The payer needs the information relayed through value codes to determine the patient's benefits and process the claim accurately.

FLs 39–41 on the UB-04 are used to report the appropriate value codes and their related dollar amounts, units, or number of visits. Completion of this field is required for Medicare billing and by most other payers when it is applicable. The codes range from 01 to 99 and A0 to ZZ. (Most of the alphanumeric value codes are reserved for national assignment.) Codes should be reported in alphanumeric order if more than one code is used.

Guidelines

Every value code must be accompanied by an amount. The amount can be expressed either as a dollar amount—for example, the cost of a semiprivate room—or as the number of visits or units—for example, the total number of physical therapy visits or the weight of a newborn in grams.

On Medicare Part A claims, which are processed through a computer system known as the Fiscal Intermediary Shared System (FISS), a nondollar amount that is reported with a value code must end with two zeros. For example, the number for thirteen therapy visits is recorded as 13.00, and the period of two grace days is recorded as 2.00. If the two zeros are not reported, the FISS will fill them in automatically. Therefore, either format, with or without the zeros, can be used. For the purposes of this text, the two zeros are used for all nondollar amounts.

FLs 39–41 can accommodate dollar amounts of up to nine digits, including the two digits for cents—for example, $1,000,000.00. Additional details on how to report amounts for particular codes are included along with the code descriptions.

Because the UB-04 contains a delimiter in FLs 39–41, decimal points do not have to be keyed. A delimiter is a character that separates one item from another; in this case, the delimiter is a dotted vertical line that separates dollars from cents. Whole numbers or nondollar amounts are right justified to the left of the delimiter, and cents are entered in the two positions to the right of the delimiter.

As shown in Figure 11.1, the UB-04 form contains four lines for reporting value codes, labeled a, b, c, and d. The top line should be filled in fully before beginning the next line, and so on. This means that FLs 39a–41a should be used first, followed by FLs 39b–41b, FLs 39c–41c, and FLs 39d–41d.

If all value code fields have been filled in, FL 81 (Code-Code field) can be used with the appropriate value code qualifier (A4) to report additional value codes and amounts (Chapter 15, "Physician Information, Remarks, and Code-Code Field," discusses FL 81).

General Codes

The available value codes are described below.

01 Most Common Semiprivate Room Rate

Code 01 reports the billing facility's most common semiprivate room rate. This code is not required for Medicare billing. If it applies, it is required for commercial and TRICARE billing.

02 Hospital Has No Semiprivate Rooms

Code 02 indicates that the provider has no semiprivate rooms available. Enter an amount of 0.00 ($0.00) in the Value Amount field when using code 02. This code is not required for Medicare billing. If it applies, it is required for commercial and TRICARE billing.

03 Reserved for National Assignment

04 Inpatient Professional Component Charges That Are Combined Billed

Value code 04 is used to report the sum of the inpatient professional component charges that are being combined billed. The professional component charges refer to the charges of the physician, which are normally billed separately from the hospital's charges. This code is required for Medicare billing when applicable. It is used by some all-inclusive rate hospitals only. Medicare uses this information in internal processes and also in the CMS (Centers for Medicare and Medicaid Services) notice of utilization sent to the patient to explain that the beneficiary is responsible for the Part B coinsurance on the professional component.

05 Professional Component Included in Charges and Also Billed Separately to Carrier

Code 05 indicates that the charges related to the professional fee are included in the Total Charges field (FL 47), but that a separate billing for them will also be made. Value code 05 is therefore used to subtract professional component charges from the total covered charges listed on inpatient claims. This amount is deducted when calculating the reimbursement amount.

FYI

Medicare Blood Deductible

Medicare beneficiaries must pay for the first three pints of blood they use in a given year. This is called the **Medicare blood deductible.** Any additional pints of blood are paid by Medicare. The three-pint deductible applies to both Part A and Part B benefits, which means that it can be satisfied under either Part A benefits or Part B benefits.

The blood product benefits under Part B vary somewhat from those under Part A. Under Part B, there is a cash deductible in addition to the three-pint deductible. Also, as with other Part B benefits, Medicare pays for 80 percent of the approved amount, and the patient is responsible for the remaining 20 percent.

Instead of paying for the first three pints of blood used, beneficiaries may replace the blood used with their own blood (or with the blood another person donated on their behalf). In this case, the hospital cannot charge them for the blood they used, although it may charge them for storing and processing their replacement blood. This is done by reporting revenue code 0390 (Administration, processing, and storage for blood and blood components) in FL 42.

The patient may also meet the blood deductible by paying for one or two pints and replacing the rest. A combination of value codes is required in most cases to cover the different possibilities.

The professional charges to Medicare, which are being billed separately, should be billed on the CMS-1500. Code 05 is used in instances when the professional charges have been reported on both claim forms. Code 05 can also be used on Medicaid claims and is required for TRICARE billing if applicable.

06   Medicare Blood Deductible

Value code 06 is used to report the total cash blood deductible amount paid by the beneficiary. The amount reported is calculated by multiplying the number of pints of blood supplied to the patient by the charge per unit. This code is required for Medicare when applicable.

Revenue code 038X (Blood and blood components) is used in FL 42 to charge the patient for the blood, and value code 06 is used to report how much the patient paid for blood on the claim. Note that it is not necessary to use code 06 if the patient has replaced all deductible pints. Code 06 is used only when the beneficiary is paying for blood used rather than replacing it.

Value code 37 (Pints of blood furnished) should be used in combination with value code 06 to keep track of the number of blood deductible pints furnished (up to three total) for which the patient is responsible.

07   Reserved for National Assignment

08   Medicare Lifetime Reserve Amount in the First Calendar Year

Value code 08 is used to report the Medicare lifetime reserve amount charged in the first calendar year of the billing period—the year of admission—for an inpatient bill that spans two calendar years. This amount is calculated by multiplying the number of lifetime reserve days by the applicable lifetime reserve coinsurance rate. The code is required for Medicare billing for Part A claims only.

09   Medicare Coinsurance Amount in the First Calendar Year in Billing Period

Value code 09 is used to report the Medicare coinsurance amounts charged in the first calendar year of the billing period—the year of admission—for an inpatient bill that spans two calendar years. This amount is calculated by multiplying the number of coinsurance days by the applicable coinsurance rate. This code is required for Medicare billing for Part A claims only.

10   Medicare Lifetime Reserve Amount in the Second Calendar Year in Billing Period

Value code 10 indicates the Medicare lifetime reserve amount charged in the year of discharge for a bill that spans two calendar years. This amount is calculated by multiplying the number of lifetime reserve days used in the second calendar year of the billing period by the applicable lifetime reserve coinsurance rate. This code is required for Medicare billing for Part A claims only.

11   Medicare Coinsurance Amount for Second Calendar Year

Value code 11 indicates the Medicare coinsurance amount charged in the year of discharge for a bill that spans two calendar years. This amount is calculated by multiplying the number of coinsurance days used in the second calendar year of the billing period by the applicable coinsurance rate. This code is required for Medicare billing for Part A claims only.

12 Working Aged Beneficiary/Spouse with EGHP

Value code 12 reflects the portion of the EGHP (employer group health plan) payment made for a working aged beneficiary that the provider is applying to covered Medicare charges on the bill. This code indicates that the EGHP is the primary payer and Medicare the secondary payer (see Billing Tip on page 218). Code 12 is required for Medicare billing if it applies.

13 ESRD Beneficiary in a Medicare Coordination Period with an EGHP

Code 13 shows the EGHP payment made on behalf of an ESRD beneficiary. This code is an MSP value code. It is required for Medicare billing when applicable. If the beneficiary's age (FL 10, Birth Date) is over sixty-four, code 13 is not valid.

When this value code is reported, occurrence code 33 (First day of the Medicare coordination period for ESRD beneficiaries covered by an EGHP) and its corresponding date must also be used.

14 No-Fault, Including Auto/Other

Code 14 shows the no-fault (including auto or other) insurance payment made on behalf of the patient or insured. This MSP value code is required for Medicare billing when applicable. The provider applies this amount to the Medicare-covered services on the bill for a Medicare beneficiary. For auto accidents, use value code 14 only if the state is a no-fault state. In a liability state, use value code 47 (Any liability insurance).

When value code 14 is used, occurrence code 02 (No-fault insurance involved—including auto accident/other) must also be used, with the corresponding date of the accident (FLs 31–34).

15 Workers' Compensation

Code 15 shows the workers' compensation payment made on behalf of the patient or insured. This MSP value code is required for Medicare billing when applicable. The provider applies this amount to the Medicare-covered services on the bill for a Medicare beneficiary. When value code 15 is used, occurrence code 04 (Accident—employment-related) and the corresponding date of the accident must also be used.

16 Public Health Service (PHS) or Other Federal Agency

Code 16 shows payment made on behalf of a Medicare beneficiary by the PHS or other federal agency that the provider is applying to Medicare-covered services on the bill. This MSP value code is required for Medicare billing when applicable.

17–20 Reserved for Payer Use Only

Providers do not report these codes.

Note

Codes 21–24 pertain to Medicaid eligibility requirements to be determined at the state level.

FYI

Billing Over a Two-Year Span

Two different codes are used when reporting Medicare lifetime reserve days (LRDs) or coinsurance days on the UB-04 when the billing period spans two years. One code is used for the first calendar year, or the year of admission, and the second code is used for the second calendar year, or the year of discharge (see value codes 08 through 11).

The two sets of codes are used because the rates for LRDs or coinsurance days vary from year to year. The LRD rate is always one-half of the annual inpatient deductible, and the coinsurance rate is always one-fourth of the annual inpatient deductible. Because the annual inpatient deductible changes each year, the rates for the LRDs and coinsurance days vary as well.

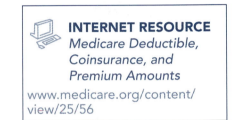

INTERNET RESOURCE
Medicare Deductible, Coinsurance, and Premium Amounts

www.medicare.org/content/view/25/56

$ $ Billing Tip $ $

Part A Versus Part B Coinsurance Value Codes

Value codes 09 and 11 are used for reporting Medicare Part A coinsurance amounts (the third digit in the TOB code in FL 4 must be 1, for inpatient). For reporting Part B coinsurance amounts when required, value codes A2, B2, or C2, described at the end of the chapter, are used.

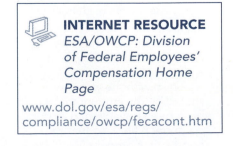

INTERNET RESOURCE
ESA/OWCP: Division of Federal Employees' Compensation Home Page

www.dol.gov/esa/regs/compliance/owcp/fecacont.htm

$$ Billing Tip $$

MSP Value Codes

There are nine value codes, referred to as **MSP value codes,** that identify the primary payers when Medicare is the secondary payer. The MSP value codes and their corresponding amounts indicate the amount paid on behalf of the beneficiary by the primary payer. In each case, Medicare is being billed as secondary for the Medicare-covered services on the claim.

The MSP value codes are as follows:

12 Working aged beneficiary/ spouse with an EGHP
13 ESRD beneficiary in a Medicare coordination period with an EGHP
14 No-fault, including auto/other
15 Workers' compensation
16 Public Health Service (PHS) or other federal agency
41 Black lung
42 Veterans Affairs
43 Disabled beneficiary under age sixty-five with LGHP
47 Any liability insurance

Note the following points that apply to all claims containing MSP value codes:

- The patient account specialist must make sure that document-ation in the patient account substantiates the MSP development.

- If an MSP value code is used with a Medicare Conditional Payment request because the primary payer has denied coverage or there has been a substantial delay in payment, enter six zeros (0000.00) in the amount field.

- The amount reported with any of the MSP value codes will be subtracted from the total reported charges to determine the amount Medicare owes the beneficiary on the claim.

- In cases where no payment or a reduced payment has been re-ceived because of failure to file a proper claim, the amount reported with the value code should be the amount that would have been payable had a proper claim been filed, so that the appropriate amount Medicare owes may be determined.

21 Catastrophic

22 Surplus

23 Recurring Monthly Income

24 Medicaid Rate Code

Note

Codes 25–29, and 33–35 below, are used to report the amounts that were paid out of the funds of a long-term care facility resident during the billing period on the claim (FL 6, Statement Covers Period) for various services, such as for prescription drugs, hearing and ear services, and podiatric services.

25 Offset to the Patient-Payment Amount— Prescription Drugs

26 Offset to the Patient-Payment Amount—Hearing and Ear Services

27 Offset to the Patient-Payment Amount—Vision and Eye Services

28 Offset to the Patient-Payment Amount—Dental Services

29 Offset to the Patient-Payment Amount— Chiropractic Services

30 Preadmission Testing

Value code 30 is used to report charges for preadmission outpatient testing (diagnostic services) that were done in preparation for a previously scheduled admission. This code is not valid for Medicare billing. It is required for Blue Cross, commercial, and TRICARE billing if it applies.

31 Patient Liability Amount

Code 31 shows the charges to be billed to the beneficiary for days of inpatient care that were considered unnecessary (noncovered accommodations, diag-nostic procedures, or treatments). This code is required for Medicare and TRICARE billing when applicable. Charges connected with this code should be listed in FL 48 (Noncovered Charges). For Medicare claims, this code indicates that the fiscal intermediary (FI) has approved the amount.

32 Multiple Patient Ambulance Transport

Code 32 is used to report the total number of patients transported if more than one patient is transported in a single ambulance trip.

33 Offset to the Patient-Payment Amount—Podiatric Services

34   Offset to the Patient-Payment Amount—Other Medical Services

35   Offset to the Patient-Payment Amount—Health Insurance Premiums

36   Reserved for National Assignment

37   Pints of Blood Furnished

Code 37 indicates the total number of pints of whole blood or units of packed red cells furnished, whether they were replaced or not, for which the patient is responsible (up to three pints annually). This code is required by Medicare and all other third-party payers when applicable.

On Medicare claims, the total pints of blood furnished to the patient, both replaced (value code 39 below) and not replaced, should be reported with this value code. Blood should be reported in terms of complete pints only, rounded up. For example, 1 1/4 pints is shown as 2 pints.

38   Blood Deductible Pints

Code 38 is used to report the number of unreplaced pints of whole blood or units of packed red cells furnished for which the patient is responsible. This code is required for Medicare and Medicaid billing if it applies. The value reported with code 38 cannot be greater than three, since the beneficiary is responsible for no more than three deductible pints of blood annually. If the beneficiary replaces all three pints or makes arrangements for the replacement, this code should not be used.

39   Pints of Blood Replaced

Code 39 indicates the total number of pints of blood or units of packed red cells that were donated by the patient or by someone else on the patient's behalf. Every donated pint is considered a replaced pint. In addition, if arrangements have been made for replacement, pints are shown as replaced. This code is required for Medicare billing when applicable.

40   New Coverage Not Implemented by HMO (for Inpatient Service Only)

Value code 40 is used to report inpatient charges covered by a Medicare-participating HMO. This code is used when the bill includes inpatient charges for newly covered services that are not paid by the HMO because the HMO has not yet implemented them. This information is reported so that Medicare will consider paying the balance that the HMO did not cover. Condition codes 04 (Information only bill) and 78 (New coverage not implemented by managed care plan) should also be reported. This code is required for Medicare billing when applicable.

41   Black Lung

Code 41 reflects the federal black lung program payment made on behalf of a Medicare beneficiary. This MSP value code is required for Medicare billing when applicable.

$ $ Billing Tip $ $

Value Code 31

Value code 31 should be used with occurrence code 31 (Date beneficiary notified of intent to bill) (FLs 31–34), and occurrence span code 76 (Patient liability) (FLs 35–36). The patient should already have signed a notice for denial of a continued stay of inpatient care.

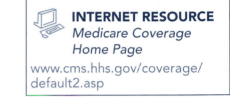

INTERNET RESOURCE
Medicare Coverage Home Page
www.cms.hhs.gov/coverage/default2.asp

$ $ Billing Tip $ $

Value Codes 38 and 39

If the pints of blood replaced (value code 39) do not equal the blood deductible reported with value code 38 (Blood deductible pints) then value code 06 (Medicare blood deductible) must also be reported. Code 06 indicates that the beneficiary is being charged for the furnished blood that was not replaced in order to meet the requirement of paying for and/or replacing three pints annually.

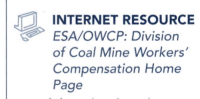

INTERNET RESOURCE
ESA/OWCP: Division of Coal Mine Workers' Compensation Home Page
www.dol.gov/esa/regs/compliance/owcp/bltable.htm

42   Veterans Affairs

Code 42 reflects the Veterans Affairs (VA) payment made on behalf of a Medicare beneficiary. This MSP value code is required for Medicare billing, when applicable. The primary payer in FL 50 (Payer Name), line A, must be described as "Veterans Affairs" or "VA."

43   Disabled Beneficiary Under Age Sixty-Five with LGHP

Code 43 shows the LGHP (large group health plan) payment made on behalf of a Medicare beneficiary. This MSP value code is required for Medicare billing, when applicable. It is not valid if the beneficiary's age (FL 10, Birth Date) is greater than sixty-four years.

44   Amount Provider Agreed to Accept from Primary Payer When This Amount Is Less Than Charges but Higher Than Payment Received

Code 44 shows the amount the provider was obligated or required to accept from a primary payer as payment in full (that is, the expected allowed amount). A secondary payment (MSP or TRICARE) may be due because the amount received is less than the total charges and less than the expected allowed amount.

Use value code 44 to report the amount the provider is obligated to accept from the primary payer (the allowed amount) and MSP value codes 12–16, 41–43, or 47 to show the amount the primary payer actually paid. For this code to be applicable, the allowed amount should always be greater than or equal to the amount paid.

45   Accident Hour

Code 45 is used to report the time of the accident that necessitated medical treatment. This code is not required for Medicare billing, but is often used. It is required for commercial billing if applicable.

Hours are indicated by a two-digit code, as listed in Table 11.1. The appropriate code is entered to the left of the delimiter in FLs 39–41; the cents area to the right of the delimiter should contain two zeros.

Table 11.1

Hour Codes

Code	A.M.	Code	P.M.
00	12:00 (midnight)–12:59	12	12:00 (noon)–12:59
01	1:00–1:59	13	1:00–1:59
02	2:00–2:59	14	2:00–2:59
03	3:00–3:59	15	3:00–3:59
04	4:00–4:59	16	4:00–4:59
05	5:00–5:59	17	5:00–5:59
06	6:00–6:59	18	6:00–6:59
07	7:00–7:59	19	7:00–7:59
08	8:00–8:59	20	8:00–8:59
09	9:00–9:59	21	9:00–9:59
10	10:00–10:59	22	10:00–10:59
11	11:00–11:59	23	11:00–11:59
		99	hour unknown

EXAMPLES: If the accident occurred at 2:15 in the morning or at 3:45 in the afternoon, FL 39 would look like this:

Time	Code	Amount
2:15 A.M.	45	02.00
3:45 P.M.	45	15.00

When value code 45 is used to report the accident hour, one of the accident-related occurrence codes (codes 01–06 in FLs 31–34) must also be reported on the claim to report the accident date.

46 Number of Grace Days

Code 46 indicates the number of days needed to arrange for postdischarge care as determined by the QIO/UR. This code is required for Medicare and all other payers if it applies.

If either condition code C3 (Partial approval) or C4 (Admission/services denied) is reported in FLs 18–28, indicating that the QIO denied all or part of the billing period, this value code must be used to report the number of days—either one, two, or three—that the QIO has determined are to be covered while arrangements are made for the patient's postdischarge care. The number of days is entered to the left of the delimiter in FLs 39–41, and the cents area to the right of the delimiter should contain two zeros.

47 Any Liability Insurance

Value code 47 reflects the portion of the payment from any liability insurer made on behalf of a Medicare beneficiary that the provider is applying to covered Medicare charges on the bill. It indicates that the liability insurer is a higher priority payer than Medicare as well as how much the liability insurer has paid. This MSP value code is required for Medicare billing when applicable.

48 Hemoglobin Reading

Code 48 indicates the patient's most recent hemoglobin reading taken before the start of this billing cycle. This code is required for Medicare billing when applicable.

A hemoglobin reading is measured as a percentage and is usually limited to two digits. The two digits are reported to the left of the delimiter. If a third-digit decimal amount is included, that amount is reported to the right of the delimiter in the cents area.

49 Hematocrit Reading

Code 49 indicates the patient's most recent hematocrit reading taken before the start of this billing cycle. This code is required for Medicare billing when applicable.

A hematocrit reading is measured as a percentage and is usually limited to two digits. The two digits are reported to the left of the delimiter. If a third-digit decimal amount is included, that amount is reported to the right of the delimiter in the cents area.

50 Physical Therapy Visits

Code 50 indicates the number of physical therapy visits provided by this billing provider from the onset of treatment through the billing period on the

$ $ Billing Tip $ $

Value Code 47 and Accident-Related Occurrence Codes

When value code 47 is reported, the appropriate accident-related occurrence code, code 01 or 03, must also be used. In the case of a car accident, occurrence code 01 (Accident/medical coverage) should be reported in a liability state. (In a no-fault state, value code 14, rather than 47, is used.) For nonwork accident situations involving liability insurance, such as medical malpractice or "slip and fall" cases, occurrence code 03 (Accident—tort liability) should be used. Occurrence code 05 (Other accident) should not be used with value code 47.

Figure 11.2

Sample Bill for Physical Therapy Using Value Code 50

31 OCCURRENCE CODE	DATE	32 OCCURRENCE CODE	DATE	33 OCCURRENCE CODE	DATE	34 OCCURRENCE CODE	DATE	35 CODE OCCURRENCE SPAN	FROM	THROUGH	36 CODE OCCURRENCE SPAN	FROM	THROUGH	37
a 11	021010	29	030110	35	030210									a
b														b

38			39 CODE VALUE CODES	AMOUNT	40 CODE VALUE CODES	AMOUNT	41 CODE VALUE CODES	AMOUNT
		a	50	5 00				
		b						
		c						
		d						

	42 REV. CD.	43 DESCRIPTION	44 HCPCS / RATE / HIPPS CODE	45 SERV. DATE	46 SERV. UNITS	47 TOTAL CHARGES	48 NON-COVERED CHARGES	49	
1	0421	PHYS THERP/VISIT	97110GP	030210	1	28 05			1
2	0421	PHYS THERP/VISIT	97110GP	030410	1	28 05			2
3	0421	PHYS THERP/VISIT	97140GP	030610	1	29 30			3
4	0421	PHYS THERP/VISIT	97140GP	030710	1	29 30			4
5	0421	PHYS THERP/VISIT	97140GP	031410	1	29 30			5
6	0424	PHYS THERP/EVAL	97001GP	030110	1	154 98			6
7									7
8									8
9									9
10									10
11									11
12									12
13									13
14									14
15									15
16									16
17									17
18									18
19									19
20									20
21									21
22									22
23	0001	PAGE 1 OF 1	CREATION DATE	033110	TOTALS ▶	298 98			23

claim. This code is required for Medicare billing when applicable. Figure 11.2 shows the use of code 50 in a bill containing five physical therapy visits.

51   Occupational Therapy Visits

Code 51 indicates the number of occupational therapy visits provided by this billing provider from the onset of treatment through the billing period on the claim. This code is required for Medicare billing, when applicable.

52   Speech Therapy Visits

Code 52 indicates the number of speech therapy visits provided by this billing provider from the onset of treatment through the billing period on the claim. This code is required for Medicare billing when applicable.

53   Cardiac Rehabilitation Visits

Code 53 indicates the number of cardiac rehabilitation visits provided by this billing provider from the onset of treatment through the billing period on the claim. This code is required for Medicare billing when applicable.

54   Newborn Birth Weight in Grams

Code 54 indicates the newborn's actual weight at birth or, in the case of an extramural birth, the weight at the time of admission. This code is required on all claims containing code 4 (Newborn) in FL 14 (Type of Admission) and on other claims as required by state law.

55 Eligibility Threshold for Charity Care

Code 55 is used to report the amount at which a health care facility determines the eligibility threshold for charity care.

Home Health-Specific and Payer-Specific Codes

With the exception of several miscellaneous codes, the remaining numeric value codes, from 56 to 99, relate specifically to home health care services or are payer-only codes.

56 Skilled Nurse—Home Visit Hours (HHA Only)

Code 56, which shows the number of hours of skilled nursing provided during the billing period, may be required for Medicare home health agencies (HHA) only when applicable. The provider should report the hours spent in the home only; travel time is not included. The number of hours should be rounded to the nearest whole hour and reported to the left of the delimiter, followed by two zeros in the cents area to the right of the delimiter.

57 Home Health Aid—Home Visit Hours (HHA Only)

Code 57, which shows the number of hours provided by a home health aid during the billing period, may be required for Medicare HHA only when applicable. The HHA should report the hours spent in the home only; travel time is not included. The number of hours should be rounded to the nearest whole hour and reported to the left of the delimiter, followed by two zeros in the cents area to the right of the delimiter.

58 Arterial Blood Gas (PO$_2$/PA$_2$)

Code 58 indicates the arterial blood gas value at the beginning of each reporting period for oxygen therapy. This code is required for Medicare billing when applicable.

This value or the value reported with value code 59 below is required on the initial bill for oxygen therapy and on the fourth month's bill. For the fourth month, a physician's recertification based on retesting is required to support the continued need for oxygen therapy.

Unlike most other nonmonetary values, the value associated with the arterial blood gas reading is reported in the cents area to the right of the delimiter. The percentage should be rounded to two decimals or the nearest whole number.

EXAMPLE: For an arterial blood gas reading of 56.5 percent, FL 39 would look like this:

Code	Amount
58	.57

For a reading of 100 percent, FL 39 would look like this:

Code	Amount
58	1.00

COMPLIANCE GUIDE
Medicare-Allowed Therapy Visits

Note that value code 50 represents the cumulative number of visits from the start of care up through the billing period on the current claim, not just the number of visits for the current billing period. Therefore, when therapy visits span more than one bill, the number of visits reported with value code 50 may be greater than the number of units reported in FL 46 (Service Units). The cumulative number is used to keep track of the total number of visits when there is a limit on the total number allowed.

For example, Medicare generally allows only thirty-six cardiac rehabilitation therapy visits. Therefore, if the number of visits exceeds thirty-six, the claim may be suspended for medical review or denied. The proper medical documentation must be in place in order to support the need for additional visits.

$ $ Billing Tip $ $

HCPCS Modifiers and Outpatient Therapy

Outpatient therapy services require the following modifiers on Medicare claims.
- GN Speech therapy
- GO Occupational therapy
- GP Physical therapy

Notice the use of modifier GP to indicate OP PT services after codes 97110, 97140, and 97001 in FL 44 of Figure 11.2.

59   Oxygen Saturation (O$_2$ SAT/Oximetry)

Code 59 indicates the oxygen saturation at the beginning of each reporting period for oxygen therapy. This code is required for Medicare billing, when applicable.

This value or the value reported with value code 58 above is required on the initial bill for oxygen therapy and on the fourth month's bill. For the fourth month, a physician's recertification based on retesting is required to support the continued need for oxygen therapy.

As with the arterial blood gas reading for code 58, the oxygen saturation reading is reported in the cents area to the right of the delimiter. The percentage should be rounded to two decimals or the nearest whole number, as shown in the examples for code 58 above.

60   HHA Branch MSA

Code 60 is used to report the number of the metropolitan statistical area (MSA) in which the HHA branch is located. This code is needed only when the branch location is different from the location of the HHA. The number of the MSA is entered to the left of the delimiter, with two zeros to the right in the cents area. This code is required for Medicare billing when applicable.

61   Location Where Service Is Furnished (HHA and Hospice)

Code 61 is used to report the MSA number or Core Based Statistical Area (CBSA) number (or rural state code) of the location where the home health or hospice service is delivered. Code 61 is used to report the site of service, not the agency location. The number is entered to the left of the delimiter, with two zeros to the right in the cents area. This code is required for Medicare billing for home health and hospice care.

62–65   Reserved for Payer Use Only

Providers do not report these codes.

66   Medicaid Spenddown Amount

This code indicates the dollar amount that was used to meet the recipient's spenddown liability for the claim.

67   Peritoneal Dialysis

Code 67 is used to report the number of hours of peritoneal dialysis provided during the billing period. It is required for Medicare billing when applicable. The code pertains to ESRD benefits. The provider should report the hours spent in the home only; travel time is not included. The number of hours is rounded to the nearest whole number and reported to the left of the delimiter, with two zeros to the right in the cents area.

68   EPO—DRUG

Code 68 indicates the number of units of EPO administered and/or supplied for self-administration in the billing period. This code is required for Medicare billing when applicable. Units are reported in whole number amounts to the left of the delimiter; the cents area to the right of the delimiter should contain two zeros.

INTERNET RESOURCE
Medicaid Eligibility Information
www.cms.hhs.gov/home/
MedicaidEligibility/

EXAMPLE: For an amount of 31,060 units supplied, FL 39 would look like this:

Code	Amount
68	31060.00

69   State Charity Care Percent

Code 69 indicates the percentage of charity care eligibility for the patient. The percentage is reported to the left of the delimiter, with fractional amounts to the right in the cents area.

EXAMPLE: For an eligibility rate of 10.5 percent, FL 39 would look like this:

Code	Amount
69	10.50

70–79 Payer Codes

Providers do not report these codes.

Codes for Covered and Noncovered Days

Value codes 80–83 are used to report the number of covered, noncovered, coinsurance, and lifetime reserve days within the claim's billing period (FL6, Statement Covers Period). These value codes were newly introduced for use on the UB-04. On the UB-92, this information was reported in FLs 7–10. To create additional space on the form, these form locators were deleted from the UB-04, and the data were assigned to value codes 80–83. The number of days is entered to the left of the delimiter, with two zeros to the right in the cents area.

80   Covered Days

Code 80 is used to report the total number of inpatient days (including hospitalization, coinsurance, and lifetime reserve days) covered by the primary payer in the claim's billing period. This code is required for inpatient billing by Medicare. Most Medicaid claims also require the code. Commercial payers require it when Medicare is listed as one of the payers on the bill. Blue Cross may require the code, depending on the plan. It is not required for TRICARE claims.

For hospitals, the number of covered days will not exceed 150:

60 days of hospitalization

30 coinsurance days

60 lifetime reserve days (if the patient elects to use them for this billing period)

For inpatient SNF claims, this number will not exceed 100:

20 days of hospitalization

80 coinsurance days

> **837I aler✚**
>
> **Value Codes 80–83 Not Available**
>
> Value codes 80–83 are not available for use with the 837I (electronic HIPAA claim). The corresponding information (covered days, noncovered days, coinsurance days, and LRDs) is reported under Claim Quantity on the 837I (Loop ID 2300, QTY01). Codes 80–83 are available for use on paper claims only.

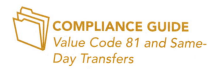
In general, the date of discharge or death is not counted as a covered day unless a patient is admitted and discharged on the same day.

81 Noncovered Days

Code 81 is used to report the total number of noncovered days in the claim's billing period. **Noncovered days** are inpatient days of care not covered by the primary payer. For Medicare beneficiaries, these days are not claimable as Medicare patient days. Beneficiaries will not be charged for utilizing Medicare Part A services.

This code is required for inpatient billing by Medicare. Most Medicaid claims also require this code. Commercial payers require it when Medicare is listed as one of the payers on the bill. Blue Cross may require it, depending on the plan. It is not required for TRICARE claims.

Noncovered days may include, for example, a hospital stay in which the patient refuses to use Medicare lifetime reserve days, leave-of-absence days when the patient is temporarily discharged from the hospital, or days for which no Part A payment can be made because benefits are exhausted or because the services are no longer considered medically necessary. Note that the day of discharge or death is not counted as either a covered day or a noncovered day.

82 Coinsurance Days

Code 82 is used to report the number of coinsurance days in the claim's billing period. Under Medicare, coinsurance days are inpatient hospital days occurring after the 60th day and before the 91st day in a single benefit period or spell of illness—or, for inpatient SNF claims, after the 20th day and before the 101st day. The number reported with this code should not exceed thirty hospital days (or eighty inpatient SNF days).

This code is required for inpatient billing only by Medicare. Medicaid claims may require this code, and commercial payers require it when Medicare is listed as one of the payers on the bill. The code is not required for Blue Cross and TRICARE claims.

Report the Medicare coinsurance amount using value codes 09 (Coinsurance amount in the first calendar year) or 11 (Coinsurance amount in the second calendar year) along with this code.

83 Lifetime Reserve Days

Code 83 is used to report the number of lifetime reserve days the patient elected to use during the claim's billing period. A Medicare patient who has used both the sixty covered hospital days and the thirty coinsurance days allowed during a benefit period may elect to use a lifetime reserve of an additional sixty days of inpatient hospital services during a spell of illness. The number of days reported with this code should not exceed sixty.

This code is required for inpatient billing only by Medicare. Commercial payers require the code when Medicare is listed as one of the payers on the bill. It is not required for Medicaid, Blue Cross, or TRICARE claims.

Report the Medicare coinsurance amount using value codes 08 (Lifetime reserve amount in the first calendar year) or 10 (Lifetime reserve amount in the second calendar year) along with this code.

84–99 Reserved for National Assignment

Alphanumeric Value Codes

A0 Special ZIP Code Reporting

Code A0 indicates the five-digit ZIP code of the location from which the beneficiary is initially placed on board the ambulance. This code is required for Medicare billing when applicable. It must be reported on every ambulance claim. More than one trip can be reported on the same claim as long as the pickup locations for the beneficiary all contain the same ZIP code.

A1 Deductible Payer A*

Code A1 is used to report the amount assumed by the provider to be applied to the patient's policy deductible for payer A (FL 50A; see Chapter 13, "Payer, Insured, and Employer Information"). This code is required for Medicare billing when applicable. It is also required for Medicaid and Blue Cross claims if applicable.

A2 Coinsurance Payer A*

Code A2 is used to report the amount assumed by the provider to be applied to the patient's coinsurance for payer A (FL 50A). This code is required for Medicare billing when applicable. It is also required for Medicaid and Blue Cross claims if applicable.

A3 Estimated Responsibility Payer A

Code A3 is used to report the amount estimated by the provider to be paid by payer A (FL 50A).

A4 Covered Self-Administrable Drugs—Emergency

Code A4 is used to report the covered charge amount for self-administrable drugs administered to the patient in an emergency situation. The only covered Medicare charge for an ordinarily noncovered, self-administrable drug is for insulin administered to a patient in a diabetic coma.

A5 Covered Self-Administrable Drugs—Not Self-Administrable in Form and Situation Furnished to Patient

Code A5 is used to report the covered charge amount for self-administrable drugs administered to the patient because the drug was not self-administrable in the form and situation in which it was furnished to the patient.

A6 Covered Self-Administrable Drugs—Diagnostic Study and Other

Code A6 is used to report the covered charge amount for self-administrable drugs administered to the patient because the drug was necessary for diagnostic study or for other reasons—for example, the drug was specifically covered by the payer.

A7 Copayment Payer A*

Code A7 is used to report the amount assumed by the provider to be applied toward the patient's copayment for payer A (FL 50A).

---

*837I aler+

Value Codes A1–A2, A7, B1–B2, B7, C1–C2, and C7 Not Available

The value codes for reporting the deductible, coinsurance, and copayment amounts for payers A, B, and C are not available for use with the 837I (electronic HIPAA claim). The corresponding information is reported on the 837I in Loop 2320 CAS segment (Claim Adjustment Group Code "PR"). These nine alphanumeric codes, each of which has been marked with an asterisk (*), are available for use on paper claims only.

$ $ Billing Tip $ $
Value Code A1: Part A Cash Deductible

Value code A1 is used to indicate the Part A cash deductible only. To report the blood deductible, use value code 06 (Blood deductible).

$ $ Billing Tip $ $
Value Code A2: Part B Coinsurance

Value code A2 is used to indicate Part B coinsurance amounts. To report Part A coinsurance amounts, use value codes 8–11 (Lifetime reserve amount in the first calendar year, Coinsurance amount in the first calendar year, Lifetime reserve amount in the second calendar year, Coinsurance amount in the second calendar year).

$ $ Billing Tip $ $
Codes A4–A6 and Revenue Code 0637

Value codes A4 through A6, which deal with covered self-administrable drugs, are used in conjunction with revenue code 0637 (Self-administrable drugs, not requiring detailed coding).

A8   Patient Weight

Code A8 conveys the weight of the patient in kilograms. This information is reported only when the patient's weight affects reimbursement due to a pre-defined change in the health plan. (For reporting a newborn's weight, use value code 54.)

A9   Patient Height

Code A9 conveys the height of the patient in centimeters. This information is reported only when the patient's height affects reimbursement due to a predefined change in the health plan.

AA   Regulatory Surcharges, Assessments, Allowances, or Health Care Related Taxes Payer A

This code is used to report the amount of regulatory surcharges, assessments, allowances, or health care related taxes pertaining to payer A (FL 50A).

AB   Other Assessments or Allowances (Such as Medical Education) Payer A

This code is used to report the amount of other assessments or allowances (for example, medical education) pertaining to payer A (FL 50A).

AC–AZ Reserved for National Assignment

B0   Reserved for National Assignment

B1   Deductible Payer B*

Code B1 is used to report the amount assumed by the provider to be applied to the patient's policy deductible for payer B (FL 50B; see Chapter 13). When applicable, this code is required for Medicare billing and also for Medicaid and Blue Cross claims.

B2   Coinsurance Payer B*

Code B2 is used to report the amount assumed by the provider to be applied to the patient's coinsurance for payer B (FL 50B). When applicable, the code is required for Medicare billing and also for Medicaid and Blue Cross claims.

B3   Estimated Responsibility Payer B

Code B3 is used to report the amount estimated by the provider to be paid by payer B (FL 50B).

B4–B6 Reserved for National Assignment

B7   Copayment Payer B*

Code B7 is used to report the amount assumed by the provider to be applied toward the patient's copayment for payer B (FL 50B).

B8–B9 Reserved for National Assignment

BA Regulatory Surcharges, Assessments, Allowances, or Health Care Related Taxes Payer B

This code is used to report the amount of regulatory surcharges, assessments, allowances, or health care related taxes pertaining to payer B (FL 50B).

BB Other Assessments or Allowances (Such as Medical Education) Payer B

This code is used to report the amount of other assessments or allowances (for example, medical education) pertaining to payer B (FL 50 B).

BC–BZ Reserved for National Assignment

C0 Reserved for National Assignment

C1 Deductible Payer C*

Code C1 is used to report the amount assumed by the provider to be applied to the patient's policy deductible for payer C (FL 50C; see Chapter 13). This code is required for Medicare billing when applicable. It is also required for Medicaid and Blue Cross claims if applicable.

C2 Coinsurance Payer C*

Code C2 is used to report the amount assumed by the provider to be applied to the patient's coinsurance for payer C (FL 50C). Medicare, Medicaid, and Blue Cross require this code if applicable.

C3 Estimated Responsibility Payer C

Code C3 is used to report the amount estimated by the provider to be paid by payer C (FL 50C).

C4–C6 Reserved for National Assignment

C7 Copayment Payer C*

Code C7 is used to report the amount assumed by the provider to be applied toward the patient's copayment for payer C (FL 50C).

C8–C9 Reserved for National Assignment

CA Regulatory Surcharges, Assessments, Allowances, or Health Care Related Taxes Payer C

This code is used to report the amount of regulatory surcharges, assessments, allowances, or health care related taxes pertaining to payer C (FL 50C).

CB Other Assessments or Allowances (Such as Medical Education) Payer C

This code is used to report the amount of other assessments or allowances (for example, medical education) pertaining to payer C (FL 50C).

CC–CZ Reserved for National Assignment

D0–DZ Reserved for National Assignment—Except D3 and DR

D3   Patient Estimated Responsibility

Code D3 is used to indicate the amount estimated by the provider to be paid by the patient named on the claim.

DR   Reserved for Disaster Related Value Code

E0–OZ Either Discontinued or Reserved for National Assignment

P0–PZ Reserved for Public Health Data Reporting

Q0–Y0 Reserved for National Assignment

Y1–Y4 Value Codes Pertaining to Medicare Demonstration Programs

Y1	Part A Demonstration Payment
Y2	Part B Demonstration Payment
Y3	Part B Coinsurance
Y4	Conventional Provider Payment Amount for Non-Demonstration Claims

Y5–ZZ Reserved for National Assignment

1 FLs 39–41 on the UB-04 are used for reporting value codes—two-digit numeric or alphanumeric codes that identify monetary data that affect the processing and payment of the claim. For example, if Medicare is a secondary payer on a claim, the amount received from the primary payer is indicated with the use of a value code. The value code indicates who the payer is (such as a liability insurer, the Department of Veterans Affairs, an EGHP, a public health service, or another federal agency). The dollar amount entered in the form locator along with the code indicates the exact amount of the payment received. This amount is then subtracted from the total reported charges on the claim to determine the final payment due on the claim.

2 Every value code must be accompanied by an amount. The amount is most often a dollar amount. Nondollar amounts are expressed as units, such as days, hours, or the number of visits. In order to process UB-04 forms efficiently, the patient account specialist must be familiar with the relationship between each value code and the type of data (dollar amount, unit, or number of visits) it represents.

3 Certain value codes bring up complicated billing scenarios because they require the use of other value codes. Examples are the use of MSP value codes and the value codes for physical, occupational, speech, or cardiac rehabilitation therapy services.

4 Many value codes contain data that must be coordinated with data in several other fields on the UB-04. For example, certain MSP value codes must be used in conjunction with accident-related occurrence codes 01–06 (FLs 31–34) as well as with the value code required for reporting the hour of the accident (value code 45). In addition, if an MSP value code is used in conjunction with a request for a conditional primary payment, the appropriate payer, insured, and employer information must be used in FLs 50–65 and the appropriate occurrence code (usually code 24) in FLs 31–34. UB-04 condition codes, occurrence codes, value codes, and revenue codes are designed to interact so that they communicate a number of billing situations to the payer.

✔ **CHECK YOUR UNDERSTANDING**

1. Define *value code,* and specify the form locators it occupies on the UB-04. _____

_____

_____

2. True or False: If you needed to report four value codes on a UB-04 claim form (FLs 39–41), you would fill in FL 39a first, followed by FLs 39b, 39c, and 39d. _____

3. Which entries would be considered valid for a value code and its corresponding amount on the UB-04?

	Code	Amount
a.	08	3840.00
b.	4	350.00
c.	A3	390.50
d.	38	4.00
e.	59	61.10
f.	80	175.00
g.	51	9.00
h.	12	0000.00

4. True or False: When value code 02 (Hospital has no semiprivate rooms) is used, an amount of 0.00 should be reported in the value code amount field. _____

5. A patient was admitted for a covered inpatient stay on January 5 and discharged on January 15. How many days should be reported with value code 80 (Covered days)? _____

6. On which type of claim is value code 56 (Skilled nurse—home visit hours) used?
   a. Medicaid
   b. commercial
   c. inpatient
   d. Medicare HHA

7. True or False: Depending on the situation, a hospital can charge a Medicare beneficiary who has used three pints of unreplaced blood in a given year both for the blood (revenue code 038X, Blood and blood components) and for the storage and processing of the blood (revenue code 0390, Administration, processing, and storage for blood and blood components). _____

8. The patient is a Medicare beneficiary who was admitted to the hospital on October 8 and discharged on November 30. She was hospitalized for fifty-eight days during August and September for the same spell of illness and was charged with using fifty-eight hospitalization days. The November billing, covering the months of October and November, is being prepared. Fill in the amounts for the value codes listed below. She has elected to use her lifetime reserve days for the first time.

Value Code	Amount
80	_____ . ___
82	_____ . ___
83	_____ . ___

9. Report the value code and corresponding amount that applies in each of the following situations. In some cases, more than one value code and amount may apply. When reporting any amount, dollar or nondollar, remember to use the correct format.

   a. A public health service pays $2,900 on behalf of a beneficiary. The provider is billing Medicare as secondary for covered services on this claim.

   UB-04 Form—FLs 39–41

39 CODE	VALUE CODES AMOUNT	40 CODE	VALUE CODES AMOUNT	41 CODE	VALUE CODES AMOUNT
a					
b					
c					
d					

b. During this billing period, which covers the month of April, the patient has used thirty covered days—ten coinsurance days and twenty lifetime reserve days. Assume that the coinsurance rate is $256 per day and that the LRD rate is $512 per day.

UB-04 Form—FLs 39–41

39 CODE	VALUE CODES AMOUNT	40 CODE	VALUE CODES AMOUNT	41 CODE	VALUE CODES AMOUNT
a					
b					
c					
d					

c. The patient was involved in an auto accident in a no-fault state. The accident occurred at 7:30 A.M. on the first day of the year. The patient has received $10,500 from the auto insurer. The provider is billing Medicare as secondary.

UB-04 Form—FLs 39–41

39 CODE	VALUE CODES AMOUNT	40 CODE	VALUE CODES AMOUNT	41 CODE	VALUE CODES AMOUNT
a					
b					
c					
d					

d. The provider estimates that the primary payer will pay $3,998.00 for the services being billed on the claim.

UB-04 Form—FLs 39–41

39 CODE	VALUE CODES AMOUNT	40 CODE	VALUE CODES AMOUNT	41 CODE	VALUE CODES AMOUNT
a					
b					
c					
d					

e. After a car accident, two patients are being transported in a single ambulance trip.

UB-04 Form—FLs 39–41

39 CODE	VALUE CODES AMOUNT	40 CODE	VALUE CODES AMOUNT	41 CODE	VALUE CODES AMOUNT
a					
b					
c					
d					

f. On the last day of the month, a Medicare beneficiary has just completed his tenth speech therapy visit for the month and his fifteenth visit since the onset of care.

UB-04 Form—FLs 39–41

39 CODE	VALUE CODES AMOUNT	40 CODE	VALUE CODES AMOUNT	41 CODE	VALUE CODES AMOUNT
a					
b					
c					
d					

g. A Medicare patient has elected to use twenty of her lifetime reserve days. The first five days fall in the year of admission, and the last fifteen days fall in the year of discharge. Assume that the LRD rate is $496 per day in the first calendar year and $512 per day in the second calendar year.

UB-04 Form—FLs 39–41

39 CODE	VALUE CODES AMOUNT	40 CODE	VALUE CODES AMOUNT	41 CODE	VALUE CODES AMOUNT
a					
b					
c					
d					

h. The provider estimates that the patient's responsibility on the claim is $820.50.

UB-04 Form—FLs 39–41

39 CODE	VALUE CODES AMOUNT	40 CODE	VALUE CODES AMOUNT	41 CODE	VALUE CODES AMOUNT
a					
b					
c					
d					

10. Report the appropriate condition code, occurrence code, occurrence span code, and/or value code requested for the billing situation described. Remember to use the correct format for each type of code.

a. On April 8, 2007, the QIO notified the patient of the hospital's intention to bill for accommodations starting on April 10, based on the determination that the patient no longer required a covered level of inpatient care. The patient remained in the hospital as an inpatient until April 13 at a rate of $800 per day. Record the appropriate occurrence code, occurrence span code, and value code indicating the patient's liability for the continued stay.

UB-04 Form—FLs 10–41

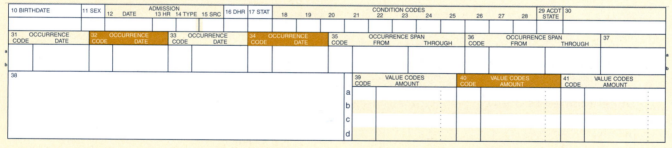

b. A patient is admitted to a PPS hospital and is transferred out on the same day. Report the required condition code and value code to indicate covered or noncovered care.

UB-04 Form—FLs 10–41

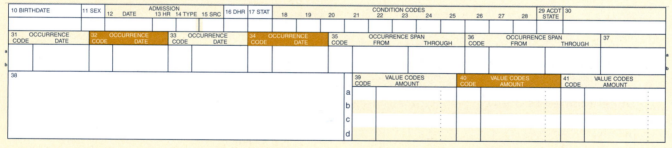

c. A patient was hospitalized after a work-related accident on June 9, 2010, at 3:30 P.M. The payment from a workers' compensation plan has been substantially delayed due to lengthy arbitration, and a

Medicare Conditional Payment request is being made. Report the required MSP value code and amount as well as the required codes to indicate the date and hour of the accident.

UB-04 Form—FLs 10–41

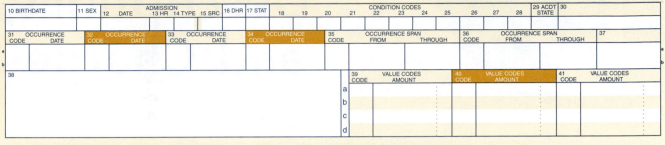

COMPUTER EXPLORATION

UB-04 Activity: Claim Analysis

Working with Value Codes: FLs 39–41

Open the file **Sample02.pdf** in Adobe Reader, and answer the following questions:

1. What are the two value codes reported on the claim? Are these codes listed in the correct order numerically? Should the second value code be listed in FL 39b instead of 40a?

2. What does the value code in FL 40 indicate? Does the TOB reflect an inpatient bill to correspond with this information?

3. How many covered days are reported with value code 80?

4. Compare this amount with the dates reported in FL 6 (Statement Covers Period). Verify that the admission date is the same as the from date in FL 6. Based on this information, does the day of discharge count as a covered day?

5. Value codes 80–83 are used primarily on Medicare claims to report covered, noncovered, coinsurance, and lifetime reserve days in the claim's billing period. Codes 80 and 81 can be used to report the number of covered and noncovered days by other payers as well. Locate a copy of the ICD-9-CM codebook, and look up the diagnosis code reported in FL 67 to determine the patient's principal diagnosis. Do you think CIGNA covers a three-day stay for a normal delivery?

6. What does the value code reported in FL 39 indicate?

7. In the list of services, locate the patient's accommodation charge. How does this rate compare with the most common rate?

8. Most deliveries result in two bills—one for the mother and one for the newborn. In some cases, the charges are combined. Are there any indications of newborn charges on this claim? Are there any nursery accommodation charges?

9. What type of admission code would be reported in FL 14 on the newborn's claim?

10. What value code would be used to report the birth weight of the newborn on the newborn's claim?

When finished viewing the claim, click Exit on the File menu.

Revenue Codes, Descriptions, and Charges

LEARNING OUTCOMES

After completing this chapter, you will be able to define the key terms and:

1. Describe the use of the two types of revenue codes that are reported in FL 42 (Revenue Code) on the UB-04: accommodation revenue codes and ancillary service revenue codes.

2. Become familiar with the narrative description or standard abbreviation that accompanies each revenue code for FL 43 (Revenue Description).

3. Understand the use of FL 44 (HCPCS/Rate/HIPPS Code) for reporting either the required HCPCS codes on outpatient claims or the charge for accommodations on inpatient claims.

4. Understand how to report the date of service in FL 45 (Service Date) and the units of measure in FL 46 (Service Units).

5. Understand how to report total charges and noncovered charges in FL 47 (Total Charges) and FL 48 (Noncovered Charges).

KEY TERMS

- accommodation revenue code
- all-inclusive rate
- ancillary service revenue code
- Durable Medical Equipment Regional Carriers (DMERCs)
- HIPPS (Health Insurance Prospective Payment System) rate code
- observation services
- revenue code series
- subcategory code
- transitional pass-through payment

All medical services provided to patients, whether inpatients or outpatients, have costs associated with them. This chapter covers form locators 42–49, lines 1–23, which are used for recording and totaling the cost of each service received for the billing period reflected on the claim (see Figure 12.1). To help the payer understand what services were received by the patient, how much each service costs, and when each service was received, the billing provider must fill in FLs 42–49 carefully and precisely.

According to the current revenue code system defined by the National Uniform Billing Committee (NUBC) for the UB-04 claim form, every service is assigned a revenue code and description. Each revenue code and corresponding description reflects an item, accommodation, or service that is billable by providers. Because revenue codes and descriptions provide the exact details of the service received, they play a key role in determining the final reimbursement amount.

The original NUBC revenue code system used three-digit codes numbered from 001 to 999. To accommodate the need for more codes, the coding system was expanded to a four-digit system. A leading zero was added to the original three-digit codes to make them four-digit codes.

Revenue codes are grouped into major categories, such as Room and Board—Private (011X), Pharmacy (025X), and Physical Therapy (042X). This chapter lists all revenue codes. Descriptions and usage guidelines are provided for the major revenue code categories. Billing tips help explain revenue codes that are often reported incorrectly. For quick reference, Appendix A contains a numerical list of all revenue codes as well as an alphabetical list of selected codes.

Figure 12.1

UB-04 Form—FLs 42–49, Lines 1–23

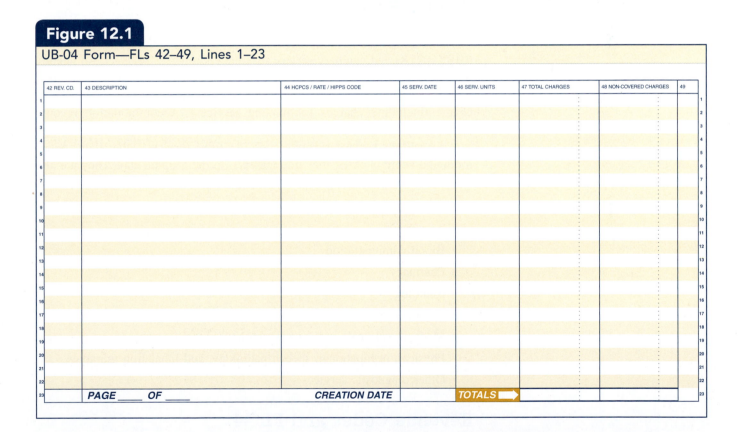

FL 42 Revenue Code

Lines 1–23 of FL 42 are used to report numeric codes, called revenue codes, that identify specific services being billed on the UB-04 claim. The associated charge for each revenue code is reported on the adjacent line in FL 47 (Total Charges). Charges are stored in the facility's charge description master (CDM), which is updated regularly.

Revenue code series are described with the use of an X in the last position (instead of a number from 0 to 9). For example, revenue code 013X stands for the revenue code series Room and board—three and four beds. For billing purposes, however, the X must be replaced with a **subcategory code,** indicated by the numbers 0 through 9. A 0 in the last position indicates a general code. Numbers 1 through 8 stand for specific subcategories. A last digit of 9 always means other.

EXAMPLE:

035X   CT scan

0350	General classification
0351	CT—head scan
0352	CT—body scan
0353–0358	Reserved
0359	CT—other

Accommodation and Ancillary Service Revenue Codes

Two major types of revenue codes are used: accommodation revenue codes (010X–021X) and ancillary service revenue codes (022X–099X). An **accommodation revenue code** is used to identify the type of routine hospital bed, room accommodation (such as private, semiprivate, and ward), and board charge (including charges for nursing services). Accommodation revenue codes apply to inpatient claims only.

An **ancillary service revenue code** identifies services, other than routine room and board charges, that are incidental to the hospital stay. They are also used on all outpatient claims. Ancillary services include:

- Operating room
- Anesthesia
- Blood administration
- Pharmacy
- Radiology
- Laboratory
- Medical, surgical, and central supplies
- Physical, occupational, speech pathology, and inhalation therapies
- Other diagnostic services

Revenue Codes and FL 44 (HCPCS/Rate/HIPPS Code)

Depending on whether the revenue code being reported is for an inpatient or outpatient claim, FL 44 may contain a HCPCS code, a room rate, or a HIPPS rate code. Inpatient claims require a room rate in FL 44 for all accommodation revenue codes (010X–021X). For all other services on inpatient claims (ancillary services), FL 44 may be left blank.

Outpatient claims, on the contrary, require a HCPCS code in FL 44 for almost all ancillary services (HCPCS codes are covered in Chapter 4,

"Medical Coding Basics"). On outpatient claims, the HCPCS code is used as the basis for payment and therefore must be reported. For claims associated with the SNF and home health Prospective Payment Systems, a HIPPS rate code is used as the basis for payment and therefore must be reported in FL 44.

Guidelines

Completion of the revenue code field is required for Medicare billing and for all other payers. Providers determine the codes and charges based on the services they provide to patients. The codes and charges stored in the facility billing system are updated as needed.

For non-Medicare claims, depending on the health plan's requirements, the general classification revenue code, usually a 0, may be used rather than one of the other, more specific subcategory codes. However, when a specific subcategory code is both applicable and available, providers are encouraged to use it to ensure accurate and quick processing of the claim.

With regard to Medicare claims, the general revenue code, usually a 0, should be used with all revenue code categories except the following, which require detailed codes (1–9):

029X	DME (durable medical equipment), rental/purchase
0304	Laboratory—nonroutine dialysis
033X	Radiology—therapeutic and/or chemotherapy administration
0367	Operating room services—kidney transplant
042X	Physical therapy
052X	Freestanding clinic, outpatient visits
055X–059X	Home health services
0624	Medical/surgical supplies—FDA investigational devices
0636	Pharmacy—drugs requiring detailed coding
080X–085X	ESRD services (080X, 082X–085X); Acquisition of body components for transplantation (081X)

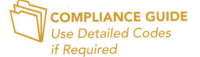

COMPLIANCE GUIDE
Use Detailed Codes if Required

The use of zero as the fourth digit when a detailed code is required may cause a delay in the claim's processing. Similarly, the use of subcategory code 9 (Other), when not appropriate, may cause a delay as well. Other revenue codes are often reserved for future assignment.

On a single UB-04 claim form, 22 lines are available for listing revenue codes and charges; line 23 is reserved for listing a claim total on the final claim page (see Figure 12.1 on page 237). If more lines are needed, additional pages are attached. (The paper claim can be up to nine pages long.) With the exception of revenue code 0001, which is reserved for line 23, applicable revenue codes should be listed in ascending numeric order by date of service.

List of Revenue Codes

0001   Total Charge

Revenue code 0001, which is reported in line 23 on the last page of a paper claim, is used to report the total of all revenue code charges on the claim. Code 0001 includes a total of all revenue code charges listed in the column associated with FL 47 (Total Charges) as well as a total of revenue code charges listed in

Figure 12.2

Example of Revenue Code 0001 in Line 23 to Report Claim Totals

	42 REV. CD.	43 DESCRIPTION	44 HCPCS / RATE / HIPPS CODE	45 SERV. DATE	46 SERV. UNITS	47 TOTAL CHARGES	48 NON-COVERED CHARGES	49	
1	0120	ROOM-BOARD/SEMI	390 00		2	780 00			1
2	0270	MED-SUR SUPPLIES			1	82 00			2
3	0301	CHEMISTRY TESTS			1	35 25			3
4	0320	DX X-RAY			1	550 00			4
5									5
6									6
7									7
8									8
9									9
10									10
11									11
12									12
13									13
14									14
15									15
16									16
17									17
18									18
19									19
20									20
21									21
22									22
23	0001	**PAGE** 1 **OF** 1	**CREATION DATE** 121509	**TOTALS** ➡		1447 25			23

8371 aler➕

The electronic HIPAA claim does not use revenue code 0001. Instead, the total claim charge is reported in the appropriate data segment/field (Loop ID 2300/CLM02).

the column associated with FL 48 (Noncovered Charges). Figure 12.2 illustrates the use of revenue code 0001 on a sample UB-04 claim form.

001X   Reserved for Internal Payer Use

002X   Health Insurance—Prospective Payment System (HIPPS)

Revenue code 002X indicates that the health insurance Prospective Payment System (HIPPS) applies to the claim. HIPPS is a procedural coding system used in association with the SNF (skilled nursing facility), home health, and inpatient rehabilitation facility Prospective Payment Systems. The code indicates which system the claim is being paid under and must be reported with a five-digit HIPPS rate code in FL 44 (HCPCS/Rate/HIPPS Code).

Code	Subcategory	Standard Abbreviation
0	Reserved	
1	Reserved	
2	Skilled nursing facility—Prospective Payment System	SNF PPS (RUG)
3	Home health—Prospective Payment System	HH PPS (HRG)
4	Inpatient rehabilitation facility—Prospective Payment System	IRF PPS (CMG)
5–9	Reserved	

Accommodation Revenue Codes

When an accommodation revenue code is reported in FL 42, a room rate must always be reported in FL 44 (HCPCS/Rate/HIPPS Code). The service unit for an accommodation revenue code, specified in FL 46 (Service Units) of the revenue line, is always number of days. For example, in Figure 12.2, revenue code 0120 (Room-Board/Semi) shows the room rate in FL 44 as $390.00 per day and the number of service units in FL 46 as two days.

010X   All-Inclusive Rate

Revenue code 010X indicates a flat fee charge incurred on either a daily basis or a total stay basis for services rendered and referred to as an **all-inclusive rate.** The charge may include room and board (R&B) plus ancillary services, or room and board only.

Code	Subcategory	Standard Abbreviation
0	All-inclusive room and board plus ancillary	ALL INCL R&B/ANC
1	All-inclusive room and board	ALL INCL R&B
2–9	Reserved	

011X   Room and Board—Private (One Bed)

Revenue code 011X indicates routine service charges incurred for accommodations in a private room (a room with a single bed).

Code	Subcategory	Standard Abbreviation
0	General classification	ROOM-BOARD/PVT
1	Medical/surgical/GYN	MED-SURG-GY/PVT
2	Obstetrics (OB)	OB/PVT
3	Pediatric	PEDS/PVT
4	Psychiatric	PSYCH/PVT
5	Hospice	HOSPICE/PVT
6	Detoxification	DETOX/PVT
7	Oncology	ONCOLOGY/PVT
8	Rehabilitation	REHAB/PVT
9	Other	OTHER/PVT

012X   Room and Board—Semiprivate (Two-Beds)

Revenue code 012X indicates routine service charges incurred for accommodations in a semiprivate room (a room with two beds). For most health plans, the fourth-digit subcategory code is required.

$ $ Billing Tip $ $

Billing for a Private Room

Most health plans do not cover private rooms except when medically necessary. If a patient requests a private room even when his or her plan does not cover it, the cost of the room is reported on the UB-04 form as follows:

FL 44	HCPCS/ Rate/ HIPPS Code	Rate for private room ($900/day)
FL 47	Total Charges	Amount due at the semiprivate rate ($840/day)
FL 48	Noncovered Charges	Difference between rates ($60/day)

FYI

Revenue Code 012X

Revenue code 012X is the most commonly used revenue code for inpatient room charges; most plans cover semiprivate rooms.

Code	Subcategory	Standard Abbreviation
0	General classification	ROOM-BOARD/SEMI
1	Medical/surgical/GYN	MED-SURG-GY/SEMI
2	Obstetrics (OB)	OB/SEMI-PVT
3	Pediatric	PEDS/SEMI-PVT
4	Psychiatric	PSYCH/SEMI-PVT
5	Hospice	HOSPICE/SEMI-PVT
6	Detoxification	DETOX/SEMI-PVT
7	Oncology	ONCOLOGY/SEMI
8	Rehabilitation	REHAB/SEMI-PVT
9	Other	OTHER/SEMI-PVT

013X   Room and Board—Three and Four Beds

Revenue code 013X indicates routine service charges incurred for rooms with three or four beds.

Code	Subcategory	Standard Abbreviation
0	General classification	ROOM-BOARD/3&4BED
1	Medical/surgical/GYN	MED-SURG-GY/3&4BED
2	Obstetrics (OB)	OB/3&4BED
3	Pediatric	PEDS/3&4BED
4	Psychiatric	PSYCH/3&4BED
5	Hospice	HOSPICE/3&4BED
6	Detoxification	DETOX/3&4BED
7	Oncology	ONCOLOGY/3&4BED
8	Rehabilitation	REHAB/3&4BED
9	Other	OTHER/3&4BED

014X   Room and Board—Deluxe Private

Revenue code 014X indicates service charges incurred for accommodations with amenities substantially in excess of private room services.

Code	Subcategory	Standard Abbreviation
0	General classification	ROOM-BOARD/DLX PVT
1	Medical/surgical/GYN	MED-SURG-GY/DLX PVT
2	Obstetrics (OB)	OB/DLX PVT
3	Pediatric	PEDS/DLX PVT
4	Psychiatric	PSYCH/DLX PVT
5	Hospice	HOSPICE/DLX PVT
6	Detoxification	DETOX/DLX PVT
7	Oncology	ONCOLOGY/DLX PVT
8	Rehabilitation	REHAB/DLX PVT
9	Other	OTHER/DLX PVT

015X   Room and Board—Ward

Revenue code 015X indicates routine service charges incurred for accommodations with five or more beds, which are considered wards.

Code	Subcategory	Standard Abbreviation
0	General classification	ROOM-BOARD/WARD
1	Medical/surgical/GYN	MED-SURG-GY/WARD
2	Obstetrics (OB)	OB/WARD
3	Pediatric	PEDS/WARD
4	Psychiatric	PSYCH/WARD
5	Hospice	HOSPICE/WARD
6	Detoxification	DETOX/WARD
7	Oncology	ONCOLOGY/WARD
8	Rehabilitation	REHAB/WARD
9	Other	OTHER/WARD

016X   Room and Board—Other

Revenue code 016X indicates any routine service charges for accommodations that cannot be included in the specific revenue code categories.

Code	Subcategory	Standard Abbreviation
0	General classification	R&B
1–3	Reserved	
4	Sterile environment	R&B/STERILE
5–6	Reserved	
7	Self-care	R&B/SELF
8	Reserved	
9	Other	R&B/OTHER

017X   Nursery

Revenue code 017X indicates accommodation charges for nursing care provided to newborns and premature infants.

Code	Subcategory	Standard Abbreviation
0	General classification	NURSERY
1	Newborn—level I	NURSERY/LEVEL I
2	Newborn—level II	NURSERY/LEVEL II
3	Newborn—level III	NURSERY/LEVEL III
4	Newborn—level IV	NURSERY/LEVEL IV
5–8	Reserved	
9	Other nursery	NURSERY—OTHER

Subcategory codes 1 through 4 are used by facilities with nursery services designed around distinct areas and/or levels of care, as described below. State regulations or other statutes that define similar levels of care supersede the following guidelines.

- *Level I (newborn nursery):* Routine care of apparently normal full-term or preterm neonates
- *Level II (continuing care):* Low-birth-weight neonates who are not sick, but require frequent feeding, and neonates who require more hours of nursing than do normal neonates
- *Level III (intermediate care):* Sick neonates who do not require intensive care, but require six to twelve hours of nursing each day
- *Level IV (intensive care):* Constant nursing and continuous cardiopulmonary and other support for severely ill infants (*Guidelines for Perinatal Care,* Second Edition, American Academy of Pediatrics and the American College of Obstetricians and Gynecologists, 1988)

When assigning a fourth-digit subcategory code, the level of care should correspond to the intensity of medical care provided to the infant, not to the facility certification level assigned by the state. Also, the level of care must be evaluated on a daily basis. Because the level of care likely fluctuates from day to day, several codes are often required to cover the infant's stay.

018X   Leave of Absence (LOA)

Revenue code 018X is used to report routine service charges for holding a room while the patient is temporarily away. Depending on the situation and the health plan, zero charges may be billed. For Medicare, charges are billable for codes 2 through 5.

Code	Subcategory	Standard Abbreviation
0	General classification	LEAVE OF ABSENCE OR LOA
1	Reserved	
2	Patient convenience	LOA/PT CONV
3	Therapeutic leave	LOA/THERAPEUTIC
4	Reserved	
5	Nursing home (for hospitalization)	LOA/NURS HOME
6–8	Reserved	
9	Other LOA	LOA/OTHER

019X   Subacute Care

Revenue code 019X indicates accommodation charges for subacute care (less than acute care) to inpatients in hospitals or skilled nursing facilities.

Code	Subcategory	Standard Abbreviation
0	General classification	SUBACUTE
1	Subacute care—level I	SUBACUTE/LEVEL I
2	Subacute care—level II	SUBACUTE/LEVEL II
3	Subacute care—level III	SUBACUTE/LEVEL III
4	Subacute care—level IV	SUBACUTE/LEVEL IV
5–8	Reserved	
9	Other subacute care	SUBACUTE/OTHER

Subcategory codes 1 through 4 reflect different degrees to which nursing intervention is required, as follows:

- *Level I (skilled care):* This level is marked by minimal nursing intervention. Comorbidities—coexisting conditions—do not complicate the treatment plan. An assessment of vitals and body systems is required one to two times per day.

- *Level II (comprehensive care):* This level is marked by moderate nursing intervention. Active treatment of comorbidities is required. An assessment of vitals and body systems is required two to three times per day.

- *Level III (complex care):* This level is marked by moderate to extensive nursing intervention. Active medical care and treatment of comorbidities is required. There is potential for the comorbidities to affect the treatment plan. An assessment of vitals and body systems is required three to four times per day.

- *Level IV (intensive care):* This level is marked by extensive nursing and technical intervention. Active medical care and treatment of comorbidities is required. There is the potential for the comorbidities to affect the treatment plan. An assessment of vitals and body systems is required four to six times per day.

020X   Intensive Care

Revenue code 020X indicates routine service charges for medical or surgical care provided to patients who require a more intensive level of care than is rendered in the general medical or surgical unit. These seriously ill patients usually receive care in the facility's intensive care unit (ICU), sometimes called the critical care unit (CCU), where specially trained staff members using special equipment provide immediate and continuous attention.

Code	Subcategory	Standard Abbreviation
0	General classification	INTENSIVE CARE (ICU)
1	Surgical	ICU/SURGICAL
2	Medical	ICU/MEDICAL
3	Pediatric	ICU/PEDS
4	Psychiatric	ICU/PSYCH
5	Reserved	
6	Intermediate ICU	ICU/INTERMEDIATE
7	Burn care	ICU/BURN CARE
8	Trauma	ICU/TRAUMA
9	Other intensive care	ICU/OTHER

021X   Coronary Care

Revenue code 021X indicates routine service charges for medical care provided to patients with coronary illness who require a more intensive level of care than is rendered in the general medical care unit. This code is reported when a distinct coronary care unit (CCU) provides such services. Patients in a CCU require specialized care from many staff members, as well as specialized equipment.

Code	Subcategory	Standard Abbreviation
0	General classification	CORONARY CARE (CCU)
1	Myocardial infarction	CCU/MYO INFARC
2	Pulmonary care	CCU/PULMONARY
3	Heart transplant	CCU/TRANSPLANT
4	Intermediate CCU	CCU/INTERMEDIATE
5–8	Reserved	
9	Other CCU	CCU/OTHER

Ancillary Service Revenue Codes

There are many ancillary service revenue codes. Figure 12.3 is an example of the way they appear on a UB-04 outpatient claim.

Ancillary service revenue codes may appear on inpatient or outpatient claims. On an inpatient claim, FL 44 (HCPCS/Rate/HIPPS Code) may remain blank when ancillary service revenue codes are reported. Almost all ancillary

Figure 12.3

Examples of Ancillary Service Revenue Codes on an Outpatient Claim

42 REV. CD.	43 DESCRIPTION	44 HCPCS / RATE / HIPPS CODE	45 SERV. DATE	46 SERV. UNITS	47 TOTAL CHARGES	48 NON-COVERED CHARGES	49
0250	PHARMACY		031609	1	1 10		
0270	MED-SUR SUPPLIES		031609	1	28 30		
0360	OR SERVICES	64721RT	031609	1	283 50		
0370	ANESTHESIA		031609	25	58 75		
0761	TREATMENT RM		031609	3	132 00		
0001	PAGE 1 OF 1	CREATION DATE	032509	TOTALS ➡	503 65		

service revenue codes on outpatient claims, however, require corresponding HCPCS codes in FL 44. An outpatient claim also requires the date of service in FL 45.

When ancillary service revenue codes are reported in FL 42, the number of service units must also be reported in FL 46. The service units for ancillary service revenue codes vary depending on the services received. Some examples of units include the number of tests performed, the miles traveled by an ambulance, the hours of respite care received, the number of emergency room visits, and the number of renal dialysis sessions.

The sequence of ancillary service revenue codes and descriptions follows. TRICARE requires the use of a detailed code rather than a general code for many ancillary services. Other payers may also require detailed codes.

022X   Special Charges

Revenue code 022X indicates charges incurred for services received during an inpatient stay or on a daily basis for certain services. This code is available for hospitals that prefer to identify the components of the services being provided in greater detail. The codes can be used to break down or itemize charges that would normally be considered part of routine services.

Code	Subcategory	Standard Abbreviation
0	General classification	SPECIAL CHARGE
1	Admission charges	ADMIT CHARGE
2	Technical support charge	TECH SUPPORT CHG
3	UR service charge	UR CHARGE
4	Late discharge, medically necessary	LATE DISCH/MED NEC
5–8	Reserved	
9	Other special charges	OTHER SPEC CHG

023X   Incremental Nursing Charge

Revenue code 023X indicates extraordinary charges incurred for nursing services assessed in addition to the normal nursing charge associated with room and board.

Code	Subcategory	Standard Abbreviation
0	General classification	NURSING INCREM
1	Nursery	NUR INCR/NURSERY
2	OB	NUR INCR/OB
3	ICU (includes transitional care)	NUR INCR/ICU
4	CCU (includes transitional care)	NUR INCR/CCU
5	Hospice	NUR INCR/HOSPICE
6–8	Reserved	
9	Other	NUR INCR/OTHER

024X   All-Inclusive Ancillary

Revenue code 024X indicates a flat-rate charge incurred on either a daily basis or a total-stay basis for ancillary services only. Subcategory codes 1, 2, and 3 are intended for use by special residential facilities only (TOB 086X).

Code	Subcategory	Standard Abbreviation
0	General classification	ALL INCL ANCIL
1	Basic	ALL INCL BASIC
2	Comprehensive	ALL INCL COMP
3	Specialty	ALL INCL SPECIAL
4–8	Reserved	
9	Other all-inclusive ancillary	ALL INCL ANCIL/OTHER

025X   Pharmacy

Revenue code 025X indicates charges for medication that was produced, manufactured, packaged, controlled, assayed, dispensed, and distributed under the direction of a licensed pharmacist. (See also 063X, an extension of 025X.)

Code	Subcategory	Standard Abbreviation
0	General classification	PHARMACY
1	Generic drugs	DRUGS/GENERIC
2	Nongeneric drugs	DRUGS/NONGENERIC
3	Take-home drugs	DRUGS/TAKEHOME
4	Drugs incident to other diagnostic services	DRUGS/INCIDENT ODX
5	Drugs incident to radiology	DRUGS/INCIDENT RAD
6	Experimental drugs	DRUGS/EXPERIMT
7	Nonprescription	DRUGS/NONPSCRPT
8	IV solutions	IV SOLUTIONS
9	Other pharmacy	DRUGS/OTHER

Correct Reporting of Units for Drugs

When a HCPCS code must be reported with a drug, it is important to review the full HCPCS code descriptor for the drug in order to determine the unit amount to be reported on the claim. The short HCPCS descriptors, often used in charge masters, are limited to twenty-eight positions and therefore may not always contain the dosage information required for determining the unit amount (FL 46) on the UB-04.

The correct reporting of the unit of a drug can affect reimbursement considerably. For example, if the description for the drug code is 8 mg,

$ $ Billing Tip $ $

Pharmacy Charges

This code must be used when billing for drugs on an inpatient claim (PPS or non-PPS). The code may also be used on outpatient claims. However, most drugs on outpatient claims are packaged into the ambulatory payment classification (APC) rate under Medicare's Outpatient Prospective Payment System (OPPS) and, therefore, are paid as part of the service with which they are billed. Most payers accept revenue code 0250 for most pharmacy services. IV solutions, however, are often reported with detailed code 0258.

In some cases, a revenue code alone is sufficient when billing for a drug. In other cases, whether for inpatient or outpatient claims, payers require a revenue code together with the HCPCS code for the drug. When a pharmacy revenue code is reported on an outpatient claim, if the general revenue code 0250 is used, a HCPCS code is not required in FL 44; however, all other detailed revenue codes under 025X require the use of a HCPCS code in FL 44 for outpatient claims. Generally, the hospital's computer system is programmed to keep track of which revenue codes require a HCPCS code and for which payers.

and 8 mg is also the amount administered to the patient, then the unit reported is 1. However, if the description for the drug code is 25 mg and the patient is administered 100 mg, then the unit reported is 4: the hospital should be reimbursed for four units of the drug instead of one. When entering the units for the drug, therefore, billers need to check the full HCPCS descriptors to ensure that the correct number of units is being reported on the claim.

It is also important to not bill the units based on the way a drug is packaged or stocked. For example, assume that a drug is packaged in a 5 mg vial and that the patient receives one vial. If the HCPCS descriptor for the drug code specifies 1 mg, then the patient has received five units even though only one vial was administered.

"Incident-to" Charges

The following three revenue codes are referred to as "incident-to-other-diagnostic-services revenue codes."

• 0254	Pharmacy	Drugs incident to other diagnostic services
• 0371	Anesthesia	Anesthesia incident to other diagnostic services
• 0622	Medical/surgical supplies	Supplies incident to other diagnostic services

These codes can be used by providers that bill drugs, anesthesia, or medical/surgical supplies used for other diagnostic services (such as EEGs or gastrointestinal services) separately from charges for diagnostic services. Parallel to these codes are the "incident-to-radiology revenue codes."

• 0255	Pharmacy	Drugs incident to radiology
• 0371	Anesthesia	Anesthesia incident to radiology
• 0621	Medical/ surgical supplies	Supplies incident to radiology

These codes can be used by providers that bill drugs, anesthesia, or medical/surgical supplies used for radiology separately from radiology procedure charges. For example, the radiology APC payment, which includes pharmacy charges incident to radiology services (revenue code 0255), covers the cost of contrast materials used during the procedure (except for low osmolar contrast material—LOCM—which requires a different revenue code). Nonetheless, a provider may want to separate the cost of the contrast material from the cost of the procedure for accounting purposes. To do so, the provider would use revenue code 0255.

If revenue code 0255 is used to separate the cost of the drugs incident to the radiology procedure, those charges must appear on the same claim as the radiology procedure. Furthermore, if the hospital's charge for the radiology procedure includes the amount for the contrast material, the hospital must

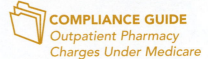

COMPLIANCE GUIDE
Outpatient Pharmacy Charges Under Medicare

According to Medicare, 025X pharmacy-related charges are not always covered and often are not properly supported by medical records. Payment for outpatient pharmacy services is allowable as long as the medication described on the claim matches the medical record. The Medicare rules require the charges to reflect reasonable costs (charges greater than $499.99 may come under medical review) and the documentation in the medical record (physician's orders, medication administration records, progress notes, and an itemized list of pharmacy charges) to justify the treatment provided. Billing only for services that are properly and fully documented in patients' medical records is critical in claims containing outpatient pharmacy services.

adjust the radiology procedure charge accordingly so that the cost of the contrast material is not included twice on the bill.

These billing principles apply to both sets of incident-to codes above.

026X IV Therapy

Revenue code 026X indicates the charge for equipment or administration of an IV solution by specially trained personnel to individuals requiring such treatment. For outpatient billing, this revenue code category usually requires HCPCS codes in FL 44. For home IV therapy equipment, the type of pump must be indicated with the appropriate HCPCS code, as the actual cost for each type of pump is factored into the basic per diem fee schedule.

Code	*Subcategory*	*Standard Abbreviation*
0	General classification	IV THERAPY
1	Infusion pump	IV THER/INFSN PUMP
2	IV Therapy/pharmacy services	IV THER/PHARM SVC
3	IV Therapy/drug/ supply delivery	IV THER/DRUG/SUPPLY/DEL
4	IV Therapy/supplies	IV THER/SUPPLIES
5–8	Reserved	
9	Other IV therapy	IV THERAPY/OTHER

027X Medical/Surgical Supplies and Devices

Revenue code 027X indicates the charges for supply items required for patient care. Medicare and other payers require a specific detail code for outpatient billing when one is available, rather than the general revenue code 0270. (See also 062X, an extension of 027X.)

Unlike most revenue codes, the revenue codes in the 027X series, except for 0278 (Other implant), do not require the use of HCPCS codes in FL 44 for Medicare outpatient billing. Most medical/surgical supplies and devices are packaged into the APC payment rate and, therefore, are paid as part of the surgical procedure or diagnostic or other service with which they are billed. When reporting packaged supplies, a HCPCS code is not required in FL 44. (*Note:* This is similar to the general pharmacy revenue code, 0250, above, for drugs that are usually considered packaged into the APC payment rate.)

Revenue code 0278 (Other implant) may require the use of a HCPCS code in FL 44 in Medicare outpatient billing to identity the implantable device, such as implantable orthotic and prosthetic devices or implantable DME. This code is also used with the appropriate HCPCS in code in FL 44 to bill for implants that have been granted pass-through status under OPPS.

On Medicare claims, only nonroutine items and services should be billed with this revenue code. For this reason, if supplies billed under revenue code 0270 are high-volume items, have high costs, and have a high potential for being noncovered, they may be selected by the FI for medical review.

Code	Subcategory	Standard Abbreviation
0	General classification	MED-SUR SUPPLIES
1	Nonsterile supply	NON-STER SUPPLY
2	Sterile supply	STERILE SUPPLY
3	Take-home supplies	TAKEHOME SUPPLY
4	Prosthetic/orthotic devices	PROSTH/ORTH DEV
5	Pacemaker	PACEMAKER
6	Intraocular lens	INTRA OC LENS
7	Oxygen—take-home	02/TAKEHOME
8	Other implant	SUPPLY/IMPLANTS
9	Other supplies/devices	SUPPLY/OTHER

028X   Oncology

Revenue code 028X indicates charges for the treatment of tumors and related diseases. This code is used in combination with revenue code 0636 (Drugs requiring detailed coding).

Code	Subcategory	Standard Abbreviation
0	General classification	ONCOLOGY
1–8	Reserved	
9	Other oncology	ONCOLOGY OTHER

029X   Durable Medical Equipment (Other Than Renal)

Revenue code 029X indicates charges for medical equipment that can withstand repeated use (excluding renal equipment). All payers require a detailed code rather than the general revenue code 0290.

Code	Subcategory	Standard Abbreviation
0	General classification	DME
1	Rental	DME-RENTAL
2	Purchase of new DME	DME-NEW
3	Purchase of used DME	DME-USED
4	Supplies/drugs for DME	DME-SUPPLIES/DRUGS
5–8	Reserved	
9	Other equipment	DME-OTHER

030X   Laboratory

Revenue code 030X indicates charges for the performance of diagnostic and routine clinical laboratory tests. The units are the number of tests. It is one of the most commonly used codes.

For Medicare claims, the general revenue code 0300 can be used to report all laboratory charges in this category except the charge for nonroutine dialysis, which requires detailed code 0304. The other subcategory codes

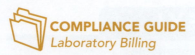
Many laboratory billing compliance issues involve charging Medicare for services not rendered, for unbundled tests, or for tests that were deemed to be medically unnecessary. Some problems stem from inaccurate physicians' orders or incomplete documentation of patients' diagnoses. These problems are serious, because an incomplete lab bill can hold up an entire claim for other care rendered to the patient. Facilities need to have procedures in place to avoid these situations.

are available to meet individual hospital needs or third-party billing requirements for more detailed coding. As with most revenue codes, code 030X requires the use of HCPCS codes in FL 44 on outpatient claims.

Code	Subcategory	Standard Abbreviation
0	General classification	LAB
1	Chemistry	CHEMISTRY TESTS
2	Immunology	IMMUNOLOGY TESTS
3	Renal patient (home)	RENAL-HOME
4	Nonroutine dialysis	NON-RTNE DIALYSIS
5	Hematology	HEMATOLOGY TESTS
6	Bacteriology and microbiology	BACT & MICRO TESTS
7	Urology	UROLOGY TESTS
8	Reserved	
9	Other laboratory	OTHER LAB TESTS

031X   Laboratory Pathology

Revenue code 031X indicates charges for diagnostic and routine laboratory tests on tissues and cultures. The units are the number of tests.

Code	Subcategory	Standard Abbreviation
0	General classification	PATHOLOGY LAB
1	Cytology	CYTOLOGY TESTS
2	Histology	HISTOLOGY TESTS
3	Reserved	
4	Biopsy	BIOPSY TESTS
5–8	Reserved	
9	Other laboratory pathology	PATH LAB OTHER

032X   Radiology—Diagnostic

Revenue code 032X indicates charges for diagnostic radiology services provided for the examination and care of patients. It includes the taking, processing, examining, and interpreting of radiographs and fluorographs. The units are the number of tests.

Code	Subcategory	Standard Abbreviation
0	General classification	DX X-RAY
1	Angiocardiology	DX X-RAY/ANGIO
2	Arthrography	DX X-RAY/ARTHO
3	Arteriography	DX X-RAY/ARTER
4	Chest X-ray	DX X-RAY/CHEST
5–8	Reserved	
9	Other radiology—diagnostic	DX X-RAY/OTHER

033X Radiology—Therapeutic and/or Chemotherapy Administration

Revenue code 033X indicates charges for therapeutic radiology services and chemotherapy administration provided for the care and treatment of patients. This code includes therapy by injection and/or ingestion of radioactive substances. The units are the number of tests. Medicare requires the use of detailed codes with this revenue code category.

While code 033X is used to charge for chemotherapy administration, the actual chemotherapy drugs are reported under pharmacy revenue codes 025X or 063X. Revenue codes 0331, 0332, and 0335 require the use of code 0636 (Drugs requiring detailed coding) with the appropriate HCPCS code.

Code	Subcategory	Standard Abbreviation
0	General classification	RADIOLOGY THERAPY
1	Chemotherapy administration—injected	RAD-CHEMO-INJECT
2	Chemotherapy administration—oral	RAD-CHEMO-ORAL
3	Radiation therapy	RAD-RADIATION
4	Reserved	
5	Chemotherapy administration—IV	RAD-CHEMO-IV
6–8	Reserved	
9	Other radiology—therapeutic	RADIOLOGY OTHER

034X Nuclear Medicine

Revenue code 034X indicates charges for procedures, tests, and radiopharmaceuticals performed by a department handling radioactive materials as required for diagnosis and treatment of patients. The units are the number of tests.

Code	Subcategory	Standard Abbreviation
0	General classification	NUCLEAR MEDICINE
1	Diagnostic	NUC MED/DX
2	Therapeutic	NUC MED/RX
3	Diagnostic radiopharmaceuticals	NUC MED/DX RADIOPHARM
4	Therapeutic radiopharmaceuticals	NUC MED/RX RADIOPHARM
5–8	Reserved	
9	Other nuclear medicine	NUC MED/OTHER

035X CT (Computed Tomographic) Scan

This code indicates charges for CT scans of the head and other parts of the body. The units are the number of tests. Because of coverage limitations, many payers require identifying each test with a HCPCS code, service date, and number of units for outpatient billing.

Code	Subcategory	Standard Abbreviation
0	General classification	CT SCAN
1	CT—head scan	CT SCAN/HEAD
2	CT—body scan	CT SCAN/BODY
3–8	Reserved	
9	CT—other	CT SCAN/OTHER

<table>
<tr><td>

$ $ Billing Tip $ $

Outpatient Surgery Charges

When an outpatient surgery procedure code (CPT code range 10021–69990) is reported in FL 44, one of the following revenue codes, reflecting the treatment site, is usually reported:

036X   Operating room services
045X   Emergency room
051X   Clinic

</td></tr>
</table>

Code	Subcategory	Standard Abbreviation
0	General classification	CT SCAN
1	CT—head scan	CT SCAN/HEAD
2	CT—body scan	CT SCAN/BODY
3–8	Reserved	
9	CT—other	CT SCAN/OTHER

036X   Operating Room Services

Revenue code 036X indicates charges for services provided to patients by specially trained nursing personnel who assist physicians with surgical and related procedures during and immediately following surgery. Medicare requires the use of a detailed code when reporting operating room services for a kidney transplant (revenue code 0367).

Code	Subcategory	Standard Abbreviation
0	General classification	OR SERVICES
1	Minor surgery	OR/MINOR
2	Organ transplant—other than kidney	OR/ORGAN TRANS
3–6	Reserved	
7	Kidney transplant	OR/KIDNEY TRANS
8	Reserved	
9	Other OR services	OR/OTHER

037X   Anesthesia

Revenue code 037X indicates charges for anesthesia services in the hospital. An anesthesia charge should be billed with a recovery room charge (revenue code category 071X).

Subcategory code 4 is used to identify acupuncture, as some payers, including Medicare, do not cover it. The patient may be billed for noncovered services if appropriate.

Code	Subcategory	Standard Abbreviation
0	General classification	ANESTHESIA
1	Anesthesia incident to radiology	ANESTH/INCIDENT RAD
2	Anesthesia incident to other DX services	ANESTH/INCIDNT OTHR DX
3	Reserved	
4	Acupuncture	ANESTH/ACUPUNC
5–8	Reserved	
9	Other anesthesia	ANESTH/OTHER

038X   Blood and Blood Components

Revenue code 038X indicates charges for blood and blood components. Private payers require these charges to be separately identified. The unit, when appropriate, is the number of pints of blood. Currently many states do not charge for blood because it is donated by organizations such as the Red Cross. Even when there are no charges for the blood because it has been donated, charges for the processing and storage of the blood still apply.

When revenue code 038X is used, the appropriate value codes must be used in FLs 39–41 (Value Codes and Amounts; see Chapter 11) to describe the blood cash deductible paid by the patient (value code 06), the pints furnished (value code 37), the pints the patient is responsible for (value code 38), and/or the pints the patient has replaced (value code 39).

Code	Subcategory	Standard Abbreviation
0	General classification	BLOOD & BLOOD COMP
1	Packed red cells	BLOOD/PKD RED
2	Whole blood	BLOOD/WHOLE
3	Plasma	BLOOD/PLASMA
4	Platelets	BLOOD/PLATELETS
5	Leukocytes	BLOOD/LEUKOCYTES
6	Other blood components	BLOOD/COMPONENTS
7	Other derivatives (cryoprecipitate)	BLOOD/DERIVATIVES
8	Reserved	
9	Other blood and blood components	BLOOD/OTHER

039X   Administration, Processing, and Storage for Blood and Blood Components

Revenue code 039X indicates charges for the administration, processing, and storage of whole blood and blood components. The units, when appropriate, are the number of pints of blood.

Code	Subcategory	Standard Abbreviation
0	General classification	BLOOD/ADMIN/STOR
1	Administration (e.g., transfusion)	BLOOD/ADMIN
2	Processing and storage	BLOOD/STORAGE
3–8	Reserved	
9	Other blood handling	BLOOD/ADMIN/ STOR/OTHER

A diagnostic mammography is paid at a higher rate than a screening mammography. Therefore, if revenue code 0401 (Diagnostic mammography) is billed, the diagnosis reported in FL 67 (Principal Diagnosis Code) must match the diagnosis for a diagnostic mammography. For Medicare, a diagnostic mammography may be provided to someone with a high risk of breast cancer, for example, which would include a personal history of breast cancer (diagnosis code V10.3), a family history of breast cancer (V16.3), or a personal history of biopsy-proven benign breast disease (V15.89). If the ordering physician records the diagnosis code for a screening mammography (for example, V76.12), but the revenue code billed is for diagnostic mammography, which is paid at a higher rate, the service may not be covered or the claim may be rejected.

FYI

Outpatient Rehabilitation Charges

Medicare payment for outpatient rehabilitation services, including physical therapy, occupational therapy, and speech-language pathology (revenue code categories 042X, 043X, and 044X), is made under the Medicare Physician Fee Schedule (MPFS). Payments are based on the HCPCS code reported. Selection of the HCPCS code is based on the amount of time the provider spends actually treating the patient. The units are time increments of approximately fifteen minutes. Recurring outpatient services billed under these revenue code categories are billed as a series at the end of each month or at the end of treatment. (When billing these services on an inpatient claim, only the revenue code and amount are required.)

040X Other Imaging Services

Revenue code 040X indicates charges for specialty imaging services for body structures. The units are the number of tests.

Code	Subcategory	Standard Abbreviation
0	General classification	IMAGING SERVICE
1	Diagnostic mammography	DIAG MAMMOGRAPHY
2	Ultrasound	ULTRASOUND
3	Screening mammography	SCRN MAMMOGRAPHY
4	Positron emission tomography	PET SCAN
5–8	Reserved	
9	Other imaging services	OTHER IMAGE SVCS

041X Respiratory Services

Revenue code 041X indicates charges for administering oxygen and certain potent drugs through inhalation or positive pressure, and other forms of rehabilitative therapy. The units are the number of treatments.

Code	Subcategory	Standard Abbreviation
0	General classification	RESPIRATORY SVC
1	Reserved	
2	Inhalation services	INHALATION SVC
3	Hyperbaric oxygen therapy	HYPERBARIC 02
4–8	Reserved	
9	Other respiratory services	OTHER RESPIR SVCS

042X Physical Therapy

Revenue code 042X indicates charges for therapeutic exercises, massage, and utilization of effective properties of light, heat, cold, water, electricity, and assistive devices for diagnosing and rehabilitating patients who have neuromuscular, orthopedic, and other disabilities. The service units correlate with HCPCS codes that define the amount of time the provider actually treats the patient. Medicare requires the use of detailed codes with this revenue code category.

Code	Subcategory	Standard Abbreviation
0	General classification	PHYSICAL THERP
1	Visit	PHYS THERP/VISIT
2	Hourly	PHYS THERP/HOUR
3	Group	PHYS THERP/GROUP
4	Evaluation or reevaluation	PHYS THERP/EVAL
5–8	Reserved	
9	Other physical therapy	OTHER PHYS THERP

043X Occupational Therapy

Revenue code 043X indicates charges for services provided by a qualified occupational therapy practitioner for therapeutic interventions to improve, sustain, or restore an individual's level of function in performance of activities of daily living and work. Services include such activities as therapeutic exercises, sensorimotor processing, psychosocial skills training, training in the use of orthotics and prosthetic devices, and adaptation of environments. The service units correlate with HCPCS codes that define the amount of time the provider actually treats the patient.

Code	Subcategory	Standard Abbreviation
0	General classification	OCCUPATION THER
1	Visit	OCCUP THERP/VISIT
2	Hourly	OCCUP THERP/HOUR
3	Group	OCCUP THERP/GROUP
4	Evaluation or reevaluation	OCCUP THERP/EVAL
5–8	Reserved	
9	Other occupational therapy	OCCUP THER/OTHER

044X Speech Therapy—Language Pathology

Revenue code 044X indicates charges for services provided by a qualified speech therapist to persons with impaired functional communications skills. The service units correlate with HCPCS codes that define the amount of time the provider actually treats the patient.

Code	Subcategory	Standard Abbreviation
0	General classification	SPEECH THERAPY
1	Visit	SPEECH THERP/VISIT
2	Hourly	SPEECH THERP/HOUR
3	Group	SPEECH THERP/GROUP
4	Evaluation or reevaluation	SPEECH THERP/EVAL
5–8	Reserved	
9	Other speech therapy	OTHER SPEECH THERP

045X Emergency Room

Revenue code 045X indicates charges for emergency treatment to ill and injured persons who require immediate unscheduled medical or surgical care. The units are the number of visits. The patient's reason for visit diagnosis code or codes should be reported in FL 70 (Patient's Reason for Visit) in conjunction with 045X.

Code 0450 should not be used in conjunction with any other revenue code in the 045X series. Note that the sum of codes 0451 and 0452 is the equivalent of 0450. Payers that do not require a breakdown should roll these two codes into code 0450. When a hospital performs an initial screening only, code 0451 may be used alone; however, stand-alone usage of code 0452 is not acceptable.

$$ Billing Tip $$

Relating Revenue Codes 042X, 043X, and 044X to Value and Occurrence Codes

Report therapy charges with the corresponding value code (50, 51, or 52) for the number of physical, occupational, or speech therapy visits from the onset of treatment through the current billing period in FLs 39–41 (Value Codes and Amounts). Also report the appropriate occurrence codes and corresponding dates in FLs 31–34 (Occurrence Codes and Dates) for the date symptoms started, the date the therapy plan was established, and the date therapy was started.

$$ Billing Tip $$

HCPCS Modifiers

Remember to use the following modifiers with outpatient therapy services on Medicare claims:

- GN Speech therapy
- GO Occupational therapy
- GP Physical therapy

FYI

EMTALA

EMTALA stands for the Emergency Medical Treatment and Active Labor Act. Under the provisions of EMTALA, a hospital that receives Medicare benefits must provide—upon request and within its capabilities—an appropriate medical screening examination and stabilizing treatment to any individual with an emergency medical condition and to any woman in active labor, regardless of the individual's ability to pay.

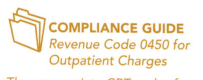

COMPLIANCE GUIDE

Revenue Code 0450 for Outpatient Charges

The appropriate CPT codes for physicians' work (evaluation and management services or procedures) are reported in FL 44 (HCPCS/Rate/HIPPS Code) on an outpatient claim with revenue code 0450. Figure 12.4 is an example of an outpatient claim showing the use of CPT codes with an emergency room visit.

Code	Subcategory	Standard Abbreviation
0	General classification	EMERG ROOM
1	EMTALA emergency medical screening	ER/EMTALA
2	ER beyond EMTALA	ER/BEYOND EMTALA
3–5	Reserved	
6	Urgent care	ER/URGENT CARE
7–8	Reserved	
9	Other emergency room	OTHER EMERG ROOM

046X   Pulmonary Function

Revenue code 046X indicates charges for tests that measure inhaled and exhaled gases, analyze blood, and evaluate the patient's ability to exchange oxygen and other exhaled gases. The units are the number of tests.

Code	Subcategory	Standard Abbreviation
0	General classification	PULMONARY FUNC
1–8	Reserved	
9	Other pulmonary function	OTHER PULMONARY FUNC

The charges may include the pharmacy, anesthesia, and supplies used in connection with the pulmonary function procedures, or providers may bill for them separately using the incident-to other diagnostic services revenue codes.

Figure 12.4

Example of CPT Code Usage with an ER Visit

42 REV. CD.	43 DESCRIPTION	44 HCPCS / RATE / HIPPS CODE	45 SERV. DATE	46 SERV. UNITS	47 TOTAL CHARGES	48 NON-COVERED CHARGES	49
0324	DX X-RAY/CHEST	71020	111909	1	159 55		
0450	EMERG ROOM	99282	111909	1	98 00		
0001	PAGE 1 OF 1	CREATION DATE	112409	TOTALS ⟶	257 55		

If billed separately, the charges must appear on the same claim with the pulmonary function procedure.

047X   Audiology

Revenue code 047X indicates charges provided by or through the supervision of a qualified audiologist for the detection and management of communication handicaps centering in whole or in part on the hearing function. The units are the number of tests.

Code	Subcategory	Standard Abbreviation
0	General classification	AUDIOLOGY
1	Diagnostic	AUDIOLOGY/DX
2	Treatment	AUDIOLOGY/RX
3–8	Reserved	
9	Other audiology	OTHER AUDIOL

048X   Cardiology

Revenue code 048X indicates charges for cardiac procedures rendered or arranged by staff from the cardiology department of the hospital. Such procedures include, but are not limited to, heart catheterization, coronary angiography, Swan-Ganz catheterization, and exercise stress tests. The units are the number of tests.

Code	Subcategory	Standard Abbreviation
0	General classification	CARDIOLOGY
1	Cardiac cath lab	CARDIAC CATH LAB
2	Stress test	STRESS TEST
3	Echocardiology	ECHOCARDIOLOGY
4–8	Reserved	
9	Other cardiology	OTHER CARDIOL

049X   Ambulatory Surgical Care

Revenue code 049X indicates charges for ambulatory surgery that are not covered by any other category.

Code	Subcategory	Standard Abbreviation
0	General classification	AMBULTRY SURG
1–8	Reserved	
9	Other ambulatory surgical	OTHER AMBL SURG

050X   Outpatient Services

Revenue code 050X indicates outpatient charges for services rendered to an outpatient who is then admitted as an inpatient before midnight of the following day. This revenue code is no longer used for Medicare billing.

Code	Subcategory	Standard Abbreviation
0	General classification	OUTPATIENT SVCS
1–8	Reserved	
9	Other outpatient	OTHER—O/P SERVICES

051X   Clinic

Revenue code 051X indicates clinic (nonemergency/scheduled outpatient visit) charges for providing diagnostic, preventive, curative, rehabilitative, and education services to ambulatory patients. The units are the number of visits.

Code	Subcategory	Standard Abbreviation
0	General classification	CLINIC
1	Chronic pain center	CHRONIC PAIN CLINIC
2	Dental clinic	DENTAL CLINIC
3	Psychiatric clinic	PSYCHIATRIC CLINIC
4	OB-GYN clinic	OB-GYN CLINIC
5	Pediatric clinic	PEDIATRIC CLINIC
6	Urgent care clinic	URGENT CARE CLINIC
7	Family practice clinic	FAMILY CLINIC
8	Reserved	
9	Other clinic	OTHER CLINIC

052X   Freestanding Clinic

Revenue code 052X indicates charges for an outpatient visit at a freestanding clinic. This code is primarily used to bill for services provided by RHCs (rural health clinics) and FQHCs (federally qualified health centers). Medicare requires the use of a detailed code with this revenue code series.

Code	Subcategory	Standard Abbreviation
0	General classification	FREESTAND CLINIC
1	Clinic visit by member to RHC/FQHC	FS-RURAL/CLINIC
2	Home visit by RHC/FQHC practitioner	FS-RURAL/HOME
3	Family practice clinic	FS-FAMILY PRACT
4	Visit by RHC/FQHC practitioner to a member in a covered Part A stay at a SNF	RHC/FQHC/SNF/COVERED
5	Visit by RHC/FQHC practitioner to a member in a SNF (not in a covered Part A stay) or NF or ICF MR or other residential facility	RHC/FQHC/SNF/NONCOVERED
6	Urgent care clinic	FR/STD URGENT CLINIC
7	Visiting nurse service(s) to a member's home when in a home health shortage area	RHC/FQHC/HOME/VIS NURSE
8	Visit by RHC/FQHC practitioner to other non-RHC/FQHC site (e.g., scene of accident)	RHC/FQHC/OTHER SITE
9	Other freestanding clinic	OTHER FS-CLINIC

053X   Osteopathic Services

Revenue code 053X indicates charges for a structural evaluation of the cranium and entire cervical, dorsal, and lumbar spine by a doctor of osteopathy. The units are the number of visits. This revenue code is designed to represent services unique to osteopathic hospitals that cannot be accommodated with existing codes.

Code	Subcategory	Standard Abbreviation
0	General classification	OSTEOPATH SVCS
1	Osteopathic therapy	OSTEOPATH RX
9	Other osteopathic services	OTHER OSTEOPATH

054X   Ambulance

Revenue code 054X indicates charges for ambulance services, usually on an unscheduled basis, necessary for the transport of ill or injured persons who require medical attention at a health care facility. The units are the number of miles, items, and services.

The point of pickup is reported on every ambulance claim in FLs 39–41 (Value Codes and Amounts) using value code A0 (Special ZIP code reporting), with the corresponding five-digit ZIP code.

EXAMPLE: RC 0540; HCPCS code A0429QNRH, where A0429 is the HCPCS code (Ambulance service, basic life support, emergency transport), QN indicates services provided directly by a provider of service, and RH (residence, hospital) indicates the pickup and destination sites. The service unit is one.

A second, separate revenue code line is reported with the HCPCS code for the mileage.

EXAMPLE: RC 0540; HCPCS code A0425 (Ground mileage); service units 18 (miles).

Each one-way ambulance trip requires the use of two separate revenue code lines. The date of service for both lines must be the same.

Code	Subcategory	Standard Abbreviation
0	General classification	AMBULANCE
1	Supplies	AMBUL/SUPPLY
2	Medical transport	AMBUL/MED TRANS
3	Heart mobile	AMBUL/HEART MOB
4	Oxygen	AMBUL/0XYGEN
5	Air ambulance	AIR AMBULANCE
6	Neonatal ambulance services	AMBUL/NEONAT
7	Pharmacy	AMBUL/PHARMAS
8	ECG transmission	AMBUL/EKG TRANS
9	Other ambulance	AMBUL/OTHER

055X   Home Health—Skilled Nursing

Revenue code 055X indicates charges for nursing services that must be provided under the direct supervision of a home health (HH) licensed nurse to ensure the safety of the patient and to achieve the medically desired result. This code may be used for nursing home services or may be a service charge

$ $ Billing Tip $ $
Ambulance Services
Revenue code series 054X requires a HCPCS code and two modifiers in FL 44 (HCPCS/ Rate/HIPPS Code) to bill for ambulance services. The modifiers indicate the type of arrangement made (whether the ambulance service was provided under arrangement by a provider or provided directly by a provider) as well as details about the pickup and destination. List the modifier describing the arrangement first, followed by the modifiers describing the origin and destination. The modifiers are reported on the same line as the HCPCS code for the transport.

As with outpatient rehabilitation services, including physical therapy, occupational therapy, and speech-language pathology (revenue code categories 042X, 043X, and 044X), any recurring outpatient services billed under home health revenue code categories 055X–059X must be billed monthly or at the conclusion of treatment. For Medicare billing, revenue codes 055X–059X also require detailed coding when applicable.

for home health billing. The units are the number of visits or, for subcategory code 2 (Hourly charge), the number of hours.

Code	Subcategory	Standard Abbreviation
0	General classification	SKILLED NURSING-HH
1	Visit charge	SKILLED NURS-VISIT
2	Hourly charge	SKILLED NURS-HOUR
3–8	Reserved	
9	Other skilled nursing	SKILLED NURS/OTHER

056X   Home Health—Medical Social Services

Revenue code 056X indicates home health agency charges for services such as counseling patients, interviewing patients, and interpreting social situation problems rendered to patients on any basis. The units are the number of visits or hours.

Code	Subcategory	Standard Abbreviation
0	General classification	MED SOCIAL-HH
1	Visit charge	MED SOC SVCS-VISIT
2	Hourly charge	MED SOC SVCS-HOUR
3–8	Reserved	
9	Other medical social services	MED SOC SVCS-OTHER

057X   Home Health Aid

Revenue code 057X indicates charges by a home health agency for aids who are primarily responsible for the personal care of a patient. The units are the number of visits or hours.

Code	Subcategory	Standard Abbreviation
0	General classification	HH AIDE
1	Visit charge	HH AIDE-VISIT
2	Hourly charge	HH AIDE-HOUR
3–8	Reserved	
9	Other HH-aid	HH AIDE-OTHER

058X   Home Health—Other Visits

Revenue code 058X indicates home health agency charges for visits other than physical therapy, occupational therapy, or speech therapy, which need to be specifically identified by their own revenue codes. The units are the number of visits or hours.

Code	Subcategory	Standard Abbreviation
0	General classification	HH-OTH VIS
1	Visit charge	HH-OTH VIS/VISIT
2	Hourly charge	HH-OTH VIS/HOUR
3	Assessment	HH-OTH VIS/ASSESS
4–8	Reserved	
9	Other HH visits	HH-OTH VIS/OTHER

059X   Home Health Units of Service

Revenue code 059X indicates charges by a home health agency that bills for services based on the units of service provided.

Code	Subcategory	Standard Abbreviation
0	General classification	HH-SVCS/UNIT
1–9	Reserved	

060X   Home Health—Oxygen

Revenue code 060X indicates home health agency charges for oxygen equipment—supplies or contents—excluding purchased equipment. The units are the number of rental months for equipment or the number of feet or pounds of oxygen for contents. Note that for this revenue code, Medicare requires detailed coding rather than the use of code 0600.

Code	Subcategory	Standard Abbreviation
0	General classification	02/HOME HEALTH
1	Oxygen—stationary equipment/supplies or contents	02/STAT EQUIP/SUPLY/CONT
2	Oxygen—stationary equipment/supplies <1 LPM	02/STAT EQP/SUPPL<1 LPM
3	Oxygen—stationary equipment/supplies >4 LPM	02/STAT EQP/SUPPL>4 LPM
4	Oxygen—portable add-on	02/PORTBLE ADD-ON
5–8	Reserved	
9	Oxygen—other	O2/OTHER

061X   Magnetic Resonance Technology (MRT)

Revenue code 061X indicates charges for magnetic resonance imaging (MRI) and magnetic resonance angiography (MRA) of the brain and other parts of the body. The units are the number of tests. Because of coverage limitations, some payers require a specific test to be identified. For Medicare billing, diagnostic services using this revenue code series may be subject to medical review by Medicare FIs because of their high cost, high usage volume, and high potential for not being covered.

Code	Subcategory	Standard Abbreviation
0	General classification	MRT
1	MRI-brain/brainstem	MRI/BRAIN
2	MRI-spinal cord/spine	MRI/SPINE
3	Reserved	
4	MRI—other	MRI/OTHER
5	MRA—head and neck	MRA/HEAD & NECK
6	MRA—lower extremities	MRA/LOWER EXTRM
7	Reserved	
8	MRA—other	MRA/OTHER
9	Other MRT	MRT/OTHER

FYI

Terminology for Oxygen Charges

Subcategory code 1 is used to report both the equipment (supply) and the oxygen (content) for a stationary system. For oxygen equipment, the number of rental months being billed should be reported in FL 46 (Units) for each piece of equipment. For oxygen content, the number of feet or pounds of oxygen used should be reported in FL 46 (Service Units). Both the equipment and the oxygen are billed on separate lines and on a monthly basis.

In subcategory codes 2 and 3, LPM refers to the amount of oxygen prescribed in liter(s) per minute. Depending on the LPM amount and several other factors, the monthly payment for stationary oxygen may be subject to an adjustment.

062X   Medical/Surgical Supplies—Extension of 027X

Revenue code 062X indicates charges for supply items required for patient care. This category is an extension of 027X and is used for reporting an additional breakdown of supply charges when needed. Medicare requires the use of a detailed code when billing for FDA investigational devices, revenue code 0624.

Providers may bill the supplies used in connection with a radiology procedure as part of the procedure itself, or they may bill them separately under revenue code 0621 in this revenue code series. If billed separately, the charge must appear on the same claim as the radiology procedure. The same rule applies to revenue code 0622 in this series (Supplies incident to other diagnostic services), which is used to bill for supplies used with other diagnostic services.

Code	Subcategory	Standard Abbreviation
0	Reserved (for general classification, use code 0270)	
1	Supplies incident to radiology	MED-SURG SUPL-INCDT RAD
2	Supplies incident to other DX services	MED-SURG SUPL-INCDT ODX
3	Surgical dressings	SURG DRESSINGS
4	FDA investigational devices	FDA INVEST DEVICE
5–9	Reserved	

063X   Pharmacy—Extension of 025X

Revenue code 063X indicates charges for medication produced, manufactured, packaged, controlled, assayed, dispensed, and distributed under the direction of a licensed pharmacist. This category is an extension of 025X and is used for reporting an additional breakdown of pharmacy drugs. The units are defined by the HCPCS codes reported in FL 44.

As with drugs reported with revenue code 025X, when a HCPCS code is required in FL 44 for drugs reported with revenue code 063X, the full HCPCS description for the drug should be checked in order to determine the unit amount. For example, the description of azithromycin, "HCPCS J0456, Injection, azithromycin, 500 mg," indicates that the dosage amount for azithromycin is 500 mg. Therefore, if the patient's medical record reports that the patient received 500 mg, the unit amount reported on the UB-04 claim would be 1, whereas if the medical record showed that the patient received 1500 mg, the unit amount reported would be 3.

Code	Subcategory	Standard Abbreviation
0	Reserved (for general classification, use code 0250)	
1	Single source drug	DRUG/SINGLE
2	Multiple source drug	DRUG/MULTIPLE
3	Restrictive prescription	DRUG/RESTRICT
4	Erythropoietin (EPO) < 10,000 units	DRUG/EPO<10,000 UNITS
5	Erythropoietin (EPO) ≥ 10,000 units	DRUG/EPO≥10,000 UNITS
6	Drugs requiring detailed coding	DRUG/DETAIL CODE
7	Self-administrable drugs	DRUG/SELF ADMIN
8–9	Reserved	

064X   Home IV Therapy Services

Revenue code 064X indicates a charge for IV drug therapy services performed in the patient's residence.

Code	Subcategory	Standard Abbreviation
0	General classification	IV THERAPY SVC
1	Nonroutine nursing*	NON RT NURSING/CENTRAL
2	IV site care*	IV SITE CARE/CENTRAL
3	IV start/care**	IV STRT CARE/PERIPHRL
4	Nonroutine nursing**	NONRT NURSING/PERIPHRL
5	Training patient/caregiver*	TRNG PT/CAREGVR/CENTRAL
6	Training disabled patient*	TRNG DSBLPT/CENTRL
7	Training patient/caregiver**	TRNG/PT/CARGVR/PERIPHRL
8	Training disabled patient**	TRNG/DSBLPT/PERIPHRL
9	Other IV therapy services	OTHER IV THERAPY SVC

*central line   **peripheral line

$$ Billing Tip $$

064X and HCPCS Codes

For home IV providers, the HCPCS code is reported for all IV equipment as well as for all types of covered therapy services.

065X   Hospice Services

Revenue code 065X indicates charges for hospice care services for a terminally ill patient who elects these services in place of other medical services for the terminal condition. The units are the number of hours or days. Revenue code 0651 (Routine home care) is used to report fewer than eight hours of care a day. Revenue code 0652 (Continuous home care) requires a minimum of eight hours of care a day, not necessarily consecutive, and must be accompanied by a physician procedure code.

Code	Subcategory	Standard Abbreviation
0	General classification	HOSPICE
1	Routine home care	HOSPICE/RTN HOME
2	Continuous home care	HOSPICE/CTNS HOME
3–4	Reserved	
5	Inpatient respite care	HOSPICE/IP RESPITE
6	General inpatient care nonrespite	HOSPICE/IP NON-RESPITE
7	Physician services	HOSPICE/PHYSICIAN
8	Hospice room and board—nursing facility	HOSPICE/R&B NURSE FAC
9	Other hospice service	HOSPICE/OTHER

066X   Respite Care

Revenue code 066X indicates charges for nonhospice respite care. The units are the number of hours or days. Revenue code 066X applies to home health billing.

Code	Subcategory	Standard Abbreviation
0	General classification	RESPITE CARE
1	Hourly charge—nursing	RESPITE/NURSING
2	Hourly charge/aid/ homemaker/companion	RESPITE/AIDE/ HMEMKR/COMP
3	Daily respite charge	RESPITE/DAILY
4–8	Reserved	
9	Other respite care	RESPITE/OTHER

067X Outpatient Special Residence Charges

Revenue code 067X indicates residence arrangements for patients requiring continuous outpatient care.

Code	Subcategory	Standard Abbreviation
0	General classification	OP SPEC RES
1	Hospital owned	OP SPEC RES/HOSP OWNED
2	Contracted	OP SPEC RES/CONTRACTED
3–8	Reserved	
9	Other special residence charge	OP SPEC RES/OTHER

068X Trauma Response

$ $ Billing Tip $ $

068X and Noncritical Care
When revenue code 068X is billed in association with services other than critical care, payment for trauma activation is bundled into the other services provided on that day.

Revenue code 068X indicates charges for the activation of a trauma team. This code is to be used by licensed trauma centers only. Activation refers to prehospital notification of key hospital personnel in response to prehospital caregivers' triage information that a trauma patient will be arriving. The various levels (I–IV) refer to designations by the state or local government authority or as verified by the American College of Surgeons.

Revenue code 068X is used to represent the trauma activation costs only and is not a replacement for the emergency room visit fee (revenue code 045X). If trauma activation occurs, both codes will normally be reported on the claim.

Code	Subcategory	Standard Abbreviation
0	Not used	
1	Level I trauma	TRAUMA LEVEL I
2	Level II trauma	TRAUMA LEVEL II
3	Level III trauma	TRAUMA LEVEL III
4	Level IV trauma	TRAUMA LEVEL IV
5–8	Reserved	
9	Other trauma response	TRAUMA OTHER

069X Reserved

070X Cast Room

Revenue code 070X indicates charges for services related to the application, maintenance, and removal of casts.

Code	Subcategory	Standard Abbreviation
0	General classification	CAST ROOM
1–9	Reserved	

071X Recovery Room

Revenue code 071X indicates a room charge for patient recovery after surgery. Under Medicare, recovery room services do not require a HCPCS code, as they are packaged with the APC payment for the HCPCS-coded medical visit or procedure.

Code	Subcategory	Standard Abbreviation
0	General classification	RECOVERY ROOM
1–9	Reserved	

072X Labor Room/Delivery

Revenue code 072X indicates charges for labor and delivery room services provided by specially trained nursing personnel to patients, including pre-natal care during labor, assistance during delivery, postnatal care in the recovery room, and minor gynecologic procedures if performed in the delivery suite. The units (for codes 0721, 0722, and 0724) are the number of days.

Code	Subcategory	Standard Abbreviation
0	General classification	DELIVERY ROOM/LABOR
1	Labor	LABOR
2	Delivery room	DELIVERY ROOM
3	Circumcision	CIRCUMCISION
4	Birthing center	BIRTHING CNTR
5–8	Reserved	
9	Other labor room/delivery	OTHER/DELIV-LABOR

073X EKG/ECG (Electrocardiogram)

Revenue code 073X indicates charges for the operation of specialized equipment to record variations in heart muscle actions for the purpose of diagnosing heart ailments. The units are the number of tests.

Code	Subcategory	Standard Abbreviation
0	General classification	EKG/ECG
1	Holter monitor	HOLTER MONT
2	Telemetry	TELEMETRY
3–8	Reserved	
9	Other EKG/ECG	OTHER EKG/ECG

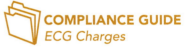

COMPLIANCE GUIDE
ECG Charges

Medicare checks that the number of units reported in the Service Units field (FL 46) for revenue code 073X does not exceed three, except for revenue codes 0730 and 0732. These two revenue codes may be reported with a HCPCS code for which the number of units cannot be greater than the number of days in the Statement Covers period (FL 6), and therefore the number of units reported may exceed three.

$ $ Billing Tip $ $

Incident-to Other Diagnostic Services

The charges for ECGs, EEGs, or GI services may include the pharmacy, anesthesia, and supplies used in connection with each procedure, or providers may bill them separately using the incident-to other diagnostic services revenue codes. If billed separately, the charges must appear on the same claim with the ECG, EEG, or GI service procedure.

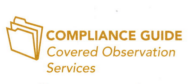

074X   EEG (Electroencephalogram)

Revenue code 074X indicates charges for operation of specialized equipment to measure impulse frequencies and differences in electrical potential in various areas of the brain to obtain data for use in diagnosing brain disorders. The units are the number of tests.

Code	Subcategory	Standard Abbreviation
0	General classification	EEG
1–9	Reserved	

075X   Gastrointestinal (GI) Services

Revenue code 075X indicates charges for GI endoscopic procedures not performed in the operating room. The units are the number of tests.

Code	Subcategory	Standard Abbreviation
0	General classification	GASTRO-INTSTL SVCS
1–9	Reserved	

076X   Specialty Room—Treatment/Observation Room

Revenue code 076X indicates charges for the use of a specialty room, such as a treatment room or observation room for outpatient observation services. Revenue code 0762 is intended for use with observation services only and should be reported together with an appropriate diagnosis code in FL 70 (Patient's Reason for Visit).

Code	Subcategory	Standard Abbreviation
0	General classification	SPECIALTY ROOM
1	Treatment room	TREATMENT RM
2	Observation room	OBSERVATION RM
3–8	Reserved	
9	Other specialty rooms	OTHER SPECIALTY RMS

077X   Preventive Care Services

Revenue code 077X is used to report charges for covered preventive care services as established by payers, including the administration of vaccines. For vaccine administration, Medicare requires detailed code 0771.

Code	Subcategory	Standard Abbreviation
0	General classification	PREVENT CARE SVCS
1	Vaccine administration	VACCINE ADMIN
2–9	Reserved	

078X   Telemedicine

Revenue code 078X indicates facility charges related to the use of telemedicine services.

Code	Subcategory	Standard Abbreviation
0	General classification	TELEMEDICINE
1–9	Reserved	

079X Extracorporeal Shock Wave Therapy (Formerly Lithotripsy)

Revenue code 079X indicates charges related to the use of extracorporeal shock wave therapy (ESWT).

Code	Subcategory	Standard Abbreviation
0	General classification	ESWT
1–9	Reserved	

080X Inpatient Renal Dialysis

Revenue code 080X indicates charges for the use of equipment designed to remove waste when the body's own kidneys have failed. The waste removal process, known as dialysis, is performed in an inpatient setting. The waste may be removed directly from the blood (hemodialysis) or indirectly from the blood by flushing a special solution between the abdominal covering and the tissue (peritoneal dialysis). The units are the number of sessions.

Code	Subcategory	Standard Abbreviation
0	General classification	RENAL DIALYSIS
1	Inpatient hemodialysis	DIALY/INPATIENT
2	Inpatient peritoneal (non-CAPD)	DIALY/IP/PER
3	Inpatient continuous ambulatory peritoneal dialysis (CAPD)	DIALY/IP/CAPD
4	Inpatient continuous cycling peritoneal dialysis (CCPD)	DIALY/IP/CCPD
5–8	Reserved	
9	Other inpatient dialysis	DIALY/IP/OTHER

081X Acquisition of Body Components

Revenue code 081X indicates charges for the acquisition and storage costs of body tissue, bone marrow, organs, and other body components not otherwise identified for use in transplantation. An organ transplant ICD-9-CM code is reported in FL 67 (Principal Diagnosis Code) to indicate the specific organ used in the transplant procedure. Detailed coding is required with this revenue code.

Code	Subcategory	Standard Abbreviation
0	General classification	ORGAN ACQUISIT
1	Living donor	LIVING DONOR
2	Cadaver donor	CADAVER DONOR
3	Unknown donor	UNKNOWN DONOR
4	Unsuccessful organ search—donor bank charges	UNSUCCESSFUL SEARCH
5–8	Reserved	
9	Other donor	OTHER DONOR

$ $ Billing Tip $ $

General Revenue Code 0770 Versus Detailed Code Use

General revenue code 0770 is appropriate with certain TOB codes for billing screening exams under Medicare, such as initial preventive physical exams for new Part B beneficiaries, screening pelvic exams, screening glaucoma services, and prostate cancer screening.

However, vaccine administration charges for influenza, pneumococcal (PPV), or hepatitis B vaccines must be billed with revenue code 0771. The charge includes the supplies used to give the vaccine, such a syringe. The vaccine products themselves are billed with revenue code 0636 (Drugs requiring detailed coding).

Both codes require the use of a HCPCS code in FL 44 (HCPCS/Rate/HIPPS Code).

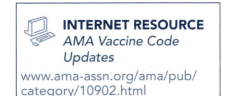 **INTERNET RESOURCE**
AMA Vaccine Code Updates
www.ama-assn.org/ama/pub/category/10902.html

FYI

ESWT

Formerly known as lithotripsy, ESWT is a method of breaking up painful bile stones and gallstones using focused shock waves so that the broken particles can then be passed in the urine.

$ $ Billing Tip $ $

Detailed Coding and ESRD Services

Medicare requires the use of detailed revenue codes 080X and 082X–085X when billing for end-stage renal dialysis (ESRD) services.

082X   Hemodialysis—Outpatient or Home Dialysis

Revenue code 082X indicates charges for a waste removal process performed in an outpatient or home setting that is necessary when the body's own kidneys have failed. Waste is removed directly from the blood. The units are the number of sessions.

Code	Subcategory	Standard Abbreviation
0	General classification	HEMO/OP OR HOME
1	Hemodialysis/composite or other rate	HEMO/COMPOSITE
2	Home supplies	HEMO/HOME/SUPPL
3	Home equipment	HEMO/HOME/EQUIP
4	Maintenance—100%	HEMO/HOME/100%
5	Support services	HEMO/HOME/SUPSERV
6–8	Reserved	
9	Other OP hemodialysis	HEMO-OTHER OP

083X   Peritoneal Dialysis—Outpatient or Home

Revenue code 083X indicates charges for a waste removal process performed in an outpatient or home setting that is necessary when the body's own kidneys have failed. Waste is removed indirectly by flushing a special solution between the abdominal covering and the tissue. The units are the number of sessions.

Code	Subcategory	Standard Abbreviation
0	General classification	PERITONEAL/OP OR HOME
1	Peritoneal/composite or other rate	PERTNL/COMPOSITE
2	Home supplies	PERTNL/HOME/SUPPL
3	Home equipment	PERTNL/HOME/EQUIP
4	Maintenance—100%	PERTNL/HOME/100%
5	Support services	PERTNL/HOME/SUPSERV
6–8	Reserved	
9	Other outpatient peritoneal dialysis	PERTNL/HOME/OTHER

084X   Continuous Ambulatory Peritoneal Dialysis (CAPD)—Outpatient or Home

Revenue code 084X indicates charges for a continuous dialysis process performed in an outpatient or home setting that uses the patient's peritoneal membrane as a dialyzer. The units are the number of days.

Codes	Subcategory	Standard Abbreviation
0	General classification	CAPD/OP OR HOME
1	CAPD/composite or other rate	CAPD/COMPOSITE
2	Home supplies	CAPD/HOME/SUPPL
3	Home equipment	CAPD/HOME/EQUIP
4	Maintenance—100%	CAPD/HOME/100%
5	Support services	CAPD/HOME/SUPSERV
6–8	Reserved	
9	Other outpatient CAPD	CAPD/HOME/OTHER

085X Continuous Cycling Peritoneal Dialysis (CCPD)—Outpatient or Home

Revenue code 085X indicates charges for a continuous dialysis process performed in an outpatient or home setting that uses a machine to make automatic exchanges at night. The units are the number of days.

Code	Subcategory	Standard Abbreviation
0	General classification	CCPD/OP OR HOME
1	CCPD/composite or other rate	CCPD/COMPOSITE
2	Home supplies	CCPD/HOME/SUPPL
3	Home equipment	CCPD/HOME/EQUIP
4	Maintenance—100%	CCPD/HOME/100%
5	Support services	CCPD/HOME/SUPSERV
6–8	Reserved	
9	Other outpatient CCPD	CCPD/HOME/OTHER

086X Reserved

087X Reserved

088X Miscellaneous Dialysis

Revenue code 088X indicates charges for dialysis services not identified elsewhere. The units are the number of sessions. Detailed coding is required with this revenue code.

Code	Subcategory	Standard Abbreviation
0	General classification	DIALY/MISC
1	Ultrafiltration	DIALY/ULTRAFILT
2	Home dialysis aid visit	HOME DIALYSIS AID VISIT
3–8	Reserved	
9	Other miscellaneous dialysis	DIALY/MISC/OTHER

FYI

Ultrafiltration

Ultrafiltration (as referred to in revenue code 0881) is the process of removing excess fluid from the blood of dialysis patients by using a dialysis machine but without the dialysate solution. The designation is used only when the procedure is not performed as part of a normal dialysis session.

089X Reserved

090X Behavioral Health Treatment/Services

Revenue code 090X indicates charges for behavioral health care services, including prevention, intervention, and treatment services in the areas of mental health, substance abuse, developmental disabilities, and sexuality. The units are the number of visits. (Also see 091X, an extension of 090X.)

The care provided is individualized, holistic, and culturally appropriate and may include ongoing care and support as well as nontraditional services.

Code	Subcategory	Standard Abbreviation
0	General classification	BH/TREATMENTS
1	Electroshock treatment	BH/ELECTRO SHOCK
2	Milieu therapy	BH/MILIEU THERAPY
3	Play therapy	BH/PLAY THERAPY
4	Activity therapy	BH/ACTIVITY THERAPY
5	Intensive outpatient services—psychiatric	BH/INTENS OP/PSYCH
6	Intensive outpatient services—chemical dependency	BH/INTENS OP/CHEM DEP
7	Community behavioral health program (day treatment)	BH/COMMUNITY
8–9	Reserved	

091X   Behavioral Health Treatment/Services—Extension of 090X

Revenue code 091X is an extension of 090X. See 090X above.

Code	Subcategory	Standard Abbreviation
0	Reserved (for general classification, use code 090X)	
1	Rehabilitation	BH/REHAB
2	Partial hospitalization—less intensive	BH/PARTIAL HOSP
3	Partial hospitalization—intensive	BH/PARTIAL INTENSV
4	Individual therapy	BH/INDIV RX
5	Group therapy	BH/GROUP RX
6	Family therapy	BH/FAMILY RX
7	Biofeedback	BH/BIOFEED
8	Testing	BH/TESTING
9	Other behavioral health treatments	BH/OTHER

Medicare does not recognize revenue codes 0912 and 0913 under its partial hospitalization program. For other payers, these codes are designed as zero-billed revenue codes (no dollars are to be reported in the amount field). They are intended to be vehicles for supplying program information as defined in the payer-provider contract.

092X   Other Diagnostic Services

Revenue code 092X indicates charges for various diagnostic services specific to common screenings for disease, illness, or medical condition. The units are the number of tests.

Code	Subcategory	Standard Abbreviation
0	General classification	OTHER DX SVCS
1	Peripheral vascular lab	PERI VASCUL LAB
2	Electromyelogram	EMG
3	Pap smear	PAP SMEAR
4	Allergy test	ALLERGY TEST
5	Pregnancy test	PREG TEST
6–8	Reserved	
9	Other diagnostic service	OTHER DX SVCS

093X Medical Rehabilitation Day Program

Revenue code 093X indicates charges for medical rehabilitation services as contracted with a payer and/or certified by the state. Services may include physical therapy, occupational therapy, and speech therapy. The units are the number of hours.

Code	Subcategory	Standard Abbreviation
0	Reserved	
1	Half day	HALF DAY
2	Full day	FULL DAY
3–9	Reserved	

094X Other Therapeutic Services

Revenue code 094X indicates charges for other therapeutic services not otherwise categorized. The units are the number of visits. (See also 095X, an extension of 094X.)

Code	Subcategory	Standard Abbreviations
0	General classification	OTHER RX SVCS
1	Recreational therapy	RECREATION RX
2	Education/training	EDUC/TRAINING
3	Cardiac rehabilitation	CARDIAC REHAB
4	Drug rehabilitation	DRUG REHAB
5	Alcohol rehabilitation	ALCOHOL REHAB
6	Complex medical equipment—routine	CMPLX MED EQUIP-ROUT
7	Complex medical equipment—ancillary	CMPLX MED EQUIP-ANC
8	Reserved	
9	Other therapeutic services	ADDITIONAL RX SVCS

095X Other Therapeutic Services—Extension of 094X

Revenue code 095X is an extension of 094X. See 094X above.

Code	Subcategory	Standard Abbreviations
0	Reserved (for general classification, use 0940)	
1	Athletic training	ATHLETIC TRAINING
2	Kinesiotherapy	KINESIOTHERAPY
3–9	Reserved	

096X Professional Fees

Revenue code 096X is generally used by critical access hospitals (CAHs) that bill both the technical and professional service components on the UB-04. Revenue code 096X separately identifies the professional fee component on the UB-04. (Most hospitals bill the professional fee component on the CMS-1500 claim form.) See also 097X and 098X.

Code	Subcategory	Standard Abbreviations
0	General classification	PRO FEE
1	Psychiatric	PRO FEE/PSYCH
2	Ophthalmology	PRO FEE/EYE
3	Anesthesiologist (MD)	PRO FEE/ANEST MD
4	Anesthesiologist (CRNA)	PRO FEE/ANEST CRNA
5–9	Reserved	
9	Other professional fee	PRO FEE/OTHER

097X Professional Fees—Extension of 096X

Revenue code 097X is an extension of 096X. See 096X above.

Code	Subcategory	Standard Abbreviation
0	Reserved (for general classification, use 0960)	
1	Laboratory	PRO FEE/LAB
2	Radiology—diagnostic	PRO FEE/RAD/DX
3	Radiology—therapeutic	PRO FEE/RAD/RX
4	Radiology—nuclear	PRO FEE/NUC MED
5	Operating room	PRO FEE/OR
6	Respiratory therapy	PRO FEE/RESPIR
7	Physical therapy	PRO FEE/PHYSI
8	Occupational therapy	PRO FEE/OCCUPA
9	Speech pathology	PRO FEE/SPEECH

098X Professional Fees—Extension of 096X and 097X

Revenue code 098X is an extension of 096X and 097X. See 096X above.

Code	Subcategory	Standard Abbreviation
0	Reserved (for general classification, use 0960)	
1	Emergency room services	PRO FEE/ER
2	Outpatient services	PRO FEE/OUTPT
3	Clinic	PRO FEE/CLINIC
4	Medical social services	PRO FEE/SOC SVC
5	ECG	PRO FEE/EKG
6	EEG	PRO FEE/EEG
7	Hospital visit	PRO FEE/HOS VIS
8	Consultation	PRO FEE/CONSULT
9	Private duty nurse	FEE/PVT NURSE

099X Patient Convenience Items

Revenue code 099X indicates charges for items that third-party payers generally consider strictly convenience items and that are therefore not covered. For Medicare billing, these noncovered charges may be billed to the beneficiary once a Medicare denial is received.

Code	Subcategory	Standard Abbreviation
0	General classification	PT CONVENIENCE
1	Cafeteria/guest tray	CAFETERIA
2	Private linen service	LINEN
3	Telephone/telecom	TELEPHONE
4	TV/radio	TV/RADIO
5	Nonpatient room rentals	NONPT ROOM RENT
6	Late discharge	LATE DISCHARGE
7	Admissions kits	ADM KITS
8	Beauty shop/barber	BARBER/BEAUTY
9	Other convenience items	PT CONV/OTHER

Other Revenue Codes

In addition to the original accommodation and ancillary service revenue codes that span code 010X to code 099X, the NUBC has created new code categories 100X–999X to cover new classifications such as alternative therapies.

100X   Behavioral Health Accommodations

Revenue code 100X indicates service charges incurred for routine accommodations at specified behavioral health facilities.

Code	Subcategory	Standard Abbreviation
0	General classification	BH R&B
1	Residential treatment—psychiatric	BH R&B RES/PSYCH
2	Residential treatment—chemical dependency	BH R&B RES/CHEM
3	Supervised living	BH R&B SUP LIVING
4	Halfway house	BH R&B HALFWAY HOUSE
5	Group home	BH R&B GROUP HOME
6–9	Reserved	

101X to 209X   Reserved

210X   Alternative Therapy Services

Revenue code 210X indicates charges for therapies not elsewhere categorized under other therapeutic service revenue codes (042X–044X, 091X, 094X–095X) or services such as anesthesia or clinic (0374, 0511). The units are the number of sessions.

   Alternative therapy is intended to enhance and improve standard medical treatment. The revenue codes in this category would be used to report services in a separately designated alternative inpatient-outpatient unit.

Code	Subcategory	Standard Abbreviation
0	General classification	ALTTHERAPY
1	Acupuncture	ACUPUNCTURE
2	Acupressure	ACUPRESSURE
3	Massage	MASSAGE
4	Reflexology	REFLEXOLOGY
5	Biofeedback	BIOFEEDBACK
6	Hypnosis	HYPNOSIS
7–8	Reserved	
9	Other alternative therapy service	OTHER ALTTHERAPY

211X–309X   Reserved

310X   Adult Care

Revenue code 310X indicates charges for personal, medical, psychosocial, and/or therapeutic services in a special community setting for adults needing supervision and/or assistance with activities of daily living (ADLs).

Code	Subcategory	Standard Abbreviation
0	Reserved	
1	Adult day care, medical and social—hourly	ADULT MED/SOC HR
2	Adult day care, social—hourly	ADULT SOC HR
3	Adult day care, medical and social—daily	ADULT MED/SOC DAY
4	Adult day care, social—daily	ADULT SOC DAY
5	Adult foster care—daily	ADULT FOSTER DAY
6–8	Reserved	
9	Other adult care	OTHER ADULT

311X–999X Reserved

FL 43 Revenue Description

FL 43 is the set of twenty-two lines adjacent to FL 42 on the UB-04 claim form that is used to report a narrative description or standard abbreviation for each corresponding revenue code reported in FL 42 (see Figure 12.5). The standard descriptions of each revenue code correspond with the revenue codes and descriptions as defined by the NUBC.

If a claim contains more than twenty-two revenue code lines, additional pages are added. Line 23 of this form locator contains the text *"PAGE ____ OF ____."* This field is used to number the pages in the claim and should be filled in on all pages.

Figure 12.5

UB-04 Form—FLs 42–49

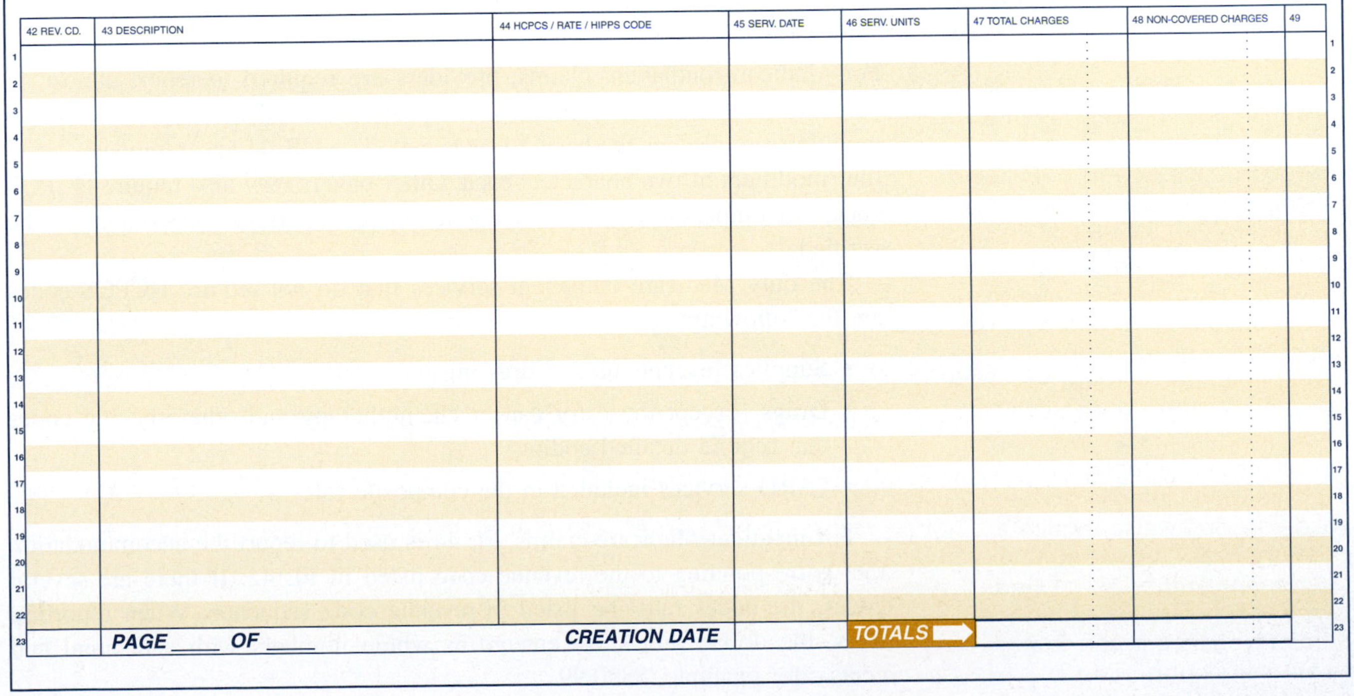

Guidelines

Completion of this field is not required on Medicare claims except for FDA investigational devices (revenue code 0624) with an exemption (IDE) and for billing certain cancer drugs (revenue code 0636, Pharmacy—drugs requiring detailed coding). Because the revenue description information is intended to assist in clerical bill review, however, this information is usually used on paper claims even when it is not required.

When subcategory codes ending in 9, referred to as "other" revenue codes, are used, they should be individually described in FL 43.

FL 44 HCPCS/RATE/HIPPS Code

FL 44 contains one of three types of information, depending on the type of claim being billed:

1. A HCPCS code when required for ancillary services on outpatient claims

2. An appropriate accommodation rate for inpatient claims

3. A HIPPS rate for claims associated with the SNF, home health, and inpatient rehabilitation facility (IRF) Prospective Payment Systems

A **HIPPS (Health Insurance Prospective Payment System) rate code** is a five-digit alphanumeric payment code that represents specific sets of patient characteristics, or case-mix groups. The Prospective Payment Systems associated with the SNFs, home health providers, and inpatient rehabilitation facilities each make payment determinations by assigning a HIPPS rate code on admission. HIPPS codes are developed and published by CMS as a means of establishing a coding system for claim submission and payment under certain Prospective Payment Systems.

Guidelines

For Medicare outpatient claims, providers are required to report almost all items and services using HCPCS codes in FL 44. The HCPCS codes and modifiers are used as the basis for payment. The UB-04 accommodates up to four modifiers of two characters each. Other payers may also require HCPCS codes for outpatient claims. The regulations of individual payers need to be verified.

The only Medicare outpatient services that do not require HCPCS codes are the following:

- Supplies (except surgical dressings)

- Drugs (except those for cancer chemotherapy and other specific codes that require detailed coding)

- ESRD services included in the composite rate

For inpatient Medicare claims, FL 44 is used to report the accommodation rate corresponding to the revenue code listed in FL 42. If there are several codes, the codes must be listed in revenue code sequence. When reporting rates, the dollar values are entered as whole numbers with a decimal and cents—for example, $890.99.

HCPCS codes and HIPPS rate codes are reported left-justified in FL 44. Accommodation rates are reported right-justified. This makes it easier to identify the type of code that is being reported at a glance.

FL 45 Service Date

The service date field (FL 45) contains the date on which the outpatient service reported in FLs 42–44 was provided in MMDDYY format. The date of service is also known as a line item date of service because each occurrence of an outpatient service requires its own revenue code line and date on the UB-04.

Guidelines

Completion of this field is required for billing outpatient Medicare claims. Depending on the specific plan requirements, other payers may also require completion of this field.

A service date must be reported on outpatient claims in FL 45 for every revenue code line. The dates must fall within the dates reported in FL 6 (Statement Covers Period). Claims submitted without the line item date of service will be returned to the provider for correction.

For therapy services, such as physical therapy, occupational therapy, speech-language pathology, and audiology services, every occurrence of the service must be repeated on a separate line along with the specific date of the service and the appropriate revenue code and HCPCS code.

Similarly, all claims for home health services must include a line item date of service for each service rendered during a visit. This means that if the billing period includes three skilled nursing visits and two home health aid visits, five separate lines with revenue codes and HCPCS codes will be reported—one for each visit.

The last line in FL 45, line 23, is labeled "CREATION DATE" and is used to report the date the claim was prepared for submission. On multiple-page claims, the creation date should appear on every page.

FL 46 Service Units

The service units field reports the quantitative measure of services rendered as specified by a given revenue code category, including items such as the number of visits, accommodation days, treatments, miles, drug dosages, and pints of blood. This field allows reporting of up to seven positions in each line.

Guidelines

Completion of this field is required for Medicare billing where appropriate, based on the requirements of each revenue code. It is also required by other payers.

For Medicare billing, units for the following revenue code categories should be reported as applicable. The unit type is shown in parentheses.

- Accommodation (days): 0100s–0150s, 0200s, 0210s
- Blood (pints): 0380s
- Clinic (HCPCS code definition for visit or procedure): 0510s and 0520s

- Dialysis treatments (sessions or days): 0800s
- Drugs and biologicals (HCPCS code definition for dosage): 0636
- Durable medical equipment (rental months): 0290s
- Emergency room (HCPCS code definition for visit or procedure): 0450, 0452, and 0459
- Orthotics/prosthetic devices (items): 0274
- Outpatient clinical diagnostic laboratory (tests): 030X–031X
- Outpatient therapy visits (the number of times the procedure or service was performed): 0410, 0420, 0430, 0440, 0480, 0910, and 0943
- Oxygen (rental months, feet, or pounds): 0600s
- Radiology (HCPCS code definition of tests or services): 032X, 034X, 035X, 040X, 061X, 0333

FL 47 Total Charges

The Total Charges field on the UB-04 is used to report the total charges for the primary payer for the current billing period (as shown in FL 6, Statement Covers Period) for each revenue code listed in FL 42, lines 1–22. Total charges include both covered and noncovered charges. Each line item, whether for a covered or a noncovered service, has its own total in FL 47. This means that the total cost of a noncovered service—for example a self-administered pill costing $4.00—would be reported in FL 47. The noncovered portion, in this case also $4.00, would be reported in FL 48 (Noncovered Services). These charges are known as line item charges.

In addition, the last line in FL 47, line 23, is labeled "TOTALS" and is used to report the sum total of all the line item charges listed in the Total Charges column—for all payers except Medicare. For Medicare, any noncovered amounts from FL 48 are first subtracted from the sum total column in FL 47, so that the sum total in FL 47 on the UB-04 actually shows the sum total of covered costs. For other payers, the sum total shows the total of all costs, covered and noncovered. Line 23 is reported on paper claims using revenue code 0001 (Total Charges) in FL 42.

Guidelines

Completion of this field is required for Medicare billing and for all other payers. Each line allows up to nine numeric digits (for example, $1,000,000.00). Excluding the dollar sign and commas, this means that seven digits are allowed for dollars and two digits for cents.

COMPLIANCE GUIDE
Fraud and Abuse Penalties

Providers who engage in fraud and abuse on claims can be sanctioned or excluded from the Medicare program. Civil monetary penalties may also be imposed. Penalties imposed by the Office of the Inspector General (OIG) include fines of $5,000 to $10,000 for each service or item falsely reported on a claim, plus triple damages under the False Claims Act. Criminal fines and/or imprisonment of up to ten years may also be imposed.

837I No Map Field
Revenue Code 0001

On the electronic HIPAA claim, revenue code 0001 is not used for reporting the total claim charge. The total claim charge is reported in Loop ID 2300, Reference Designator CLM02, data element 782.

FL 48 Noncovered Charges

Lines 1–22 in FL 48 are used to report the total noncovered charges for each revenue code line. Each noncovered item has its own total. In addition, line 23 in FL 48 is used to report the sum total of all noncovered charges for all of the line items.

Guidelines

If noncovered days are reported in FLs 39–41 (Value Codes and Amounts) using value code 81 (Noncovered days), noncovered charges must also be reported in FL 48. Charges for services or items not covered by Medicare are listed in this field. For example, the cost of self-administered drugs, such as aspirin, would be listed as a noncovered charge. The extra cost of a private room would be listed as a noncovered charge. The cost of a semiprivate room would be listed as a covered charge, and the extra cost of the private room over and above the semiprivate room rate would be listed as a noncovered charge. The cost of a noncovered service such as acupuncture would also be listed in FL 48.

Medicare requires submission of a claim for every hospital stay, even one for which no payment is made or expected. The FIs and CMS use the no-payment bill to maintain beneficiary utilization and eligibility records.

837I No Map Field

Summary of Noncovered Services

Although the electronic HIPAA claim contains a field for reporting noncovered services by line item (Loop 2400, Reference Designator SV207, data element 782), it does not have a field for reporting a total of noncovered services for all line items on a claim.

FL 49 Unlabeled Field

REVIEW AND APPLICATIONS | CHAPTER 12

CHAPTER SUMMARY

1. FLs 42–49 on the UB-04 claim are used to record and total the cost of each service received during the billing period reflected on the claim. Two main types of revenue codes are reported in FL 42: accommodation revenue codes (010X–021X) and ancillary service revenue codes (022X–099X). An accommodation revenue code is used to identify the types of routine hospital bed, room accommodation, and board charges that are being billed on an inpatient claim. Ancillary service revenue codes identify services, other than routine room and board charges, that are incidental to the hospital stay. Ancillary service revenue codes are also used on all outpatient claims. Services such as radiology, laboratory, pharmacy, and anesthesia are represented by ancillary service revenue codes. On paper claims, the last line in FL 42, line 23, is used to report revenue code 0001, Total charges.

2. The revenue description field (FL 43) is used to report the standard abbreviated text for describing each revenue code listed in FL 42. This field is also used to individually describe "other" revenue codes—codes ending in 9 and available with most revenue code categories for describing a code not otherwise listed in that category. Line 23 of FL 43 includes the text *PAGE ___ OF ___*. This should be filled in on all pages of the claim.

3. FL 44 (HCPCS/Rate/HIPPS Code) is used to report one of three types of information, depending on the type of claim. (a) On

outpatient claims, FL 44 is used to report the appropriate HCPCS codes for ancillary services. Medicare rules require using HCPCS codes when billing all hospital outpatient medical and clinical services. (b) On inpatient claims, FL 44 is used to report the appropriate accommodation rate, reflecting the type of room and board. Dollar values for accommodation rates must include whole dollars, the decimal, and cents (for example, $425.99). (c) FL 44 is also used to report the HIPPS rate code for claims associated with the SNF, home health, and inpatient rehabilitation facility Prospective Payment Systems.

④ FL 45 (Service Date) contains the line item date of service—the date on which the corresponding outpatient service listed on the same line in FL 42 was provided. For Medicare outpatient claims, a line item date of service is required for every line where a HCPCS code is required. Line 23 of FL 45 contains a field for reporting the claim's creation date (MMDDYY).

The unit of service associated with each revenue code line is reported in FL 46 (Service Units); the type of service unit used varies with different revenue code categories. Examples include the number of accommodation days, emergency room visits, renal dialysis sessions, and miles traveled in an ambulance.

⑤ The Total Charges field (FL 47) is used to report the total charges for the current billing period pertaining to each revenue code line listed in lines 1–22 of FL 42. Line 23 is used to report the sum total of all line item charges on the claim. For Medicare claims, charges for noncovered services are first subtracted from the total so that the sum total in FL 47 includes covered charges only. For all other claims, the sum total field includes covered and noncovered charges.

⑥ FL 48, Noncovered Charges, is used to indicate any noncovered charges on the claim. Lines 1–22 list noncovered charges for individual line items, and line 23 indicates the sum total of all noncovered charges from lines 1–22.

✔ CHECK YOUR UNDERSTANDING

1. Define *revenue code,* and specify which form locator it occupies on the UB-04.

_____

_____

2. Which of the following represents the correct order for listing revenue codes in FL 42 on the UB-04?
   a. 0001, 0023, 0444, 0561
   b. 0023, 0444, 0561, 0001
   c. 0561, 0444, 0023, 0001

3. For each of the following revenue codes, list the name of the revenue code category, followed by the name of the subcategory code when a subcategory is indicated. Examples are given for the first two codes.

	Revenue Code	Name of Category	Name of Subcategory
a.	020X	Intensive care unit	_____
b.	0233	Incremental nursing charge	ICU
c.	017X	_____	_____
d.	025X	_____	_____
e.	0300	_____	_____
f.	0324	_____	_____
g.	037X	_____	_____
h.	0434	_____	_____
i.	0540	_____	_____
j.	0636	_____	_____
k.	0710	_____	_____
l.	0822	_____	_____
m.	0903	_____	_____
n.	2101	_____	_____
o.	0001	_____	_____

4. For each of the following revenue codes, describe the corresponding unit of service. An example is given for the first code.

	Revenue Code	Unit of Service
a.	0180	# days
b.	0352	_____
c.	0543	_____
d.	0450	_____
e.	0410	_____
f.	0274	_____
g.	0801	_____
h.	0120	_____

5. True or False: When revenue code 019X (Subacute care) is reported on a claim, a HCPCS code should be reported in FL 44 (HCPCS/Rate/HIPPS Code). _____

6. On which kind of claims is revenue code 018X (Leave of absence) used?

a. outpatient

b. inpatient

c. home health

d. all of the above

7. For each of the following revenue codes, indicate whether a HCPCS code would be required in FL 44 on a Medicare outpatient bill by writing *Yes* if it is required and *No* if it is not required.

_____ **a.** 0480 (Cardiology, general classification)

_____ **b.** 0710 (Recovery room, general classification)

_____ **c.** 0250 (Pharmacy, general classification)

_____ **d.** 0450 (Emergency room, general classification)

_____ **e.** 0421 (Physical therapy, visit)

_____ **f.** 0270 (Medical/surgical supplies and devices)

_____ **g.** 0300 (Laboratory, general classification)

8. Fill in FLs 42–49 below for the Medicare patient whose patient services information is listed below. Remember to complete line 23.

TOB: 0131

Date of Service: 4-20-2010

Bill Processing Date: 4-24-10

Services	Units	Charges
Pharmacy	1	100.00
Lab (CPT 86001)	1	45.00
Emergency room (CPT 99282)	1	109.00
Drug/self-admin	1	8.60
Professional fee/ER (CPT 99282)	1	125.00

UB-04 Form—FLs 42–49

42 REV. CD.	43 DESCRIPTION	44 HCPCS / RATE / HIPPS CODE	45 SERV. DATE	46 SERV. UNITS	47 TOTAL CHARGES	48 NON-COVERED CHARGES	49
1							1
2							2
3							3
4							4
5							5
6							6
7							7
8							8
9							9
10							10
11							11
12							12
13							13
14							14
15							15
16							16
17							17
18							18
19							19
20							20
21							21
22							22
23	**PAGE ____ OF ____**	**CREATION DATE**		**TOTALS** ▶			23

9. Fill in FLs 42–49 below for the Medicare patient whose patient services information is listed below. Remember to complete line 23.

TOB: 0111

Dates of Service: 5-3-2010 to 5-6-2010

Bill Processing Date: 5-16-2010

Services	Units	Charges
Room-board/semi	3	500.00/day
Pharmacy	1	420.00
IV solutions	1	185.00
Med-sur supplies	1	200.00
Non-ster supplies	1	18.00
Lab	1	645.00
Respiratory svcs	1	525.00
Emerg room	1	1010.00

UB-04 Form—FLs 42–49

42 REV. CD.	43 DESCRIPTION	44 HCPCS / RATE / HIPPS CODE	45 SERV. DATE	46 SERV. UNITS	47 TOTAL CHARGES	48 NON-COVERED CHARGES	49
1							1
2							2
3							3
4							4
5							5
6							6
7							7
8							8
9							9
10							10
11							11
12							12
13							13
14							14
15							15
16							16
17							17
18							18
19							19
20							20
21							21
22							22
23	PAGE ____ OF ____		CREATION DATE	TOTALS ➡			23

10. Fill in FLs 42–49 below for a newborn admission based on the following patient services information. Remember to complete line 23.

TOB: 0111

Dates of Service: 6-1-2010 to 6-3-2010

Bill Processing Date: 6-11-2010

Services	Units	Charges
Nursery	2	380.00/day
Pharmacy	1	82.00
Med-sur supplies	1	29.50
Lab	1	178.00

UB-04 Form—FLs 42–49

42 REV. CD.	43 DESCRIPTION	44 HCPCS / RATE / HIPPS CODE	45 SERV. DATE	46 SERV. UNITS	47 TOTAL CHARGES	48 NON-COVERED CHARGES	49
1							1
2							2
3							3
4							4
5							5
6							6
7							7
8							8
9							9
10							10
11							11
12							12
13							13
14							14
15							15
16							16
17							17
18							18
19							19
20							20
21							21
22							22
23	PAGE ____ OF ____		CREATION DATE	TOTALS ➡			23

11. On April 14, 2008, a patient was administered 4 mg of the drug Lorazepam by injection. This drug requires detailed coding. The full description for the drug is "HCPCS J2060, Injection, lorazepam, 2 mg." The total cost is $13.60. Fill in the revenue code line below (FLs 42–49).

UB-04 Form—FLs 42–49

42 REV. CD.	43 DESCRIPTION	44 HCPCS / RATE / HIPPS CODE	45 SERV. DATE	46 SERV. UNITS	47 TOTAL CHARGES	48 NON-COVERED CHARGES	49
1							1

COMPUTER EXPLORATION

UB-04 Activity: Claim Analysis

Comparing IP and OP Claims: The Revenue Code Section

Open the files **Sample02.pdf** and **Sample03.pdf** in Adobe Reader, and answer the following questions:

1. Because inpatient and outpatient claims are paid under two different payment systems, the data requirements in the revenue codes sections on inpatient and outpatient claims are different. View the revenue code section in the inpatient claim, Sample02.pdf, first. Study the list of revenue codes and corresponding descriptions in FLs 42 and 43. Which revenue code makes it clear that this claim is an inpatient claim?

2. Examine the information reported in FLs 44 through 49. What does 625 00 in FL 44 represent? How is the total amount ($1875.00) for line 1 calculated?

3. For the remaining revenue codes listed (lines 2 through 8), what information is reported? Why are there no HCPCS/CPT codes or service dates reported for these lines?

4. Now view Sample03.pdf. Based on the TOB, what type of claim is shown. Sample03 is new; therefore, read over the claim to familiarize yourself with it. Note the billing period in FL 6, the patient's name, address, date of birth, and gender. Determine the admission type, the patient's point of origin, and the patient's discharge status.

5. Look through the list of services in the revenue code section. Is there an accommodation revenue code or are all the codes ancillary codes? What is the principal diagnosis code? Look up this code in the ICD-9-CM to determine the principal diagnosis.

6. Compare the data in FLs 44 and 45 on this claim with those on the previous claim. How is it different? Does every revenue code line report a service date?

7. Notice that some of the revenue code lines contain HCPCS/CPT codes in FL 44 and others do not. Make a list of each revenue code and corresponding service without a HCPCS/CPT code in FL 44. Because these items are packaged into the APC payment rate, they are paid as part of the surgical procedure(s) with which they are billed. (In Sample03, the two surgical procedures are those listed under revenue code 0360.) When reporting packaged supplies or services, A HCPCS/CPT code is not required in FL 44.

8. Make a list of each revenue code and corresponding service that is reported with a HCPCS/CPT code in FL 44. Look up each code in a CPT codebook and write down the code's definition. Note that HCPCS codes beginning with C and J are supply codes. Therefore, they are located in a HCPCS Level II codebook, and not in CPT.

9. What is the general description for the C series of HCPCS codes in the HCPCS level II book?

10. What general description is given for the J series of codes?

When finished viewing each claim, click Exit on the File menu.

Payer, Insured, and Employer Information

LEARNING OUTCOMES

After completing this chapter, you will be able to define the key terms and:

1. Explain how to correctly identify and bill the primary payer as well as a secondary and a tertiary payer, if applicable, in FL 50, lines A, B, and C, of the UB-04 form.

2. Discuss how lines A, B, and C in adjacent fields FL 51 through FL 55 contain information related to the payers reported in lines A, B, and C of FL 50.

3. Understand the importance of reporting the billing provider's National Provider Identifier (NPI) in FL 56, as well as previous legacy identifiers as required in FL 57, lines A, B, and C.

4. Describe the types of information about the insured that must be reported in FL 58 through FL 62, lines A, B, and C, on the UB-04.

5. Describe the purpose of FL 63, Treatment Authorization Codes, in reporting a course of treatment that requires prior authorization, and FL 64, Document Control Number (DCN), when filing a replacement or cancellation to a previously processed claim.

6. Discuss the use of FL 65 for reporting the name of the insured's employer when applicable.

KEY TERMS

- assignment of benefits
- carrier code
- health insurance claim number (HICN)
- National Provider Identifier (NPI)
- NPI Registry
- provider number

From locators 50–65 of the UB-04 contain detailed information about the payer and the insured, including the insured's employment. This information must be reported accurately to make a proper determination of benefits and to coordinate benefits when there is more than one payer. To ensure proper and timely reimbursement, each payer must be identified accurately in this section of the UB-04. The details of the patient's insurance, especially the insured's identification number, must also be accurate and complete. If the insurance identification number is reported incorrectly, for example, or if there is more than one payer on a claim and the payers are listed in the wrong order, the reimbursement process will be held up. If Medicare is possibly a secondary payer based on the patient's responses to Medicare Secondary Payer (MSP) program development during the admission process, the insured's employer information must be double-checked for accuracy.

With the exception of FL 56 for reporting the hospital's NPI, which contains one line only, each field in this section of the claim form contains three lines that run the full width of the form. These lines are labeled A, B, and C in the left margin of the claim form (see Figure 13.1). They are used to represent three levels of payers: line A is used to report information connected with the primary payer, line B the secondary payer if applicable, and line C the tertiary payer if applicable.

Figure 13.1

UB-04 Form—FLs 50–65

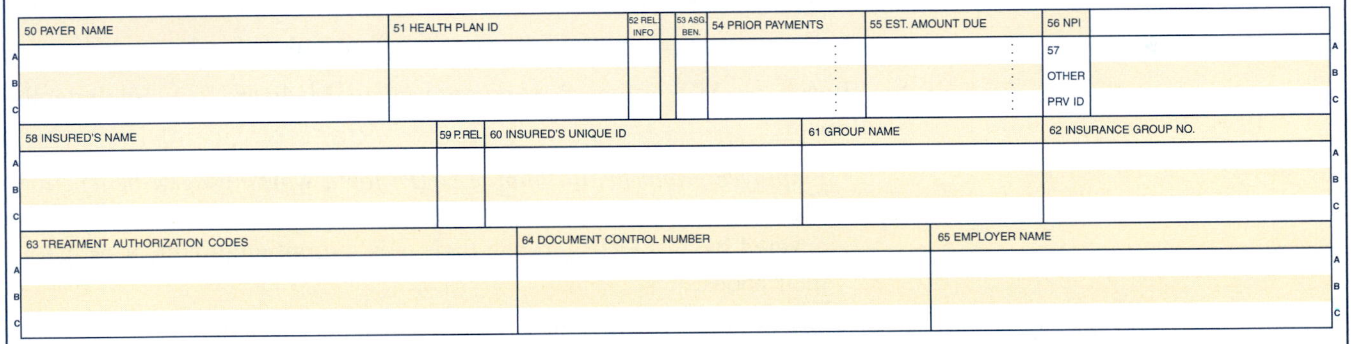

FL 50 Payer Name

The Payer Name field contains the name of the health plan from which total or partial payment for the bill is expected. Line 50A is used to report the name of primary payer, line 50B the name of the secondary payer if applicable, and line 50C the name of the tertiary payer if applicable.

Guidelines

Completion of FL 50 is required for Medicare billing as well as for most other payers. Up to twenty-three alphanumeric characters are allowed on each of lines A, B, and C.

Reporting Medicare as the primary payer on a claim (FL 50, line A) indicates that the provider has completed the MSP development questions during the admission process (usually in the form of an MSP questionnaire) and has determined that Medicare is the primary payer.

When Medicare is the primary payer and another form of insurance should be billed as well, the following form locators must be completed:

- *FL 50, line B:* Name of the other insurance
- *FL 51, line B:* Health plan ID of the other insurance

FYI

Identifying the Payer

The payer's name may be the name of an insurance company, a program, an organization, or another liable third-party payer. Examples are Medicare, TRICARE, and Blue Cross and Blue Shield. All payers who may have full or partial responsibility for payments of charges, deductibles, and/or coinsurance must be listed in lines A, B, and C in the order of the greatest to the least responsibility.

- *FL 58, line B:* Name of the insured

- *FL 59, line B:* Patient's relationship to the insured

- *FL 60, line B:* Identification number assigned to the beneficiary by the other insurance

If there is a third payer, the same form locators should be filled in on line C.

When a payer is identified on line A, B, or C, the corresponding line in FL 60 (Insured's Unique ID) must contain the unique identification number assigned by that payer to the insured.

Payers Primary to Medicare

Under certain circumstances, Medicare is the secondary rather than the primary payer. When Medicare is secondary, the primary payer must be listed in line A of FL 50 and Medicare in line B. Circumstances under which Medicare is a secondary payer may include the following:

- Another payer paid some of the charges, and Medicare is secondarily liable for the remainder.

- Another payer denied the claim.

- The provider is requesting a conditional payment.

Based on MSP rules, payers primary to Medicare may include the following:

- *Employer group health plan (EGHP) for a working aged beneficiary:* Medicare is secondary for beneficiaries sixty-five or older who are covered by an EGHP through their own current employment or that of their spouse.

- *Group health plan for an ESRD beneficiary:* Medicare is secondary for beneficiaries entitled to benefits solely on the basis of ESRD during a period of up to thirty months.

- *Automobile medical or no-fault insurance:* Medicare is secondary for beneficiaries of any age who receive medical services that are likely to be covered under automobile no-fault, automobile medical, or personal injury insurance.

- *Workers' compensation or black lung:* Medicare is secondary for beneficiaries of any age who receive services due to work-related injuries or diseases.

- *Veterans Affairs:* Medicare is secondary for beneficiaries of any age who receive services due to military-related injuries or diseases.

- *Large group health plan (LGHP) for a disabled beneficiary:* Medicare is secondary for beneficiaries younger than sixty-five years old who are entitled to benefits solely on the basis of disability. This applies to beneficiaries who are covered by an LGHP through their own current employment or that of a spouse or other family member.

- *Liability insurance:* Medicare is secondary to liability insurance, such as homeowner's or malpractice insurance, that provides payment based on legal liability for illness, injury, or property damage. However, if the liability insurer does not pay the provider within 120 days, Medicare may be billed for a conditional payment.

$ $ Billing Tip $ $

MSP Value Codes

When Medicare is billed as the secondary payer, report the applicable MSP value code and amount received from the primary insurer in FLs 39–41, Value Codes and Amounts (see value codes 12–16, 41–43, and 47 in Chapter 11). The claim should be submitted to Medicare only after a final payment or denial is received from the primary insurer.

Many fiscal intermediaries (Fls) have automatic crossover billing with other payers for coordination of benefits, so that after a claim is processed with Medicare as the primary payer, the claim data are automatically transmitted to the secondary payer. The provider should not have to bill the secondary (or tertiary) payer separately. For crossover billing, it is important to provide the appropriate source of payment code and/or plan code or other identifier for the secondary payer as required. Since Medicaid is recognized as a "payer of last resort"—liable for payments only after all other payers—a Medicaid claim should always be processed after all other payers have been billed and have responded.

FL 51 Health Plan Identification Number

Form locator 51 is used to report the number used by the health plan to identify itself. In the future, the payer's National Plan Identifier, mandated under HIPAA, will be reported here. Similar to the National Provider Identifier that is now used to identify each provider, the National Plan Identifier will be a unique number assigned to each health plan. Until CMS establishes this program, however, the legacy health plan ID number that has been set up between trading partners—in this case between the hospital and the insurance company—is reported in FL 51.

Guidelines

This field holds up to fifteen alphanumeric characters. Many health plans use a **carrier code** as the health plan ID. Carrier codes usually contain two leading zeros followed by three numbers or letters. For example, 00813 is the carrier code used to report an AARP insurance plan. Blue Cross usually has a plan code indicated on the subscriber's identification card that is the equivalent of the carrier code and is reported in FL 51.

FL 52 Release of Information Certification Indicator

FL 52 is used to report whether the patient has signed a statement permitting the provider to release medical and billing information to other parties and whether the provider has that signed statement on file.

Guidelines

This is a required field on the UB-04. It is completed by selecting one of two codes:

1. *Y (yes):* Indicates that the hospital has a signed statement permitting the release of health information for the purpose of claiming insurance benefits.
2. *I (informed consent):* Indicates that the hospital has informed consent to release health information for conditions or diagnoses regulated by federal statues. This code is required when the provider has not collected a signature, and when any state and federal laws that require a signature do not supersede the HIPAA Privacy Rule.

FL 52 must be completed on all claims and adjustments submitted to Medicare. The back page of the UB-04 form contains a certification statement by the provider that all release statements required by Medicare are on file.

FL 53 Assignment of Benefits Certification Indicator

HIPAA TIP

PHI for Other Purposes

To legally release a patient's protected health information (PHI) for purposes other than treatment, payment, or health care operations, a separate signed authorization document is required.

FYI

Assignment of Benefits

A patient who authorizes a payer to pay the provider directly for medical services signs a form known as **assignment of benefits**.

Form locator 53 indicates whether the provider has a signed form authorizing the payer to pay the provider directly for services rendered.

Guidelines

This is a required field on the UB-04. The field is completed by selecting one of three codes:

1. *N (no):* Indicates that benefits have not been assigned. The payment will be sent to the insured, who will then be responsible for paying the provider.

2. *Y (yes):* Indicates that benefits have been assigned. The benefit payment will be sent to the provider directly (rather than to the insured).

3. *W (not applicable):* Indicates that the patient has refused to assign benefits (available for use on the paper UB-04 only).

FL 54 Prior Payments—Payer

COMPLIANCE GUIDE

Assignment of Benefits Versus Release of Medical Information Authorizations

A signed assignment of benefits form does not automatically permit the release of medical information about the patient. Although they are often grouped together for administrative reasons, the assignment of benefits certification and the release of information certification are separate authorizations.

The amount the hospital has received to date from the health plan toward payment of this bill is reported in FL 54 (Prior Payments—Payer). If any amount has been received from the payers listed in FL 50 on lines A, B, or C, this amount is reported on lines A, B, or C in FL 54.

Guidelines

Completion of this field is required for Medicare outpatient claims and by all other payers. For an MSP claim, any prior payment amount received from another insurer is reported on the appropriate line in FL 54.

This field holds up to ten digits for each line. Eight positions are for dollars, and two are for cents.

FL 55 Estimated Amount Due—Payer

837I No Map Field

Code W, which is used in FL 53 on the UB-04 to indicate that the patient has refused to assign benefits, is not available for use with the 837I claim. Only Y and N can be used on an electronic claim.

The amount reported in FL 55 (Estimated Amount Due—Payer) is the hospital's estimate of the amount due from the corresponding payers indicated in lines A, B, and C of FL 50. The amount reported on any of the lines in this form locator is the estimated responsibility less any prior payments received, as indicated in FL 54 (Prior Payments—Payer).

Guidelines

Completion of this field is not required for Medicare, Medicaid, Blue Cross, or TRICARE. It may be used by commercial payers. If used, this field usually lists the total claim amount as reported with revenue code 0001 in FL 47, line 23.

The field holds up to ten digits for each line. Eight positions are for dollars, and two are for cents.

FL 56 National Provider Identifier—Billing Provider

Form locator 56 is used to report the hospital's **National Provider Identifier (NPI).** Under HIPAA mandate, all health care providers, whether individuals or organizations, were required to obtain an NPI and to begin using it to identify themselves in all HIPAA standard transactions as of May 23, 2007. The NPI is a unique ten-digit number assigned to each provider for lifetime use. It is assigned by the National Provider System.

In addition to taking applications from providers and assigning them NPIs, the National Provider System is responsible for making the NPI database available to the public by way of the Internet.

Only certain provider data contained in the NPI database can be disclosed under the Freedom of Information Act (FOIA). Some key data elements for institutional providers that may be disclosed include:

- NPI
- Entity type code (2 = organization)
- Replacement NPI
- Employer Identification Number (EIN)
- Provider organization name
- Provider other organization name (3 = doing business as name; 4 = former legal business name; 5 = other)
- Provider business mailing address
- Provider business location address
- Health care provider taxonomy code(s)
- Other provider identifier(s) and type code
- Provider enumeration date
- Last update date
- NPI deactivation reason code and date
- NPI reactivation date
- Authorized official contact information (name, title, position, phone number)

Other data elements, including Social Security numbers, IRS individual taxpayer identification numbers, and dates of birth, are not considered disclosable under FOIA.

Guidelines

On the UB-04 form, FL 56 contains the NPI of the provider submitting the bill—in this case, the hospital. The NPIs of the attending provider, the operating physician, and other provider types, such as referring providers, are also required on the UB-04 and are reported in FLs 76–79 (see Chapter 15, "Physician Information, Remarks, and Code-Code Field").

$ $ Billing Tip $ $

Caution with Blank FL 54

Certain payers' computer programs have been programmed to review a second line of data in FL 54 only when the line above it contains data. Therefore, it is recommended that FL 54 be filled with three zeros (0.00) for any line when there is a payment in the line below it, rather than leaving the field blank. The zero entry will force the computer to check the line below it in order to register any payment amounts reported there before it moves to the next form locator.

FYI

National Plan and Provider Enumeration System (NPPES)

The database containing NPI data is known as the National Plan and Provider Enumeration System (NPPES). The NPPES lists health care providers and stores their NPIs as well as information from their NPI applications and any updates to this information. In the future, once a standard unique health identifier for health plans has been adopted, the NPPES will be used to store similar information for health plans.

INTERNET RESOURCE
NPI Registry

The **NPI Registry** is a query-only portion of the NPPES database. It contains a complete list of NPIs and other provider data that can be made available to the public under the Freedom of Information Act. The NPI Registry is maintained as part of the CMS website. https://nppes.cms.hhs.gov/NPPES/NPIRegistryHome.do

FL 57 Other (Billing) Provider Identifier

Form locator 57 contains a unique number assigned to the health care provider by the payer. This number is known as the **provider number.** It is also referred to as the legacy number or proprietary number. On the UB-04 form, the provider number is assigned to the hospital by the payer indicated in FL 50.

Guidelines

The field for the provider number allows up to fifteen alphanumeric characters in each of lines A, B, and C. The provider number should not contain hyphens, spaces, or any special characters.

Following the NPI contingency period, completion of this field will not be required except when an NPI is not used and another identification number is necessary for the receiver to identify the provider. However, until the NPI system is fully tested and established, reporting of this number in conjunction with the NPI is required so that payers are able to identify providers without difficulty.

FL 58 Insured's Name

The Insured's Name field contains the name of the patient or insured individual in whose name the insurance listed in FL 50 is issued.

Guidelines

Completion of this field is required for Medicare billing and by all other payers. In general, for each payer, the name reported must correspond with the name on the insured's identification card.

This field allows twenty-five alphanumeric characters in each of lines A, B, and C corresponding to the insurance named as primary, secondary, and tertiary in FL 50. The insured or patient information reported in FL 58 should be in order of last name, first name, and middle initial. The name must be spelled exactly as it appears on the health insurance card. Following are some rules that apply to the way the name is reported in FL 58:

- Report the last name first, and use a comma or space to separate the last and first names, as in Satterfield, Louise.
- Do not leave a space between the two parts in names such as VonAllen or McCarthy.
- Retain the hyphen in names such as Geller-Brown.
- Do not use titles, such as Ms. or Dr.
- For names containing suffixes, as in III, the following format is used: Ramados III, David, J.

FLs 59–65, the remaining fields in this section of the UB-04, all pertain to the insured named in FL 58. Depending on the circumstances of the claim, completion of these fields may or may not be required, as described below.

FL 59 Patient's Relationship to Insured

FL 59 contains a two-digit code used to indicate the relationship of the patient to the insured individual identified in FL 58. The codes are listed below.

Guidelines

Completion of this field is required on Medicare claims when Medicare is the secondary or tertiary payer. This field is also required by most other payers.

Codes

01   Spouse

18   Self

19   Child

20   Employee

21   Unknown

39   Organ Donor

Code 39 indicates care given to an organ donor when the care is paid for by the receiving patient's insurance company.

40   Cadaver Donor

Code 40 indicates procedures performed on the cadaver donor when they are paid for by the receiving patient's insurance company.

53   Life Partner

G8   Other Relationship

Figure 13.2 illustrates the use of two different relationship codes in FL 59—01 (Spouse) and 18 (Self)—when a patient has two types of insurance. The primary coverage is provided through the patient's spouse, who is employed, and the secondary plan is the patient's Medicare plan. As per MSP rules, the coverage provided through the patient's working spouse is primary to Medicare. Payer information for both plans is reported—payer IDs are listed in FL 51, provider numbers in FL 57, and insured IDs in FL 60.

Figure 13.2

Insured's Information Illustrating the Use of Two Different Relationship Codes in FL 59

50 PAYER NAME	51 HEALTH PLAN ID	52 REL INFO	53 ASG BEN.	54 PRIOR PAYMENTS	55 EST. AMOUNT DUE	56 NPI	3322100065	
A CIGNA HEALTH PLAN	00524	Y	Y	0 :00	2045 :35	57	219004	A
B MEDICARE	00308	Y	Y	0 :00		OTHER	070089	B
C						PRV ID		C

58 INSURED'S NAME	59 P.REL	60 INSURED'S UNIQUE ID	61 GROUP NAME	62 INSURANCE GROUP NO.	
A TONY RAY	01	CG 60025-1	CIGNA CT	J904	A
B SHAREEN TOBIS-RAY	18	132508767			B
C					C

63 TREATMENT AUTHORIZATION CODES	64 DOCUMENT CONTROL NUMBER	65 EMPLOYER NAME	
A A4562201		SONY	A
B			B
C			C

FL 60 Insured's Unique Identifier

Form locator 60 contains the unique identification number assigned to the insured by the health plan. This field allows twenty alphanumeric characters in each of lines A, B, and C.

Guidelines

Completion of this field is required for Medicare billing and by all other payers. In general, the insurance identification card numbers assigned by the various payers are recorded in the field. When Medicare is secondary (line B) and the provider is requesting a conditional payment, Medicare requires the primary payer identification information on line A. Medicaid also requires this information on line A whenever Medicaid is secondary.

A Medicare beneficiary's unique **health insurance claim number (HICN)** must appear in this field.

The patient name reported in FL 8 on the UB-04 must match the Medicare HICN reported in FL 60 in order for the claim to be processed correctly. In addition, Medicare may reject the claim if the HICN does not match the eligibility files.

FL 61 Insured's Group Name

FL 61 contains the name of the group or plan that is providing the health insurance coverage to the insured. This field allows fourteen alphanumeric characters.

Guidelines

Completion of this field is not required for primary Medicare billing. Medicare payers do not have group names or numbers. However, when Medicare is the secondary (or tertiary) payer, Medicare requires the insured group name for the payer that is primary (or secondary).

For other payers, the group name is required if group coverage applies and a group name, rather than a group number, is available. If the identification card shows a group number, the number is reported and the name is not required.

For TRICARE beneficiaries, the branch of service that applies to the sponsor, for example, *USA* for U.S. Army or *USAF* for U.S. Air Force, should be reported here.

FL 62 Insured's Group Number

FL 62 contains the identification number, the control number, or the code that is assigned by the insurance company to identify the group under which the individual is insured. This field allows seventeen alphanumeric characters in each of lines A, B, and C.

Guidelines

Completion of this field is not required for primary Medicare billing. However, when Medicare is the secondary (or tertiary) payer, Medicare requires the insured group number for the payer that is primary (or secondary). It is required for all other third-party payers when the insured's identification card shows a group number.

For TRICARE claims, the sponsor's military status, such as *ACT* for active or *RET* for retired, and pay grade codes must be entered.

FL 63 Treatment Authorization Codes

FL 63 is used to report a number or other indicator that designates that the treatment covered by this bill has been authorized by the payer indicated in FL 50. This field allows thirty alphanumeric characters in each line.

Guidelines

Completion of this field is required for Medicare billing whenever an authorization or referral number is assigned. In addition, whenever a Quality Improvement Organization (QIO) review has been performed for outpatient preadmission, preprocedure, or inpatient preadmission, the authorization number is required for all approved admissions or services.

Completion of this field is required by other payers as well when an authorization or referral number is assigned by the payer or utilization management organization (UMO). Some payers do not require preauthorization.

COMPLIANCE GUIDE
Advance Treatment Authorization

Often, advance approval (called precertification or authorization) is needed before a hospitalization or an elective surgical procedure. The notification allows the payer to authorize payment or recommend some other course of action. For example, in the Medicare program, certain surgical procedures and scheduled inpatient services must be reviewed and approved by a QIO in advance. If this procedure is not followed and an authorization number correctly reported, the payer may charge a fine or refuse to pay the bill.

FL 64 Document Control Number (DCN)

FL 64 is used to report the document control number, also known as the internal control number (ICN), assigned to the original claim by the payer. The DCN is reported on the UB-04 only when filing a replacement or cancellation to a previously processed claim (TOB 0XX7 or 0XX8). The DCN is assigned by the payer or the payer's fiscal agent while processing the claim and can be found on the remittance advice for the processed claim.

837I No Map Field
FL 65: Employer Name

The electronic HIPAA claim does not contain a field for reporting the name of the insured's employer. This information is reported on paper claims only.

FL 65 Employer Name of the Insured

FL 65 contains the name of the employer that provides health care coverage for the insured individual identified in FL 58. This field allows twenty-five alphanumeric characters in each of lines A, B, and C.

Guidelines

Completion of this field is required for Medicare billing only when Medicare is the secondary (or tertiary) insurer—Medicare requires the employer name of the insured corresponding to the payer that is primary (or secondary). Depending on the circumstances of the claim and the type of insurance, this field may be required by other payers.

HIPAA TIP

Employer Name: Part of PHI

The name of the patient's employer, as reported in FL 65 on the UB-04, is considered a part of PHI.

CHAPTER SUMMARY

1 The section of the UB-04 claim form that contains FLs 50–65 is used to report details about the payer, the insured, and the insured's employer. Payer, insured, and employer information are required on the UB-04 to make an accurate determination of benefits as well as to coordinate benefits when there is more than one payer.

2 FLs 50–55 and FL 57 on the UB-04 contain details about the payer. Each of these fields has three lines, labeled A, B, and C, used to identify the primary, secondary, and tertiary payer, respectively.

- FL 50 contains the name for each payer.
- FL 51 contains the health plan ID for each payer.
- FL 52 indicates whether the provider has a release of information authorization from the patient.
- FL 53 indicates whether the patient has assigned the benefits directly to the provider.
- FL 54 is used to report any payment of the bill received to date from the payer(s) listed in FL 50.
- FL 55 is used to estimate the amount due from the payer(s) listed in FL 50 (the estimated responsibility less any payments received).
- FL 57 is used to report the health plan legacy number assigned to the provider by the indicated payer in FL 50; it is used as a secondary identifier to supplement the NPI when required.

3 FL 56 in this section, which contains only one line, indicates the billing provider's ten-digit National Provider Identifier (NPI), mandated by HIPAA for use as the provider's primary identifier beginning May 23, 2007. The NPI is a unique identifier assigned to each provider nationally for lifetime use. The NPI Registry is a query-only database available through the CMS website that contains a complete listing of NPIs and other provider data that are available to the public.

4 Situations in which Medicare may be listed as a secondary payer (FL 50, line B) on a claim include the following:

- Another payer paid some of the charges, and Medicare is secondarily liable for the remainder.
- Another payer denied the claim.
- The provider is requesting a conditional payment.

When Medicare is billed as a secondary payer, the applicable value code and amount received from the primary insurer must be reported in FLs 39–41 (Value Codes and Amounts) on the UB-04.

5 The insured portion of the UB-04 claim includes FLs 58–62. FL 58 (Insured's Name) contains the name of the patient or the individual in whose name the insurance listed in FL 50 is issued. This name must correspond with the name on the insured's identification card. The remaining FLs in this portion all pertain to the person identified in FL 58.

- FL 59 indicates the patient's relationship to the insured.
- FL 60 contains the insured's identification number assigned by the payer organization.
- FL 61 indicates the name of the group or plan that is providing coverage to the insured.
- FL 62 indicates the insurance group number under which the insured individual is being covered.

6 The last portion of the payer, insured, and employer information section of the UB-04 contains FLs 63–65.

- FL 63 is used to report a treatment authorization code when an authorization or referral number is assigned by the payer or utilization management organization (UMO), or in the case of Medicare by the Quality Improvement Organization (QIO).
- FL 64 is used to report the document control number (DCN), also known as the internal control number (ICN), assigned to the original bill by the indicated health plan in FL 50; it is reported on the UB-04 only when filing a replacement or cancellation to a previously processed claim (TOB 0XX7 or 0XX8).
- FL 65 contains the name of the employer who is providing health care coverage for the insured indicated in FL 58 (for use with paper claims only).

✔ CHECK YOUR UNDERSTANDING

1. Define *National Provider Identifier,* and specify which form locator(s) it occupies on the UB-04.

   _____

   _____

2. True or False: When a patient signs a statement agreeing to assign insurance benefits directly to a provider, it is understood that the patient is agreeing to allow the release of his or her medical information as well. _____

3. Which of the following form locators must be completed when Medicare is the primary payer and AARP is a supplemental insurer? (Choose all that apply).
   a. FL 50: Payer name, lines A and B
   b. FL 58: Name of the insured, lines A and B
   c. FL 59: Patient relationship to insured, lines A and B
   d. FL 60: Insured's unique ID, assigned by the health plan, lines A and B
   e. all of the above
   f. none of the above

4. Which of the following entries would be considered valid for FL 58 (Insured's Name) on the UB-04? (Choose all that apply.)

   a. Arnie J. DeGalbo

   b. Mc Gowan, Stephanie S.

   c. Teresa McCarthy

   d. Gelb, Gerrard

   e. DiNapoli III, Roger, T.

   f. Phyllis B. Owens, Sr.

   g. Cohen-Blakely, Alice, Y.

5. In each of the following billing situations, list the payers in the correct order.

   a. A three-year-old boy has a hernia and needs an operation. He is covered by Medicaid. He also has limited coverage under his father's insurance at work, American Mutual.

   50 PAYER NAME

   A _____

   B _____

   C _____

   b. A Medicare beneficiary who has met her deductible for the year has AARP supplemental insurance through her husband. She has received two months of physical therapy. Two of the last five visits this month exceed the allowed number of visits for the benefit period.

   50 PAYER NAME

   A _____

   B _____

   C _____

   c. An older man slips on a wet floor in the doorway of a store and breaks his kneecap. He is a Medicare beneficiary with a MediGap plan. The store has liability coverage through Mid Valley Insurance.

   50 PAYER NAME

   A _____

   B _____

   C _____

6. A working-aged beneficiary had a joint replacement in her left hand. She received a partial payment of $1,150.60 from her employer's benefit plan. The unpaid amount is being submitted to Medicare as the secondary payer. What value code and amount should be reported in FLs 39–41 on the claim?

   FL 39 VALUE CODES

Code	Amount
_____	_____ . ___

7. For the following scenarios, indicate what code would be reported in FL 59 (Patient's Relationship to Insured) on the lines indicated.

   a. A Medicare beneficiary receives primary coverage through his life partner's insurance with a Blue Cross and Blue Shield plan and secondary coverage through his Medicare plan.

   Line A code _____; line B code _____

   b. A daughter receives insurance coverage through her mother's insurance plan.

   Line A code _____

   c. A woman who is donating a kidney to her twin sister is covered under her sister's Medicare plan.

   Line A code _____

8. Fill in FLs 50–65 below for patient Maria Giorgo, given the following insurance and patient information. The hospital's NPI is 3322100065.

Insurance Information
Primary: Empire BC/BS
Plan ID/Carrier Code: 00444
Release of Info on File: Y
Benefits Assigned: Y
Preauthorization Number: 0022798
Provider ID: Y1002Q

Patient Information
Patient's Name: Maria Giorgo
Insured's Name: Maria Giorgo
Patient Relationship to Insured: Self
Insured's Plan ID: 99-2305
Insurance Group Name/No: 8402-S92
Employer: Towne Drug

UB-04 Form—FLs 50–65

50 PAYER NAME	51 HEALTH PLAN ID	52 REL INFO	53 ASG. BEN.	54 PRIOR PAYMENTS	55 EST. AMOUNT DUE	56 NPI	
A						57 OTHER PRV ID	A
B							B
C							C

58 INSURED'S NAME	59 P.REL	60 INSURED'S UNIQUE ID	61 GROUP NAME	62 INSURANCE GROUP NO.	
A					A
B					B
C					C

63 TREATMENT AUTHORIZATION CODES	64 DOCUMENT CONTROL NUMBER	65 EMPLOYER NAME	
A			A
B			B
C			C

9. Fill in FLs 50–65 below for patient Renee Chang, given the following insurance and patient information. Note that this is a replacement claim. The insurance carrier information on the previous claim was incorrect. The hospital's NPI is 3322100065.

Insurance Information
Primary: Medicare
Plan ID/Carrier Code: 00308
Release of Info on File: Y
Benefits Assigned: Y
Preauthorization Number:—
Provider ID: 070089
DCN: ZZ50062J3

Patient Information
Patient's Name: Renee Chang
Insured's Name: Simon Chang
Patient Relationship to Insured: Wife
Insured's Plan ID: 099256666
Insurance Group Name/No:—
Employer:—

UB-04 Form—FLs 50–65

50 PAYER NAME	51 HEALTH PLAN ID	52 REL INFO	53 ASG. BEN.	54 PRIOR PAYMENTS	55 EST. AMOUNT DUE	56 NPI	
A						57 OTHER PRV ID	A
B							B
C							C

58 INSURED'S NAME	59 P.REL	60 INSURED'S UNIQUE ID	61 GROUP NAME	62 INSURANCE GROUP NO.	
A					A
B					B
C					C

63 TREATMENT AUTHORIZATION CODES	64 DOCUMENT CONTROL NUMBER	65 EMPLOYER NAME	
A			A
B			B
C			C

10. Fill in FLs 50–65 below for patient Leo P. Trevor, given the following insurance and patient information. The hospital's NPI is 3322100065. To date, the hospital has received $1,009.00 from Aetna toward the payment of this claim.

Insurance Information	*Patient Information*
Primary: Aetna	Patient's Name: Leo P. Trevor
Plan ID/Carrier Code: 000007	Insured's Name: Lynn Trevor
Release of Info on File: Y	Patient Relationship to Insured: Husband
Benefits Assigned: Y	Insured's Plan ID: CJ88 2Y
Preauthorization Number: 98664H	Insurance Group Name/No: A5JJ
Provider ID: AE922VZ	Employer: Safeway

Insurance Information	*Patient Information*
Secondary: Medicare	Patient's Name: Leo P. Trevor
Plan ID/Carrier Code: 00308	Insured's Name: Leo P. Trevor
Release of Info on File: Y	Patient Relationship to Insured: Self
Benefits Assigned: Y	Insured's Plan ID: 197228851A
Preauthorization Number:—	Insurance Group Name/No:—
Provider ID: 070089	Employer:—

UB-04 Form—FLs 50–65

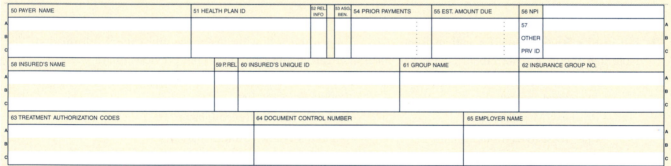

COMPUTER EXPLORATION

UB-04 Activity: Claim Analysis

Viewing FLs 50–65: Payer, Insured, and Employer Information

Open the files **Sample02.pdf** and **Sample03.pdf** in Adobe Reader, and answer the following questions:

1. Sample02 is the inpatient claim for Rose Washington. What type of insurance does Rose Washington have? What is her insurance plan's ID?

2. Does she have a release of information form on file? Does this release of information give her insurance company the right to use her PHI for pharmaceutical research purposes?

3. What is Longwood Hospital's NPI? How many digits does it contain? Are all NPIs the same number of digits?

4. Does Rose have her own insurance? Based on the information in FL 59, what is her relationship to John Washington? What is his health plan ID? Does his plan have a group name or number? Is he employed?

5. Switch to Sample03, the claim for Vera Van Husen. Look through the payer, insured, and employer section of Vera's claim. How many insurance plans does she have?

6. Is the primary plan in her name? What does code 18 in FL 59 indicate?

7. What is the name and plan ID of her secondary insurance? Based on the data in FLs 58 and 59, in whose name is the secondary plan? What does code 01 in FL 59 indicate?

8. FL 63 reports the number 123PP. What does this number represent, and who assigned it?

9. Compare the information in FL 56 (NPI) in both sample claims. Why is this information the same?

10. What is the legacy provider number for Vera's secondary plan? What is the relationship between this number and the NPI in FL 56? Which number is more important to report?

When finished viewing both claims, click Exit on the File menu.

Diagnosis and Procedure Codes

LEARNING OUTCOMES

After completing this chapter, you will be able to define the key terms and:

1. Understand how to indicate in FL 66 (Diagnosis and Procedure Code Qualifier) which version of the ICD is being used on the current claim.

2. Understand the importance of reporting an ICD-9-CM diagnosis code in FL 67 (Principal Diagnosis Code and Present on Admission Indicator) to describe the patient's principal diagnosis as well as whether the condition associated with it was present on admission (POA) or acquired during the hospital stay.

3. Discuss the difference between the principal diagnosis, reported in FL 67, and secondary or other diagnoses, reported in FLs 67 A–Q (Other Diagnosis Codes and POA Indicators).

4. Explain the use of FL 69 (Admitting Diagnosis Code) to describe the patient's diagnosis at the time of inpatient admission or the use of FL 70a–c (Patient's Reason for Visit) to describe the patient's reason for an unscheduled visit at the time of outpatient registration.

5. Explain the use of FL 71 (Prospective Payment System Code) and FL 72 (External Cause of Injury Code).

6. Understand when to report an ICD-9-CM code and corresponding date in FL 74 (Principal Procedure Code and Date) to describe the principal procedure performed during the period covered by the bill.

7. Discuss the use of FLs 74a–e (Other Procedure Codes and Dates) in reporting other significant procedures performed during the period covered by the bill.

KEY TERMS

- admitting diagnosis (ADX)
- POA exempt list

- principal procedure

orm locators 66 to 75 (Figure 14.1) play an important role on the UB-04 claim form, as these fields are used to report the clinical information related to the claim, including diagnosis and procedure codes. Most of the computer reviews (edits) performed by Medicare with the Outpatient Code Editor (OCE) and the Medicare Code Editor (MCE) check the accuracy of the codes reported in these fields. A logical connection must exist between the reported diagnoses and the procedures used to treat the problems associated with the diagnoses. Without this connection, the claim will be rejected or singled out for closer examination and correction.

The procedures performed must also be considered medically necessary, given the diagnosis reported; if they are not, third-party payers will not pay for the charges. The present on admission (POA) indicator that is reported with diagnosis codes on the UB-04 also plays an important role in this section of the claim, as it can influence the final payment received for the inpatient admission.

Patient account specialists must work closely with coders in the health information management (HIM) department to verify the accuracy and completeness of the diagnosis codes, POA indicators, and procedure codes contained in this section of the claim. Generally, the HIM staff members are responsible for assigning these codes based on the most up-to-date coding rules, the type of claim, and the patient's medical record and discharge summary.

Figure 14.1

UB-04 Claim Form—FLs 66–75

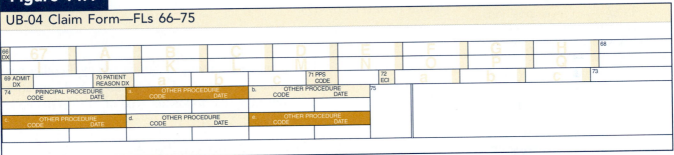

FL 66 Diagnosis and Procedure Code Qualifier (ICD Version Indicator)

FL 66 contains the qualifier code that indicates which version of the ICD (International Classification of Diseases) is being reported on the claim. Currently, 9 is the only acceptable entry, as ICD-9-CM (Ninth Revision) is the only version currently allowed under HIPAA. When ICD-10-CM is implemented in the future, code 0 will be reported in this field.

Guidelines

Completion of this field is required for Medicare and other payers when filing a paper claim. The field allows for one of the following single-digit codes:

- 9: Ninth Revision
- 0: Tenth Revision

837I No Map Field

FL 66—ICD Version Indicator

Qualifier codes 9 and 0 are not used on the electronic HIPAA claim. Although the HIPAA claim is designed to accept the expanded size of future ICD-10-CM codes (ICD-9-CM codes are three to five digits long, and ICD-10-CM codes will be up to seven digits long), currently it does not contain a field for reporting the ICD version being used. In the future, it is likely that the electronic claim will add qualifier codes for this purpose.

COMPLIANCE GUIDE
Correct Code Sets

The correct medical code sets are those valid at the time the health care is provided. The correct administrative code sets are those valid at the time the transaction—such as the claim—is started.

FL 67 Principal Diagnosis Code and Present on Admission Indicator

FL 67 contains the complete ICD-9-CM diagnosis code, either three, four, or five digits, that represents the principal diagnosis, followed by a single-digit modifier that represents the present on admission (POA) indicator. On the UB-04, this field allows for up to eight alphanumeric characters; positions 1 through 7 are used to report the ICD-9-CM diagnosis code, and position 8, which is shaded on the UB-04, is used to report the POA indicator. Although all seven positions are not currently required for reporting the diagnosis code, they will be used when the ICD-10-CM codes are introduced.

Although a decimal is used between the third and the fourth digits of a diagnosis code in the ICD-9-CM system, it is not necessary to use the decimal on the UB-04 claim form. For example, the diagnosis code 414.01 is reported as 41401, and 425.4 is reported as 4254. Also, as illustrated in the last example, zeros are not added to make a three- or four-digit code five digits long. Both of these formatting rules apply to all diagnosis codes reported on the claim form (FLs 67–72).

Guidelines

Completion of this field is required for Medicare billing and by all other payers. ICD-9-CM diagnosis codes are required for inpatient and outpatient Medicare claims. Claims containing the following type of bill (TOB) codes require a principal diagnosis code:

011X	Hospital, inpatient, Medicare Part A
012X	Hospital, inpatient, Medicare Part B
013X	Hospital, outpatient
014X	Hospital, other, Medicare Part B, including SNF diagnostic clinical laboratory services to nonpatients
018X	Hospital, swing bed

V Codes

The principal diagnosis code for a Medicare inpatient or outpatient can be a V code that is selected from the list of accepted V codes. E codes and V codes are supplementary codes found in the ICD-9-CM. V codes identify encounters for reasons other than illness or injury. E codes identify the external causes of injuries and poisoning. Because E codes describe the circumstances that caused an injury rather than the injury itself, they cannot represent a principal diagnosis code.

Depending on the condition and the code, a V code can be used as either a primary code for an encounter or as an additional code. V codes are used in various ways:

- For encounters with healthy patients who receive services other than treatments, such as annual checkups and immunizations. For example, the diagnosis code for a routine adult general medical examination is V70.0.
- For encounters with patients who have known conditions for which they are receiving one of three types of treatment: chemotherapy, radiation therapy, or rehabilitation.

- For encounters in which a problem not currently affecting the patient's health status, such as a family history of a disease, needs to be noted.
- For encounters in which patients are being evaluated preoperatively for a given condition.

POA Indicator

The POA (present on admission) indicator is a single-digit modifier that is attached to a diagnosis code on an inpatient acute-care claim. Its purpose is to indicate whether the condition associated with the diagnosis was present on admission or acquired during the hospital stay. By making hospitals financially accountable for treating certain hospital-acquired infections and conditions, POA reporting is intended to improve the quality of care in hospitals.

POA Indicator Guidelines

There are five POA indicators:

Code	Definition
Y	Yes (present at the time of inpatient admission)
N	No (not present)
U	Unknown (documentation is insufficient to determine)
W	Clinically undetermined (provider is unable to clinically determine)
1 or blank	Unreported/not used—exempt from POA reporting

Indicator 1 was created for use with the electronic claim format, as it is not advisable to leave a blank as a response on an electronic claim. On the paper claim, a blank or a 1 may be used to indicate that a diagnosis is exempt from POA reporting. Only diagnosis codes that are on the official **POA exempt list,** as specified in the ICD-9-CM *Official Guidelines for Coding and Reporting,* can be reported as exempt.

On the UB-04, the POA indicator is reported as the eighth digit in FL 67 (Principal Diagnosis Code and POA Indicator), FLs 67A–Q (Other Diagnosis Codes and POA Indicators), and FLs 72a–c (External Cause of Injury Codes). The eighth position appears as a single-digit shaded box on the far right of each of these fields. Figure 14.2 shows an example of POA indicators in FLs 67 and 67A–F.

COMPLIANCE GUIDE
Use of the Most Specific Code

ICD-9-CM codes should always be used at their highest level of specificity to avoid claim errors caused by incomplete diagnosis codes or claim rejection. If a principal diagnosis code is missing from the claim, or if the code reported is not the full ICD-9-CM code, including all five digits when applicable, the patient account specialist should contact the health information management (HIM) department to obtain the appropriate code.

$ $ Billing Tip $ $

Use V Codes to Show Medical Necessity

V codes such as family history or a patient's previous condition help demonstrate why a service was medically necessary.

$ $ Billing Tip $ $

Hospitals Exempt from POA Reporting

Critical access hospitals, Maryland waiver hospitals, long-term care hospitals, cancer hospitals, and children's inpatient facilities are exempt from POA reporting.

INTERNET RESOURCE
Official Guidelines: POA Exempt List

www.cdc.gov/nchs/datawh/ftpserv/ftpicd9/icdguide07.pdf
This version of the *Official Guidelines* is effective October 1, 2007. The POA exempt list begins on page 97.

Figure 14.2

UB-04 Form—Example of POA Indicators

Form Locators That Require POA Indicators

The POA indicator is required on the UB-04 in FL 67 for the principal diagnosis code and in FLs 67A–Q for all secondary diagnosis codes. Although the POA indicator field is available for use with E codes in FLs 72a–c (External Cause of Injury Codes), a POA indicator code is not required in this field on Medicare claims. Medicare requires a POA indicator for an E code only when it is listed as a secondary diagnosis in FLs 67A–Q. On the UB-04, according to the NUBC, the POA indicator has been made available in FLs 72a–c because of the importance of the data from a patient safety perspective. Although there are exceptions, in most cases the POA indicator for a principal diagnosis code is Y.

FLs 67A–Q Other Diagnosis Codes and POA Indicators

The Other Diagnosis Codes and POA Indicators field is used to report ICD-9-CM diagnosis codes for additional conditions that coexist at the time of admission, that develop subsequently, or that affect the patient's treatment and/or the length of stay. Diagnoses connected to an earlier episode that have no bearing on the current hospital stay are not reported. A POA code indicator is required for each code reported in this field.

The NUBC guidelines define other diagnosis codes on the UB-04 as additional conditions that affect patient care or length of stay by requiring the following: clinical evaluation, therapeutic treatment, diagnostic procedures, an extended hospital stay, or increased nursing care and/or monitoring.

Guidelines

Completion of this field is required for Medicare billing and for all other payers. In general, the same guidelines apply to this field as apply to FL 67 (Principal Diagnosis Code and Present on Admission Indicator), including the limited use of V codes and the requirement of a POA indicator for each diagnosis code. Unlike in FL 67, however, E codes can be reported in FLs 67A–Q as secondary diagnoses.

When reporting other, or secondary, diagnosis codes, each code must be followed by a POA modifier indicating whether the diagnosis was present at the time of admission. See the list of POA indicators in the instructions for FL 67 above. The POA indicator is reported as the eighth digit in the shaded area in FLs 67A–Q.

Although the UB-04 contains space for up to seventeen secondary diagnosis codes, Medicare processes up to eight secondary diagnosis codes only on both inpatient and outpatient claims. These are the codes in the top row of the form locator (FLs 67A–H). Medicare ignores data submitted in the bottom row, FLs 67 I–Q.

The principal diagnosis code provided in FL 67 may not be duplicated as a secondary diagnosis code in FLs 67A–Q.

The codes in FLs 67A–Q should be reported in order of priority based on the information in the patient's medical record. Generally the HIM staff establishes this order. Comorbidities and complications are listed before other conditions, such as those related to the patient's medical history or other factors influencing the patient's health status.

Comorbidities and Complications

Other conditions that are present at admission and have an effect on the patient's hospital stay or course of treatment are called comorbidities, meaning coexisting conditions. On the UB-04, comorbidities are indicated with POA indicator Y. Conditions that develop as a result of surgery or other treatments are coded as complications. Complications are indicated with POA indicator N. In the patient medical record, comorbidities and complications are indicated with the initials *CC*. CCs are important to report in the Other Diagnosis Codes field on the UB-04 because their presence influences the hospital's final reimbursement.

EXAMPLES: The physician's notes state that the patient needed additional care because of chronic obstructive pulmonary disease (COPD) with emphysema (a comorbidity). The principal diagnosis code is 496, COPD, which is reported in FL 67. The secondary diagnosis code is 492.8, emphysema, and is reported in FLs 67A–Q. The POA indicator in both codes is Y, present on admission.

In the same case, the physician's notes indicate a diagnosis of postoperative hypertension as a postoperative complication. The secondary diagnosis is 997.91, postoperative hypertension—complications, which is reported in FLs 67A–Q. The POA indicator in this case is N, not present on admission.

FYI

Admitting Diagnosis

The **admitting diagnosis (ADX)** is the condition identified by the physician at the time of admission to the hospital that is the main reason for the hospitalization. The admitting diagnosis may not match the principal diagnosis once a final decision has been made about the patient's medical condition. For example, the inpatient admitting diagnosis may be probable acute appendicitis, represented by diagnosis code 540.9. After the patient is admitted and evaluated, the principal diagnosis may be diverticulosis of the small intestine, represented by diagnosis code 562.00. Reporting the admitting diagnosis helps show why certain tests and procedures were performed that were not actually necessary to treat the principal diagnosis established after study.

FL 68 Unlabeled Field

837I aler✚

Admitting Diagnosis Required on All Inpatient Claims

On the electronic claim, the admitting diagnosis is required on all inpatient admission claims and encounters.

FL 69 is used to report the ICD-9-CM diagnosis code that describes the patient's diagnosis at the time of inpatient admission.

Guidelines

Completion of this field is required for Medicare billing for inpatient hospital claims that are subject to QIO review. It is also required for commercial, TRICARE, Blue Cross, and Medicaid claims, depending on the individual plan or contract.

On the UB-04, the admitting diagnosis is required for the following inpatient TOBs only: 011X, 012X, 018X, and 021X.

The NUBC guidelines include the following conditions as possibilities for the admitting diagnosis on the UB-04: a significant finding in terms of patient distress, an abnormal finding on examination, a possible diagnosis, a diagnosis established from a previous encounter or admission, an injury, a poisoning, or a reason or condition that is not an illness or injury, such as labor during pregnancy.

FL 69 allows for seven alphanumeric characters. Only one admitting diagnosis is reported, although there may be secondary reasons for the admission. The main condition is determined based on ICD-9-CM coding directives and the *Official Guidelines*.

$$ Billing Tip $$

Distinct Field for Outpatient Reason for Visit

Unlike its predecessor, the UB-92, the UB-04 contains a distinct field for reporting the patient's reason for an outpatient visit. Previously, this information was reported in the same field as the admitting diagnosis code. The new Patient's Reason for Visit field also has space for reporting up to three reasons (FL 70a–c). The separation of these two data elements and the increase in the number of subfields is designed to curtail payment delays. The new design allows payers to determine more readily whether the services provided on the claim meet medical necessity.

FL 70 is used to report the ICD-9-CM diagnosis code that describes the patient's stated reason for seeking care at the time of outpatient registration.

Guidelines

Completion of this field is required by Medicare for all unscheduled outpatient visits. It is also required for commercial, TRICARE, Blue Cross, and Medicaid claims, depending on the individual plan or contract.

This form locator allows for seven alphanumeric characters in each of subfields a, b, and c, so that up to three diagnosis codes can be reported.

The diagnosis describing the patient's stated reason for seeking care should be a condition representing patient distress, an injury, a poisoning, or a reason or condition that is not an illness or injury, such as labor during pregnancy. The condition is determined based on ICD-9-CM coding directives and the *Official Guidelines*.

A reason for visit code may also be reported for scheduled outpatient visits, such as for ancillary tests, when this information provides additional support for medical necessity.

FYI

Unscheduled Outpatient Visits

Unscheduled outpatient visits are defined as visits with the following data elements:

- Outpatient TOB code 013X or 085X

- Type of Visit (FL 14) code 1 (Emergency), 2 (Urgent), or 5 (Trauma)

- Revenue codes 045X (Emergency room), 0516 (Urgent care clinic), 0526 (Freestanding urgent care clinic), or 0762 (Observation room)

FL 71 Prospective Payment System (PPS) Code

FL 71 is used to identify the DRG associated with the claim. The DRG is based on the grouper software called for under contract with the primary payer.

Guidelines

A PPS code is required on inpatient claims if the hospital is under DRG contract with a payer and the contract stipulates that the payer be provided with this information. Completion of the field is not required for Medicare billing. Other payers may request a PPS code as part of a DRG contract with the hospital. Many workers' compensation programs require this information.

This form locator allows for four numeric characters.

837I No Map Field

837I Claim Still Uses Dual Field

Unlike the UB-04, the electronic claim does not contain distinct fields for reporting the admitting diagnosis code and the patient's reason for an outpatient visit code. Distinct fields will likely be incorporated in the next update to match the UB-04 format.

FL 72 External Cause of Injury (ECI) Codes

FL 72 contains the ICD-9-CM code for the external cause of an injury, poisoning, or other adverse effect when applicable.

Guidelines

Completion of this field is not required for Medicare billing or by any other payer. It may be required in some states when the claim contains a diagnosis code for an injury or poisoning. In practice, most claims list E codes in order of priority as part of the secondary diagnosis codes in FL 67A–Q (Other Diagnosis Codes and POA Indicators) rather than in FL 72. Medicare requires a POA indicator for an E code only when it is listed in FL 67A–Q. On Medicare claims, data entered in FL 72 are ignored.

This field allows for eight alphanumeric characters in each of subfields a, b, and c, so that up to three E codes can be reported in FL 72. The E code is reported in positions 1–7, and a POA indicator is reported in the shaded eighth position when required. See the list of POA indicators in the instructions for FL 67 above.

$ $ Billing Tip $ $
E-Codes and Liability

E-codes are used by some payers to obtain information regarding liability. For example, if code E813 (motor vehicle traffic accident involving collision with another vehicle) is reported on the claim, the payer will not pay the claim because it is likely that auto insurance is the primary payer.

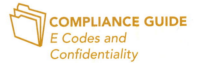

COMPLIANCE GUIDE
E Codes and Confidentiality

Special care should be given in the use of some E codes because of their sensitive nature. For example, suicide attempts and assaults are likely to be highly confidential matters.

FL 73 Unlabeled Field

FL 74 Principal Procedure Code and Date

FL 74 contains the ICD-9-CM code that identifies the inpatient principal procedure performed during the period covered by the bill and the date on which the procedure was performed.

EXAMPLE:
Inpatient principal diagnosis: Acute tonsillitis 463 (ICD-9-CM code from Volume 1)
Inpatient principal procedure: Tonsillectomy 28.2 (ICD-9-CM code from Volume 3)

Guidelines

Completion of this field is required for Medicare billing for inpatient services if a procedure is performed during the stay. However, this field is not used on Medicare outpatient claims.

Other payers also require completion of this field for inpatient claims. Although the field was used for reporting ICD-9-CM procedure codes on outpatient claims by some non-Medicare payers in the past, electronic HIPAA-compliant claims now require the use of CPT codes only for reporting outpatient surgical procedures. Therefore, FL 74 has become an inpatient-only form locator.

This field allows seven alphanumeric characters for the procedure code and six characters for the date. The date is recorded in the MMDDYY format on the UB-04. The electronic version of this field requires the CCYYMMDD format.

FLs 74a–e Other Procedure Codes and Dates

FLs 74a–e contain five subfields, labeled a through e, that are used to report up to five procedure codes for significant procedures that were performed during the billing period, other than the principal procedure, and their corresponding dates. The procedures that are most important for this episode of care, and specifically any therapeutic procedures closely related to the principal diagnosis, are reported.

Guidelines

Completion of this field is required for Medicare billing for inpatient services when additional procedures must be reported. Other payers also require completion of this field for inpatient claims. However, the field is not used on Medicare outpatient claims; nor is it used on outpatient claims for any other payer when using the electronic HIPAA claim.

The field allows seven alphanumeric characters for the procedure code and six characters for the date in each of subfields a through e. The date is recorded in the MMDDYY format on the paper version of the UB-04. The electronic version of this field requires the CCYYMMDD format.

The procedure codes in FLs 74a–e are reported in the order of importance, from most important to least important.

The dates of the procedures on Medicare inpatient claims must fall within the from and through dates reported in FL 6 (Statement Covers Period), except for outpatient surgical procedures that are reported on an inpatient claim. As allowed under the 72-hour rule, dates for these services may be prior to the admission date indicated in FL 12 (Admission, Start of Care Date) as long as they are not more than three days prior and are related to the inpatient stay.

FL 75 Unlabeled Field

1   FL 66 (Diagnosis and Procedure Code Qualifier) on the UB-04 is used to report the version of ICD being used on the claim. Currently, as per HIPAA requirements, only the ICD-9-CM version may be used. When ICD-10-CM is implemented in the future, version 10 will be reported.

2   FLs 66–75 of the UB-04 claim form contain the clinical information needed to process the claim, including diagnosis codes, POA indicators, and procedure codes. FL 67 is used to report the ICD-9-CM diagnosis code that describes the patient's principal diagnosis. Third-party payers use the principal diagnosis to determine whether the services listed on the claim are medically necessary. FL 67 also requires a POA indicator for the principal diagnosis so that the payer can determine whether the condition was present at the time of admission or developed during the stay. A POA indicator may lead to a lower reimbursement if the hospital is considered responsible for a hospital-acquired condition or infection.

3   FLs 67A–Q are used to report secondary diagnoses—other medical conditions that are listed because they have an effect on the treatment received or on the length of the patient's stay. The HIM department should make sure the appropriate secondary diagnosis codes are listed, including applicable codes for comorbidities and complications, E codes, and V codes, as their presence may increase the hospital's reimbursement. In addition, a POA indicator is required for each diagnosis code, as it is also a factor in determining reimbursement. POA indicators are always reported in the shaded box in the last position of a diagnosis code field.

4   FL 69 (Admitting Diagnosis Code) is used to report the main diagnosis code that represents the patient's diagnosis or symptoms at the time of inpatient admission. In some cases, the admitting diagnosis and the principal diagnosis are different. At the time of admission, the problem may be diagnosed as one condition; after evaluation, it may turn out to be another. Similarly, FLs 70a–c are used on outpatient claims to record the patient's reason for an unscheduled visit. FL 70 contains three fields, a–c, for reporting up to three reason-for-visit codes.

5   A new field on the UB-04, FL 71 (PPS Code), is used to identify the claim's DRG. This is required only if the hospital's DRG contract with the payer stipulates that it be provided. The field is not used for Medicare claims.

6   FL 72 is used to report the external cause of injury, poisoning, or other adverse effect, known as an E code, together with a POA indicator. On the UB-04, FL 72 contains three fields, a–c, for reporting up to three E codes and POA indicators. Completion of this field is desirable when appropriate, but it is not required by payers.

7 FL 74 (Principal Procedure Code and Date) is used to report a principal procedure on an inpatient claim. It is usually a surgical procedure and is the procedure most closely related to the principal diagnosis. FLs 74a–e (Other Procedure Codes and Dates) are used to report up to five procedure codes and corresponding dates for significant procedures that were performed during the billing period on the claim, other than the principal procedure. These procedures should reflect conditions that coexisted at the time of admission and were treated.

✔ CHECK YOUR UNDERSTANDING

1. Define the following terms, and specify which form locator each occupies on the UB-04.
   a. admitting diagnosis _____
   _____

   b. POA exempt list _____
   _____

   c. principal procedure _____
   _____

2. True or False: If the admitting diagnosis code duplicates the principal diagnosis on a Medicare claim, the Medicare Code Editor (MCE) will reject the claim. _____

3. Which of the following items are reported in FL 69? Choose all that apply.
   a. POA indicator
   b. admitting diagnosis for inpatient
   c. other procedure code and date
   d. patient's reason for unscheduled outpatient visit

4. Which of the following codes would be considered valid as principle diagnosis codes on the UB-04 (FL 67, Principal Diagnosis Code and POA Indicator)? Choose all that apply.
   a. E930
   b. 93.31
   c. V70.0
   d. 562.00

5. True or False: For inpatients, if operating room charges are listed in the Revenue Code and Description fields (FLs 42–43), a principal procedure code and date must be listed in FL 74. _____

6. A patient is referred to the hospital for evaluation of hypertension. The medical record also documents diabetes. Diabetes would be reported in FL _____. What POA indicator would be reported on the claim? _____

7. True or False: The secondary procedure codes in FLs 74a–e are reported in the order of occurrence based on the patient's medical record. _____

8. A Medicare claim with TOB code 013X contains revenue code 0360 (Operating room services) for a surgical procedure and a principal procedure code and date in FL 74 for the surgical procedure. The claim is rejected by Medicare. What mistake was made on the claim?

_____

_____

9. Completion of FL 70 (Patient's Reason for Visit) is required for all unscheduled outpatient visits. Unscheduled outpatient visits are defined as visits with the presence of certain data elements. For each data element listed below, write *Yes* to indicate that the data element described would signify an unscheduled outpatient visit on a UB-04 claim or *No* if it would not.

_____ **a.** TOB code 013X (FL 4)

_____ **b.** Revenue code 0120 (FL 42)

_____ **c.** Type of visit code 2 (FL 14)

_____ **d.** Revenue code 045X (FL 42)

_____ **e.** Type of visit code 5 (FL 14)

_____ **f.** TOB code 011X (FL 4)

_____ **g.** TOB code 085X (FL 4)

_____ **h.** Type of visit code 3 (FL 14)

10. A patient with a history of colon cancer was admitted for closure of her colostomy, which was performed under general anesthesia. Fill in FLs 66–74 below using the following diagnostic and procedure code information. The TOB on the claim is 0111.

Diagnosis: Admission for colostomy closure, history of colon cancer.

Principle Diagnosis Code: V55.2   POA: 1 (exempt from reporting)

Other Diagnosis Code: V10.05   POA: 1 (exempt from reporting)

Admitting Diagnosis: V55.2

Principal Procedure Code: 46.52 (Closure of colostomy)

Date of Procedure: May 22, 2008

UB-04 Form—FLs 66–77

UB-04 Activity: Claim Analysis

Analyzing Diagnosis and Procedure Codes: FLs 66-74

Open the files **Sample02.pdf** and **Sample03.pdf** in Adobe Reader, and answer the following questions:

1. Sample02.pdf is the inpatient claim for Rose Washington. The first field in the diagnosis and procedure codes section is FL 66. This is a single-digit field for reporting which version of the ICD was used in preparing the claim: the ICD-9-CM or the ICD-10-CM. Have both versions been approved for use? Which version is reported here?

2. Study the data in FLs 67 and 67A. If you haven't already done so, refer to the ICD-9-CM for definitions of the two diagnosis codes reported on the claim. The first code indicates the type of delivery, and the second code indicates the outcome of the delivery. Did the patient have a normal delivery? Was the baby born alive?

3. Because this is an inpatient claim, POA indicators must be reported in FL 67 (Principal Diagnosis Code) and FLs 67A-Q (Other Diagnosis Codes). Notice the POA indicator is the same for both diagnosis codes. What does it indicate? Why is this POA indicator the logical choice for the diagnosis codes on this claim?

4. What is the admitting diagnosis (FL 69) on the claim? Notice that the admitting diagnosis is the same as the principal diagnosis in this case.

5. Now look at the procedure code section. Inpatient surgical procedures are contained in Volume 3 of ICD-9-CM. Find a description of both inpatient procedures. How was the baby delivered? On what date was the baby born?

6. Switch to Sample03.pdf, the outpatient claim for Vera Van Husen. What is the principal diagnosis code on Vera's claim? Are there additional diagnosis codes? Explain why a POA indicator is not reported with the diagnosis on this claim.

7. Look up the description of the principal diagnosis code in the ICD-9-CM. What type of hernia does Vera have?

8. Since this is an outpatient claim, notice that it does not contain an admitting diagnosis code in FL 69. FL 70 is used to report the patient's reason for an unscheduled outpatient visit. Notice FL 70 is blank. What three codes in FL 14 (Type of Visit) would indicate an unscheduled visit?

9. To report a surgical procedure on an outpatient claim, the appropriate HCPCS/CPT code for the procedure is listed in FL 44 along with a surgery-related revenue code, such as 036X (OR SERVICES), which indicates the use of an operating room. Locate the two surgical procedure codes reported in FL 44.

10. Look up the descriptions for these two HCPCS/CPT codes in CPT-4. What type of implant was used in repairing the hernia? To confirm this, look up the C code listed along with revenue code 0278 (SUPPLY/IMPLANTS). C codes are found in the HCPCS-Level II codebook.

When finished viewing the claims, click Exit on the File menu.

Physician Information, Remarks, and Code-Code Field

LEARNING OUTCOMES

After completing this chapter, you will be able to define the key terms and:

1. Explain the use of FL 76 (Attending Provider Name and Identifiers) when reporting the name, the NPI, and the other identifier number of the physician who has primary responsibility for the patient's medical care and treatment.

2. Explain the use of FLs 77–79 when reporting the name, the NPI, and the other identifier numbers of the operating physician on a claim that contains a surgical procedure and/or the name, the NPI, and the other identifier numbers of other providers, such as a referring provider, if other providers were involved in the patient's care.

3. List the various types of notes that can be reported in the Remarks field (FL 80) to help payers process claims more accurately and efficiently.

4. Describe the function of the Code-Code field in reporting overflow codes from other form locators in addition to listing information represented by externally maintained codes sets, such as taxonomy codes, that have been approved by the NUBC for use with the UB-04 form.

KEY TERMS

- qualifier codes
- secondary identifiers
- taxonomy code
- UPIN (unique physician identification number)

The last section of the UB-04, FLs 76–81, contains three types of information that bring the billing process to a conclusion (see Figure 15.1). The first type of information is a set of four fields for reporting physician information (FLs 76–79). Physician information is required by all payers. The UB-04 contains separate fields for reporting the attending physician and an operating physician, and two fields for reporting other provider types who may have been involved in the patient's care.

The other two fields in this section—the field for text remarks (FL 80) and the Code-Code field (FL 81)—serve as locations for information that does not fit in other fields. The Remarks field is used to enter remarks needed to process the claim that are not shown elsewhere on the bill—for example, information needed to coordinate a claim that involves more than one payer. The Code-Code field captures information through the use of special qualifiers and code sets. It is used to report overflow codes from other form locators or codes external to the UB-04 data set. The Remarks and Code-Code fields, while not used on all claims, provide a format for reporting miscellaneous information that payers may require on a particular claim. With this closing information, the claim is complete.

Figure 15.1

UB-04 Form—FLs 76–81

				76 ATTENDING	NPI	QUAL		
				LAST		FIRST		
				77 OPERATING	NPI	QUAL		
				LAST		FIRST		
80 REMARKS	81CC a			78 OTHER	NPI	QUAL		
	b			LAST		FIRST		
	c			79 OTHER	NPI	QUAL		
	d			LAST		FIRST		

UB-04 CMS-1450 APPROVED OMB NO. 0938-0997 NUBC National Uniform Billing Committee THE CERTIFICATIONS ON THE REVERSE APPLY TO THIS BILL AND ARE MADE A PART HEREOF.

FL 76 Attending Provider Name and Identifiers

FL 76 is used to report the name, the NPI, and the secondary identifier (when required) of the attending provider. The attending provider is the licensed physician who normally would be expected to certify the medical necessity of the services rendered and/or who has primary responsibility for the medical care and treatment reported in the claim. For inpatient claims, this is the physician who has primary responsibility for the care of the patient from the beginning of the hospital episode. For outpatient claims, this is the physician who ordered the surgery, therapy, diagnostic tests, or other services received by the patient.

Guidelines

Completion of this field is required for Medicare billing and by other payers as well. As mandated by HIPAA, all providers, institutional as well as individuals, must report a ten-digit NPI. The attending provider's NPI is reported in line 1 of FL 76. Next to the NPI is a field for reporting an optional secondary identifier. The attending provider's last name and first name are reported in line 2 of FL 76.

Line 1 of FL 76 allows up to eleven positions for the NPI; two positions for a secondary identifier code qualifier, indicating the type of number being reported; and nine positions for the secondary identifier itself. Line 2 allows up to sixteen positions for the provider's last name and twelve positions for the first name (see Figure 15.2).

Figure 15.2

UB-04 Form—Close-up of FL 76 with Data

76 ATTENDING	NPI 1109110988	QUAL G2	MA22290
LAST DONOVAN		FIRST MARK	

Secondary Identifiers

In each of the provider information form locators (FLs 76–79), the UB-04 provides a field for reporting a secondary provider identifier. **Secondary identifiers** reported in these form locaters are the old legacy numbers, such as physician UPINs or state license numbers, that were considered primary identifiers prior to the implementation of NPI. Unlike an NPI, a secondary identifier is not required on the UB-04 unless specified by the payer.

When a payer requires a secondary identifier, a **qualifier code** is reported before the identifier to indicate the type of identifier being reported. The qualifier codes for the secondary identifier are:

- 0B: State license number
- 1G: Provider UPIN
- G2: Provider commercial number

Depending on the payer and the claim, secondary identifiers may or may not be required. For example, Medicaid claims sometimes require state license numbers. On Medicare claims, UPINs are required if an NPI is not reported for any reason. At present, some commercial carriers require a provider commercial number in addition to the NPI. While payers and providers test the use of the newly mandated NPI system, both CMS and the NUBC recommend that both NPI and legacy numbers be reported on claims. Eventually, UB-04 claims will require only an NPI for provider identification.

HIPAA Tip

UPINs and NPIs

Prior to NPI implementation, the **UPIN (unique physician identification number)** was a number assigned by the Centers for Medicare and Medicaid Services (CMS) to identify physicians and suppliers who provided medical services or supplies to Medicare beneficiaries. Each physician had a unique six-character alphanumeric identification number designed to track payment and utilization information. This physician numbering system was replaced in 2007 by a National Provider Identifier (NPI) system, implemented by CMS. The NPI is a ten-digit identifier. The new system is one of the requirements of the Health Insurance Portability and Accountability Act (HIPAA).

$ $ Billing Tip $ $

QIO Review

Provider information reported in FLs 76–79 is one of the main elements required for QIO review. If data are absent or incorrect in this section of the claim, the claim will be returned before payment.

FL 77 Operating Physician Name and Identifiers

FL 77 contains the name, the NPI, and the secondary identifier (when required) of the individual with the primary responsibility for performing the surgical procedure on the claim. This field should be left blank if no surgical procedure was performed.

Guidelines

Completion of this field is required for Medicare billing and by other payers when the claim contains a surgical procedure code. The operating physician's ten-digit NPI is reported in line 1 of FL 77. To the right of the NPI, a secondary identifier qualifier code and number are reported if required. The operating physician's last and first name are reported in line 2.

The format for FL 77 is identical to the format for FL 76. When secondary identifiers are required for an operating physician, choose from one of the qualifier codes listed in the instructions for FL 76 above (Attending Provider Name and Identifiers).

When the operating physician is the same as the attending physician identified in FL 76, the same information should be repeated in both form locators.

FLs 78–79 Other Provider Names and Identifiers

FLs 78–79 are used to report the name, the NPI, and the secondary identifier of up to two other provider types involved in the patient's care. In addition, when using FLs 78 and 79, the other type of provider being reported, such as a referring provider, must be indicated using the appropriate provider type qualifier code as outlined below. If no other provider type is involved in the patient's care, this field is left blank.

Guidelines

Completion of this field is required for Medicare billing and by other payers when another provider type, such as a referring provider or assisting operating physician, is involved in the patient's care. A code for the provider type is reported in a small box to the left of the NPI in line 1 of FLs 78 and 79, followed by the ten-digit NPI. To the right of the NPI, a secondary identifier and qualifier code are reported the same way as in FLs 76 and 77. The provider's last and first name are reported in line 2 (see Figure 15.3).

Provider Type Qualifier Codes

In addition to reporting the provider's NPI, name, and secondary identifier in FLs 78–79, a provider type qualifier code must be reported to indicate the type of provider being reported. FLs 78 and 79 contain a two-digit field in line 1 (to the left of the NPI) for this purpose. Provider type qualifier codes for FLs 78 and 79 are as follows:

- *DN—referring provider:* Required on outpatient claims only, when the referring provider is different from the attending provider. A referring provider is a provider who sends the patient to another provider for services. If not required by the payer, the referring provider information should not be reported.

- *ZZ—other operating physician:* Required when another operating physician is involved in the services on the claim. This refers to a physician who performs a secondary surgical procedure or who assists the operating physician reported in FL 77. If not required by the payer, other operating physician information should not be reported.

- *82—rendering provider:* Required when state or federal regulations call for both facility and professional fees to be reported on the same claim, known as a combined bill. Some states require combined bills for Medicaid clinics or critical access hospitals, for example. If not required by the payer, this information should not be reported.

Figure 15.3

UB-04 Form—Close-up of FLs 78–79 with Data

78 OTHER	ZZ	NPI	2002119888		QUAL	0B	MC00104
LAST	TAGORE			FIRST	RAVI		
79 OTHER		NPI			QUAL		
LAST				FIRST			

THE CERTIFICATIONS ON THE REVERSE APPLY TO THIS BILL AND ARE MADE A PART HEREOF.

FL 80 Remarks

The Remarks field (FL 80) is used to make notations about any outstanding details on the claim. Information that has not been reported elsewhere because of the form's limitations and that, in the judgment of the provider, is needed to substantiate the medical treatment on the claim may be entered as a remark.

Guidelines

Completion of this field is required for Medicare billing and all other payers when applicable. The field contains four lines. The first line allows nineteen alphanumeric characters. The second, third, and fourth lines allow twenty-four alphanumeric characters each.

On Medicare claims, the Remarks field should be used to explain the reason for reporting noncovered days if none of the reasons represented by occurrence codes 20, 21, or 22 apply. Notations should also be provided in this field on Medicare claims when:

- An unlisted procedure code is used on an outpatient claim. A brief narrative description of the unlisted procedure, test, drug, or service should be given.

- A trauma code is being reported but is not eligible for Medicare Secondary Payer (MSP) development. The remark should explain why MSP is not involved.

- PPS claims subsequent to the first claim are being prepared. "PPS interim bill" may be noted to alert the payer.

- Another insurance carrier denies the claim. The reason the claim was denied should be provided.

- Certain types of durable medical equipment (DME) are being billed. The rental rate, cost, and anticipated months of usage should be provided so that the fiscal intermediary (FI) may determine whether to approve the rental or purchase of the equipment.

- A replacement claim (TOB 0XX7) is being sent to correct the dates on a claim. The corrected dates may be reported in FL 80.

- A Medicare beneficiary has end-stage renal disease and is covered by an employer group health plan (EGHP). The first month of the thirty-month period during which Medicare benefits are secondary to benefits payable under the EGHP should be noted.

- A local FI or MAC requires other information not contained on the claim.

This field may be used to report an address—for example, the address of the insured when it is not the same as that of the patient, or the address of the insured's employer when a payer requires this information. This field may also be used to report the reason for a voided or cancelled claim (TOB 0XX8).

> **INTERNET RESOURCE**
> *Directory of Toll-Free Numbers for Local Medicare FI or A/B MAC*
> www.cms.hhs.gov/ MLNProducts/downloads/ CallCenterTollNumDirectory.zip

FL 81 Code-Code Field

FL 81 is used to report overflow codes from other form locators. It is also used to report data represented by externally maintained codes sets, such as taxonomy codes, that have been approved by the NUBC for use with the UB-04 form.

Guidelines

Completion of this field is required for Medicare billing and all other payers, when applicable. This form locator contains four lines labeled a through d for reporting up to four codes. Each line contains three columns with the following formatting:

Left Column	Middle Column	Right Column
2 positions	10 positions	12 positions
alphanumeric	alphanumeric	numeric
left-justified	left-justified	right-justified

EXAMPLE: | A2 | 16 | 04162009 |

The left column contains the qualifier code indicating the type of information being reported; for example, qualifier code A2 indicates an overflow occurrence code. The middle column contains the actual code being reported; for example, occurrence code 16 (Date of last therapy). The right column lists a date, a numeric value, or an amount associated with the code; for example, the date April 16, 2009, is reported in MMDDCCYY format as 04162009. Figure 15.4 illustrates this example. FL 81 is called the Code-Code field because it contains a qualifier code followed by another code.

Following are the qualifier codes currently available for use with the Code-Code field:

- 01–A0   Reserved for national assignment
- A1   NUBC condition codes (overflow from FLs 18–28)
- A2   NUBC occurrence codes (overflow from FLs 31–34)
- A3   NUBC occurrence span codes (overflow from FLs 35–36)
- A4   NUBC value codes (overflow from FLs 39–41)
- A5–B0   Reserved for national assignment
- B1   Standards for the classification of federal data on race and ethnicity (code source: ASC X12 external code source 859)
- B2   Reserved for marital status (code source: ASC X12 data element 1067)
- B3   Health care provider taxonomy code (code source: ASC X12 external code source 682, National Uniform Claim Committee)
- B4–ZZ   Reserved for national assignment

Figure 15.4

UB-04 Form—Close-up of FL 81 with Data

81CC a	A2	16		04162009
b				
c				
d				

NUBC™ National Uniform Billing Committee

Codes A1–A4, which are used for reporting overflow codes, are not used for Medicare claims but are available for other types of claims.

Codes B1 and B2 are used solely for public health data reporting. They are used only when required by state or federal law or regulations, and they are intended to promote standardized public health reporting.

For codes that are not associated with a date, a numeric value, or an amount, such as condition codes and taxonomy codes, the right column is left blank.

When reporting a dollar amount associated with a value code in FL 81, there is an implied dollars-cents delimiter separating the last two positions (positions 11 and 12) in the right column of the form locator.

EXAMPLE: $321.25 would be reported as _ _ _ _ _ _ _32125.

When reporting value codes, follow the formatting rules indicated for each value code as it would be reported in FLs 39–41. In most cases, whole number or nondollar amount value codes are right-justified to the left of the implied dollars-cents delimiter.

EXAMPLE: Nondollar amount 5005 would be reported as _ _ _ _ _ _ 5005_ _ .

Taxonomy Codes

Qualifier code B3 is used in FL 81 to report the billing provider's taxonomy code. The taxonomy code on institutional claims describes the type of hospital that is submitting the claim.

Taxonomy information is required on Medicare claims for hospitals containing distinct subparts (for example, psychiatric or rehabilitation units) for which individual NPIs have not been requested. A hospital with subparts that submits claims for both the primary facility and the subparts using a single NPI must report a taxonomy code on all Medicare claims so that the payer can identify which part of the hospital is sending the claim; the taxonomy code assists Medicare with the crosswalk from the NPI of the hospital to each of its subparts. If the hospital has applied for a unique NPI for each subpart, the taxonomy code is not required. However, to avoid confusion during the transition to the NPI system, it is recommended that all hospitals report taxonomy codes.

HIPAA Tip

Taxonomy Codes

In hospital billing, **taxonomy codes** are an administrative code set under HIPAA used to report the billing provider's type of facility. Examples of taxonomy codes for institutional providers include:

Type of Facility	Taxonomy Code
Short-term hospitals (general acute care and specialty)	282N00000X
Critical access hospitals	282NC0060X
Long-term care hospitals	282E00000X
Rehabilitation hospitals	283X00000X
Rehabilitation unit	273Y00000X
Psychiatric hospitals	283Q00000X
Psychiatric unit	273R00000X

In physician billing, taxonomy codes are used to indicate a provider's specialty.

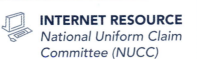

INTERNET RESOURCE
National Uniform Claim Committee (NUCC)

www.nucc.org
The NUCC is the organization that maintains and distributes the Health Care Provider Taxonomy code set. The website contains the latest updates to taxonomy codes.

CHAPTER SUMMARY

1 The UB-04 claim form contains a set of four fields for reporting physician ID information—FLs 76–79. FL 76 identifies the name, the NPI, and the secondary identifier of the licensed physician who normally would be expected to certify the medical necessity of the services rendered and/or who has primary responsibility for the patient's medical treatment. On inpatient claims this refers to the physician who is responsible for the care of the patient from the beginning of the hospital episode. For outpatient claims it refers to the physician who requested the surgery, therapy, diagnostic tests, or other services.

2 If there is a surgical procedure on the claim, FL 77 identifies the name, the NPI, and an optional secondary identifier of the licensed physician who performed the surgical procedure. If the physician identified here is the same as the attending physician, the same information is repeated in both form locators. FLs 78 and 79 are used to report the name, the NPI, and the secondary identifier of other provider types who were involved in the patient's medical care. The format for FLs 78 and 79 is similar to the format for FLs 76 and 77; however, FLs 78 and 79 require a two-digit qualifier code for specifying the type of provider being reported. For example, qualifier code DN indicates that the provider listed in FL 78 or 79 is a referring provider. The provider type qualifier code is reported in the two-digit field that precedes the NPI field in FLs 78 and 79.

3 The UB-04 also contains a text field for remarks. FL 80 (Remarks) is used to provide information that is necessary to adjudicate the claim and that is not shown elsewhere on the claim. This may be, for example, an explanation of noncovered days and charges, a description of an unlisted procedure code, a note indicating that the claim is a PPS interim bill, the reason for a denial by another insurance carrier, an explanation of why a particular trauma code is not eligible for MSP, the dates to be corrected on a replacement claim, or the rental rate and purchase information for certain equipment on Medicare DME claims.

4 FL 81, the Code-Code field, is used to report overflow codes from other form locators and/or information represented by externally maintained code sets approved by the NUBC for use with the UB-04. The qualifier code is used in the first column in FL 81 to indicate the type of code and information being reported, such as a value code or taxonomy code. The actual code itself is listed in the middle column, and the date, numeric value, or amount that may be associated with the code is reported in the right column. Up to four lines, labeled a–d, are available in FL 81 for reporting four different codes.

✔ CHECK YOUR UNDERSTANDING

1. Define the following terms, and specify the form locators they occupy.

   a. secondary identifier (for physician information) _____

   _____

   b. taxonomy code _____

   _____

2. The physician who is responsible for the patient's medical care or plan of treatment is referred to as the _____ physician.

3. True or False: Provider type qualifier code 82 is used on outpatient claims only, for reporting a rendering provider. _____

4. Which of the following form locators should be completed when the claim contains a surgical procedure code?

   a. FL 76

   b. FL 77

   c. FL 78

   d. FL 79

5. FLs 39–41 (Value Codes and Amounts) are already full on a UB-04 claim. Two other value codes and corresponding amounts need to be reported as well: value code 01, amount $480.50, and value code 16, amount $1,000.50. Enter the information in the Code-Code field below.

   UB-04 Form—FL 81

81CC a		
b		
c		
d		

   NUBC™ National Uniform Billing Committee

6. Which item would not be included in FL 80 (Remarks)?

   a. a description of an unlisted procedure

   b. the address of the person who has insurance coverage for a patient

   c. a revenue code and description

   d. information on DME equipment

7. Using the following claim data, fill in FLs 76–81 below.
   - Attending provider: Sammy Tonayoma, NPI 3322211165, BCBS Number BY2220
   - Referring provider: Theresa Green, NPI 0876599911

- Remarks: Insured's employer: Quinnlee's Outlets, 29 Grovenor Drive, Pittsburgh, PA 15215
- Fls 35–36 overflow data: Occurrence span code M2 (Inpatient respite dates), January 13–16, 2009
- Hospital taxonomy code: 282N00000X

UB-04 Form-FLs 76–81

74 PRINCIPAL PROCEDURE CODE DATE	a. OTHER PROCEDURE CODE DATE	b. OTHER PROCEDURE CODE DATE	75	76 ATTENDING	NPI		QUAL	
				LAST			FIRST	
c. OTHER PROCEDURE CODE DATE	d. OTHER PROCEDURE CODE DATE	e. OTHER PROCEDURE CODE DATE		77 OPERATING	NPI		QUAL	
				LAST			FIRST	
80 REMARKS		81CC a		78 OTHER	NPI		QUAL	
		b		LAST			FIRST	
		c		79 OTHER	NPI		QUAL	
		d		LAST			FIRST	
UB-04 CMS-1450	APPROVED OMB NO. 0938-0997	NUBC™ National Uniform Billing Committee		THE CERTIFICATIONS ON THE REVERSE APPLY TO THIS BILL AND ARE MADE A PART HEREOF.				

COMPUTER EXPLORATION

UB-04 Activity: Claim Analysis

Viewing FLs 76-81: Physician Information, Remarks, and Code-Code Field

Open the file **Sample01.pdf** in Adobe Reader, and answer the following questions:

1. Sample01.pdf is an outpatient claim for Owen Murdock. What is the name of Owen Murdock's attending physician?

2. What is the attending physician's NPI?

3. Qualifier code 1G is reported in FL 76. What does 1G indicate?

4. An operating physician must be reported in FL 77 whenever a surgical procedure is reported on the claim. Who is the operating physician on Owen's claim?

5. On an inpatient claim, the principal procedure code reported in FL 74 represents the surgical procedure. On an outpatient claim, a surgery-related revenue code and corresponding HCPCS/CPT surgery code represent the surgical procedure. What revenue code and HCPCS/CPT code represent the surgical procedure on this claim?

6. Are there any other physician types reported on the claim? In what form locator would a referring provider be reported?

7. The Remarks field in FL 80 is used to report important information that is not contained elsewhere on the claim. Give an example of the type of information that might be reported in the Remarks field in this claim.

8. Based on the qualifier code reported in the Code-Code field on this claim, what information is being reported?

9. What type of facility does the number 28N00000X represent?

10. Another function of the Code-Code field is to report overflow codes from other form locators. What qualifier code would be used in the Code-Code field to report an overflow in FLs 35-36?

When finished viewing the claim, click Exit on the File menu.

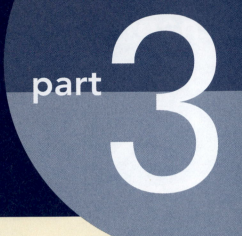

part 3

Simulation

chapter 16

Using the Simulated UB-04 Form

Chapter 16 introduces you to the interactive simulated UB-04 form that was created for use with this text. The simulated UB-04 form is a pdf file that can be used with Adobe Reader to view, create, edit, and print UB-04 claims. You will work with the simulated form in the Computer Exploration exercises at the end of each chapter in Part 2, as well as in Chapter 17 when creating claims for the case studies.

The first part of this chapter, "Introduction to the Simulated Form," shows you the basics of using the form. After downloading the blank form and three sample claims from the text's Online Learning Center, you learn how to open one of the sample claims in Adobe Reader, navigate through the form, and print it. This section should be reviewed before completing the Computer Exploration exercises in Part 2.

The second part of the chapter, "Completing a UB-04 Claim," takes you through the steps of completing a hospital claim using the simulated form. By going through the claim completion steps once, you will be prepared to complete the claims required for the case studies in Chapter 17 on your own.

Introduction to the Simulated Form

To use the simulated form with this text, you will need a computer with the following system requirements:

- Microsoft Windows 2000 or XP operating system
- 128 MB of RAM minimum, 256 MB or greater recommended
- Up to 100 MB of available hard-disk space
- Microsoft Internet Explorer 5.5 or higher
- Adobe Reader version 7 or 8 (version 8 is recommended)
- Printer
- Active Internet connection to access the Online Learning Center

Tip

Adobe Reader

If you do not have the Adobe Reader program on your computer, you can download a free copy from the Adobe website at: www.adobe.com/products/acrobat/readstep2.html

Downloading the UB-04 Form and Sample Claims from the Online Learning Center

A copy of the simulated form (UB04.pdf) and three sample claims created with the form (Sample-01.pdf, Sample-02.pdf, and Sample-03.pdf) are stored on the text's Online Learning Center (OLC). To download these files:

1. Create a folder on your computer under My Documents for storing the files you will be working with in this text (for example, C:\ . . . \ My Documents\Hospital Billing).
2. Go to the text's OLC at www.mhhe.com/MagovernHospitalBilling2.
3. Access the Student Center.
4. Under the Student Resources section, click on the link "Simulated UB-04 Form (UB04.pdf) and Sample Claims."
5. Follow the instructions for copying the UB04.pdf file and the three sample claims to the folder you created in step one above.
6. Exit the OLC.

Opening a Sample Claim in Adobe Reader

1. From the Windows desktop, click the Start button and then click All Programs to display the directory of programs on your computer.
2. Locate Adobe Reader in the list of programs, and then click on it to open it.
3. Open the File menu at the top of the screen, and then click on the Open option.
4. In the Open dialog box that appears, locate the folder where you stored the simulated form and three sample claims.
5. Double click on the folder to open it. Notice the files contained in it (Sample-01, Sample-02, Sample-03, and UB04).
6. Double click the file **Sample-01** to open it.
7. The sample claim appears on the screen.

Navigating through the Form

1. Use the scroll bar or the up and down arrows in the right margin of the screen to scroll through the file. Notice that the first page contains

Auto-Complete Feature Off

When you use the simulated form, if a message appears asking you if you would like to turn the Auto-Complete feature on, click No. The Auto-Complete feature is not required for the purposes of this text.

the front of the UB-04 form, and the second page contains the back of the form. Return to the first page.

2. Open the Zoom option on the View menu to display the available zoom options. If it is not already selected, select the Fit Width option to show the full width of the form on the screen. Because the type on the form is small, the Fit Width option is the recommended viewing option.

3. Without clicking inside the field, let the cursor hover over the data in FL 12 (Admission Date) until the following rollover text appears.

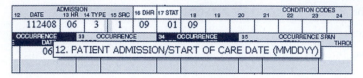

4. Rollover text describing the contents of the field is supplied for each field on the form.

5. Click inside FL 3a to orient the cursor. The following Cannot Save Form Information message may appear, informing you that you need to print out the completed form to save a record of your work. Click the Don't Show Again option and then the Close button to continue.

Cannot Save Form Information

Cannot Save Form Information

Please Note: You cannot save a completed copy of this form on your computer. If you would like a copy for your records, please fill it in and print it

☐ Don't show again

Close

6. After clicking inside FL 3a, press TAB five times. The TAB key moves the cursor forward through each field on the claim in numeric order. Press SHIFT TAB to move the cursor backwards through the same fields. You can also move the cursor to any field on the form simply by clicking inside the field.

FYI

Adobe Reader Versus Adobe Acrobat

In Adobe Reader, form data can be viewed, entered, edited, and printed, but it cannot be saved to a pdf file. To save form data to a pdf file, the form must be opened in Adobe Acrobat, version 8—a full-scale software program that is purchased separately. Although the claim exercises in this text can be completed with either program, because of the high cost of the Adobe Acrobat software, the exercises are designed to be completed using Adobe Reader.

Printing a Claim

It is important to know how to print a claim in Adobe Reader. Because you cannot save any data you have entered in the form when you exit the program, you must print the claim to have a record of your work. Follow the steps below to practice printing Sample-01.pdf.

1. To print Sample-01.pdf, click the Print option on the File menu.

2. The Print dialog box appears, as shown on page 331.

3. In the Printer section, verify the correct printer is selected in the Name box.

4. In the Print Range section, if you do not want a copy of page 2 (the back of the claim form), change the print range to print page 1 only, or click the Current Page option. To print both pages, leave the print range setting as it is.

5. In the Page Handling section, set the Page Scaling option either to Shrink to Printable Area or Fit to Printable Area. (Depending on your printer, the line numbers in the far right and left margins of the claim may be cut off if the None option is selected.)

6. Click the OK button at the bottom of the dialog box to print the claim.

Using the Save as Text Option

As an alternative to saving the data in a form, Adobe Reader provides a Save as Text option that enables you to save the data that is on-screen into a separate text file. You lose the layout of the form, but the data itself is saved. The text file, a Windows Notepad file, lists the names of the 81 form locators together with the data currently displayed in them. Follow the steps below to practice using the Save as Text option with Sample-01.pdf:

1. Open the File menu and select Save as Text. The Save As dialog box appears, as shown on page 332.

2. In the File Name field at the bottom of the dialog box, notice that the original name of the pdf file (Sample-01) is displayed. The Save as Type field should display the new default extension (.txt), to indicate the file is being saved as a text file.

3. Click the Save button to save the text file under the suggested name and extension.

4. The Save As dialog box closes. To view the text file, you must open it while in Windows Explorer. First exit Adobe Reader by clicking the Exit option on the file menu.

5. Open Windows Explorer, and locate the folder where you are storing your work for this text. The text version of the file (Sample-01.txt) should now be displayed in the same folder. Double click on the file name to open it.

6. The file opens in Windows Notepad, as shown here.

```
(1. BILLING PROVIDER NAME) LONGWOOD HOSPITAL
(1. BILLING PROVIDER STREET ADDRESS) 3290 ALBANY AVE
(1. BILLING PROVIDER CITY, STATE, ZIP) KINGSTON, NY 12401
(1. BILLING PROVIDER COUNTRY CODE, PHONE NUMBER) 845-340-2200
(2. PAY-TO NAME)
(2. PAY-TO STREET ADDRESS)
(2. PAY-TO CITY, STATE, ZIP)
(2. PAY-TO COUNTRY CODE, PHONE NUMBER)
(3a. PATIENT CONTROL NUMBER) 90038761
(3b. MEDICAL/HEALTH RECORD NUMBER) S119066
(4. TYPE OF BILL) 0131
(5. FEDERAL TAX NUMBER) 35-9287761
(6. STATEMENT COVERS PERIOD FROM DATE) 112408
(6. STATEMENT COVERS PERIOD TO DATE) 112408
(7. RESERVED)
(8a. PATIENT IDENTIFIER)
(8b. PATIENT NAME) MURDOCK, OWEN
(9a. PATIENT STREET ADDRESS) 23 WALL ST
(9b. PATIENT CITY) KINGSTON
(9c. PATIENT STATE) NY
(9d. PATIENT ZIP CODE) 12401
(9e. PATIENT COUNTRY CODE)
(10. PATIENT BIRTH DATE (MMDDYYYY)) 02181940
(11. PATIENT SEX) M
(12. PATIENT ADMISSION/START OF CARE DATE (MMDDYY)) 112408
(13. PATIENT ADMISSION HOUR) 06
```

7. Notice that each field name and number is listed in parentheses. Any data that was in the fields at the time the file was saved as text is listed after the parentheses. When finished viewing the text file, click the X in the upper right corner of the window to close the Notepad screen.

This completes the introduction to the simulated UB-04 form. You now have the instructions and files that you need to complete the Computer Exploration exercises at the end of each chapter in Part 2. The second half of this chapter provides step-by-step instructions for using the simulated form to create a claim. The step-by-step instructions should be followed after completing Part 2, and before starting Chapter 17, "Case Studies."

Completing a UB-04 Claim

This section contains a step-by-step guide for using the simulated UB-04 form to complete a claim. The claim is for patient Gail Astore. Her case study information, which includes patient information, insurance information, and patient services data, precedes the completion guide. The billing information for the hospital where the services were performed is also provided. This section is designed to give you practice in creating a hospital claim so that you can complete the claims in Chapter 17, "Case Studies," on your own.

About the Hospital:

Name: Hanover Regional Hospital

Address: 2600 Record Street

City/State/ZIP: Hanover, CT 06783

Telephone: 860-376-2000

Federal Tax ID: 07-1282340

NPI: 1288561733

Medicare Provider ID: 070089

Taxonomy Code: 282N00000X

ASTORE'S CASE

PATIENT INFORMATION

Patient Name: Gail Astore

Patient Address: 8 River Road

City/State/Zip: Hartford, CT 06516

Telephone Number: 203-555-2211

Social Security Number: 102-12-3712

Patient Control Number: 53820705

Medical Record Number: 3496815

Date of Birth: 08-05-1936

Occupation: Husband retired 6-1-03

Sex: F

Marital Status: M

Employer: ---------

INSURANCE INFORMATION

Primary Insurance

Insured's Name: Gail Astore

Patient's Relationship to Insured: self

Insured's ID Number: 102123712B

Health Plan: Medicare

Health Plan ID/Carrier Code: 00308

Group Name/No.: ---------

Secondary Provider No.: 070089

Release of Information on File Y/N: Y

Accepts Assignment Y/N: Y

Preauthorization Number: 01916931

Copayment: --------- **HMO Y/N:** N

PATIENT SERVICES

Date of Service: Admitted 3-4-10, 12:15 P.M. / Discharged 3-9-10, 4:45 P.M.

Date Claim Created: 3-12-10

Notes: QIO medical review to be completed after claim is paid. Patient discharged to home under care of Wellday Home Health Care.

PATIENT SERVICES (cont.)

Services	Units	Charges
Emergency room	2	481.50
IV therapy		101.90
EKG		47.32
Bacteriology & Micro. Tests		44.18
Chemistry Tests		1858.01
Supplies-Sterile		42.39
Pharmacy		102.85
CT Scan/Head	1	485.66
Radiology-Diagnostic (X ray)	1	809.25
Hematology Tests		184.82
Semiprivate Room–2 Bed/Surgical	5	@ 1080.00
Physical therapy evaluation		154.21
Physical therapy		177.74

Principal Dx: Hyposmolality (276.1), **POA:** yes

Secondary Dx: Drug withdrawal syndrome (292.0) **POA:** yes

Esoinophilic fascitis (728.89) **POA:** yes

Essential hypertension (401.9) **POA:** yes

Anxiety disorder (300.00) **POA:** yes

Depressive disorder (311) **POA:** yes

Accidental fall (E888.8) **POA:** yes. *Note:* Patient fell at home on 3-3-10 at about 11 P.M.

Admitting Dx/Reason for Visit: Asthenia (780.79)

Procedures: --------- **Date of Surgery:** ---------

Attending Provider ID: John Wood, NPI 1233281192

Secondary Provider ID: B18642 (UPIN)

Completion Guide

1. If you have not already done so, read the first part of this chapter, "Introduction to the Simulated Form," including the instructions on downloading the form from the Online Learning Center, so that you have a copy of the form on your computer. The file name of the form is UB04.pdf.

2. Open Adobe Reader, and then open UB04.pdf. A blank UB-04 form is displayed on the screen, as illustrated on page 335.

3. Notice that the first two form locators, FL 1 and FL 2, are unlabeled. Let the cursor hover over each field to display the rollover text. FL 1 contains the billing provider's name, address, and phone number, and FL 2 contains

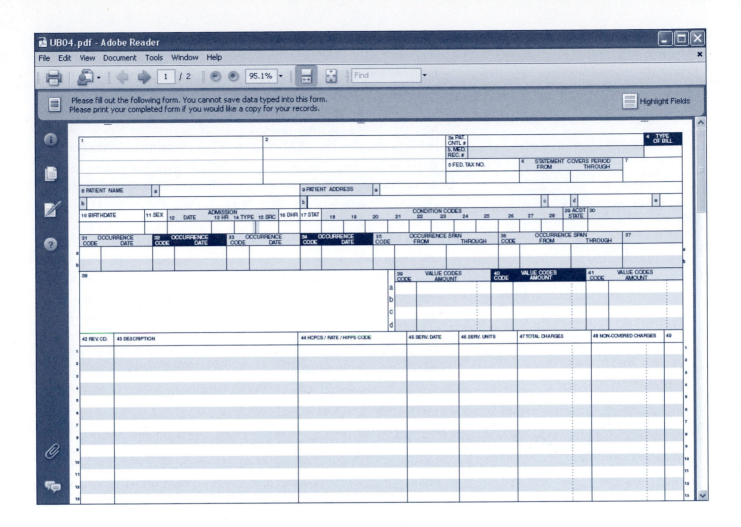

the pay-to address for the billing provider. (FL 2 should be filled in only if the billing provider has a separate mailing address for payments.)

4. Click inside the first line in FL 1. (If a Cannot Save Form Information message appears, reminding you that you must print the completed form to save a copy of your work, click the Don't Show Again option and then the Close button to continue.)

5. In the first line of FL 1, enter the hospital's name as provided above (on page 333). Common practice is to use all capital letters when filling in the form (for example, HANOVER REGIONAL HOSPITAL). The use of all capital letters is a standard practice on the UB-04. The larger letters are also easier to read, given the size of the form.

6. Press TAB to move to line 2, and enter the hospital's street address. Continue to fill in the rest of the address and phone number in lines 3 and 4.

7. Press TAB to move to FL 2. The billing provider does not have a separate billing address, so no information is required in FL 2. Press TAB to move through each line in FL 2 until you reach FL 3a (Patient Control Number), or simply click inside FL 3a to move to that field.

8. Refer to Gail Astore's patient information data to locate her Patient Control Number. Key the number (*53820705*) in FL 3a. Press TAB.

9. FL 3b (Medical Record Number) is used to report the number assigned by the provider to the patient's medical or health record. Locate this number in Astore's patient information data, and key it (*3496815*) in FL 3b. Press TAB.

> **Tip**
>
> *Appendix A: UB-04 Codes*
>
> Appendix A provides lists of the following UB-04 codes for quick reference:
>
> - Type of Bill Codes
> - Occurrence Codes
> - Value Codes
> - Revenue Codes: Numerical Order
> - Revenue Codes: Alphabetical Order

10. The cursor moves to FL 4 (Type of Bill). Refer to Astore's patient services data to determine the TOB code for this case study. Key *0111* in FL 4, for "Hospital," "Inpatient," "Admit through discharge claim," and then press TAB.

11. FL 5 (Federal Tax Number) requires the hospital's TIN. Refer to the hospital's billing information above to locate this number. Key *07-1282340* in FL 5, and then press TAB to go to FL 6 (Statement Covers Period).

12. Refer to Astore's date-of-service information in her patient services data to determine the from and through dates (Admitted 3-4-10; Discharged 3-9-10). Key the dates in FL 6 using the MMDDYY format (*030410* and *030910*). Press TAB.

13. Leave FL 7 (Unlabeled Field, reserved for national assignment) blank, and press TAB.

14. Notice that FL 8 (Patient Name) contains two lines. FL 8b, the bottom line, is used to report the patient's name. This field must be completed on all claims. FL 8a, the top line, is only used under certain circumstances when the patient and the insured are not the same person. In Gail Astore's claim, since the insured and the patient are the same person, no data is reported in FL 8a. Press TAB to move to FL 8b.

15. Key the patient's full name in FL 8b, last name first (*ASTORE, GAIL*). Press TAB.

16. Refer to Astore's patient information data. Using this data, key her address, birth date, and gender code in FLs 9 through 11, respectively. Use the rollover text in FL 9 to determine the various parts of the address that are reported in fields 9a, b, c, and d. In FL 10 (Patient Birth Date), remember to use the MMDDCCYY format (*08051936* for 08-05-1936).

17. In FL 12 (Admission, Start of Care Date), key the admission date for this visit as recorded in Astore's patient information data (*030410* for 3-4-10). Press TAB.

18. Refer to Astore's patient services data to determine her admission time (12:15 P.M.). Although completion of this field is not required for Medicare, as it is for most other payers, the admission time is usually reported for information purposes. Look up the appropriate hour code in Table 8-1 on page 162 to report the time in FL 13 (Admission Hour). Key the two-digit code (*12*) and press TAB.

19. The cursor moves to FL 14 (Type of Admission or Visit). Refer to Astore's patient services information and the Type of Admission Codes listed in Chapter 8 (codes 1–9) to determine the correct code. In this instance, 1 (Emergency) fits the patient services information. Key *1* in FL 14 and press TAB.

20. In FL 15 (Point of Origin for Admission or Visit), possible point of origin codes include 1–9, A–F, and, for newborns, 5–6. Refer to the codes listed in Chapter 8 to decide which of these codes fits Astore's patient services data. In this case, 7 (Emergency room) is the appropriate code. Key *7* in FL 15 and press TAB.

21. For FL 16 (Discharge Hour), locate the time of Astore's discharge in the patient services information. Look up the appropriate hour code in Table 8-1 on page 162 (hour code 16 for 4:45 P.M.). Key *16* in FL 16 and press TAB.

22. Look back at the information in Chapter 8 to learn whether FL 17 (Patient Discharge Status) is required for Medicare inpatient billing. As

a patient discharge status code *is* required, read through the list of status codes (01–99) in Chapter 8 to locate the appropriate code based on Astore's case study data. *Hint:* Her patient services data notes, "Patient discharged to home under care of Wellday Home Health Care." Therefore, patient status code 06 (Discharged and transferred to home under care of organized home health service organization in anticipation of covered skilled care) is required. Key *06* in FL 17 and press TAB.

23. The cursor moves to FL 18. The next three sections of the claim are used to report three types of codes: condition codes (FLs 18–28), occurrence codes and dates (FLs 31–36), and value codes (FLs 39–41). Study Astore's case to identify any special conditions, particular occurrences and dates, or value amounts a payer may need to know that affect the processing and payment of the claim.

24. In Astore's insurance information data, notice there is a preauthorization number, and that one of the notes under the patient services data states, "QIO medical review to be completed after claim is paid." Look through the categories of codes in Chapter 9, "Condition Codes." Under "Other Special Codes," locate the category. "QIO Approval Indicator Services." Within this category, condition code C5 (Postpayment review applicable) is required. Key *C5* in the first condition code box, FL 18.

25. Since this is the only condition code required on the claim, press TAB until you reach FL 29 (Accident State). FL 29 is only used when there is an accident involved in the claim and the accident is an automobile accident. Although this claim involves an accident, it does not involve an automobile accident. Therefore press TAB to continue.

26. FL 30 (Unlabeled Field, reserved for national assignment) should also be left blank. Press TAB to move the cursor to FL 31 (Occurrence Code and Date).

27. Research the different categories of occurrence codes in Chapter 10, "Occurrence Codes and Dates," or in Appendix A, while referring to Astore's case study information to locate any required occurrence codes. Two codes and their corresponding dates are required. Under the Diagnoses section of Astore's patient services data, there is a secondary diagnosis code for an "Accidental fall," on 3-3-10. Under the accident-related occurrence codes, 05 (Accident/No Medical or Liability Coverage) needs to be reported. Key *05* and the date of the accident (*030310*) in FL 31 (line a). Press TAB.

28. The cursor moves to FL 32. In the patient information data, under occupation, it is noted "Husband retired 6-1-03." From the insurance-related occurrence codes, 19 (Date of retirement of spouse) needs to be reported. Key *19* and the date of her husband's retirement (*060103*) in FL 32 (line a). Since there are no more occurrence codes or occurrence span codes that need to be reported, move the cursor to the next field, FL 37.

29. FL 37 (Unlabeled Field, reserved for national assignment) can be left blank. FL 38 (Responsible Party Name and Address) is also not required for this claim. Move the cursor to FL 39 (Value Codes and Amounts).

30. Refer to the list of value codes in Chapter 11, "Value Codes and Amounts," or in Appendix A to locate any value codes relevant to Astore's case study. Notice value code 45 (Accident hour) applies. Key *45* in FL 39, line a. In the corresponding Amount box, key the hour code for the accident hour followed by a space for the decimal position and two zeros (*23 00* for 11:00 P.M.), and then press TAB.

Tip

When to Use FL 38

FL 38 (Responsible Party Name and Address) is not a required field. On some paper claims, when a window envelope is used for mailing the bill, the name and mailing address of the responsible party are reported here to show through the window. For Medicare claims, the five blank lines may be used to report the name and address of the other payer when a claim involves a payer that is primary to Medicare.

31. The cursor moves to FL 40. A second value code must be reported—code 80 (Covered days). This value code is listed among the codes for covered and noncovered days in Chapter 11 and is required on all inpatient paper claims to report the number of days within the claim's billing period that are covered by the primary payer (on electronic claims, this information is reported in a different field). Review Astore's patient services data to determine how many days she was in the hospital (five days). Because the data does not report any noncovered days, assume all of these days are covered days. Key *80* in FL 40, line a. In the corresponding Amount box, key the number of covered days followed by a space (for the decimal position) and two zeros (*5 00* for 5 days), and then press TAB. This completes the condition, occurrence, and value code sections of the claim.

32. The next section of the claim, FLs 42–49, is used to report transaction data. Click inside FL 42 (Revenue Code), line 1. Refer to Astore's patient services data for the list of services Astore received during her hospitalization. Notice that the units and charges are also recorded for each service. Revenue codes must be listed in ascending numeric order on the UB-04. Therefore, you need to assign a revenue code beside each item listed in the patient services data *before* entering the codes into FL 42 so that you can put the codes into the correct numeric order while keying them into the form.

    Refer to Chapter 12, "Revenue Codes, Descriptions, and Charges," or to the two lists of revenue codes in Appendix A (Revenue Codes: Alphabetical Order and Revenue Codes: Numerical Order), to look up the corresponding revenue code and standard abbreviated description for each service received. Enter the appropriate revenue codes and descriptions in FLs 42 and 43, respectively. Check your work against Figure 16-1 on page 342, which illustrates the revenue codes in the required order (FL 42) along with their standard abbreviated descriptions (FL 43).

33. In FL 44 (HCPCS/Rate/HIPPS Code), line 1, key the daily rate that corresponds to the accommodation revenue code in FL 42, as recorded in the patient services data (*1080 00*). This is the only rate code required.

34. Leave the column labeled FL 45 (Service Dates) blank, as service dates are not required on inpatient Medicare claims. (Note that service dates *are* required on outpatient claims.)

35. To complete FL 46 (Service Units), refer to the Units column in Astore's patient services data. Report units for any units listed in the patient services data. (There are four services that require a units entry.)

36. Locate the total charge for each revenue code in the patient services data, and key the amount for each line in the column labeled FL 47 (Total Charges). There are thirteen charges in all. (For the accommodation charge in line 1, you will need to multiply the units by the daily rate to obtain the total charge.)

37. Enter the data for the totals line (line 23) in the transaction section to summarize the thirteen transactions just listed: Move the cursor to FL 42, line 23, and enter revenue code *0001* to indicate total charges. In FL 43, indicate that this is page 1 of 1. Look up the creation date for the claim, and key the date in FL 45 (*031210*). In FL 47, add the total charges column, and key the result (*9889 83*). As there are no noncovered charges listed in the patient services data, leave the column labeled FL 48 (Non-Covered Charges) blank. This completes the transaction section.

38. Move the cursor to FL 50 (Payer Name), line A. FL 50 is the first field in the Payer, Insured, and Employer Information section of the claim,

which includes FLs 50-65. Because Gail Astore does not have a secondary insurance plan, only line A will need to be completed for FLs 50–65.

39. Refer to Astore's insurance information data to locate the name and carrier code for her primary insurance. Key this information in FLs 50 and 51 (*MEDICARE, 00308*).

40. In FL 52 (Release of Information Certification Indicator) and FL 53 (Assignment of Benefits Certification Indicator), key *Y* for Yes, as indicated in Astore's insurance information data, under the headings "Release of Information on File Y/N" and "Accepts Assignment Y/N."

41. Leave FL 54 (Prior Payments—Payer) and FL 55 (Estimated Amount Due—Payer) blank as these are not required fields for this claim.

42. In FL 56 (National Provider Identifier—Billing Provider), key the hospital's ten-digit NPI as listed in the hospital's billing information (*1288561733*). This is the primary identifier for the hospital. FL 57 (Other Provider ID) provides a field for reporting a secondary legacy identifier when required. Once the transition to the NPI system is complete, a secondary identifier will not be required. As a secondary identifier on this claim, key the legacy Medicare provider ID in FL 57 (*070089*). Move the cursor to FL 58 (Insured's Name).

43. Key the name of the patient in whose name the insurance is issued, in this case, Gail Astore. Remember to key the last name first (*ASTORE, GAIL*). Press TAB to move to FL 59 (Patient's Relationship to Insured).

44. Refer to Astore's insurance information data to determine the patient's relationship to the insured. In this instance, "Self" is indicated. Look up the appropriate two-digit code in Chapter 13, "Payer, Insured, and Employer Information," under FL 59 (Patient's Relationship to Insured). Code 18 is used to indicate self. Key *18* in FL 59 and press TAB.

45. The cursor moves to FL 60 (Insured's Unique Identifier). Locate Astore's Insurance ID Number in her insurance information data, and key the number in FL 60 (*102123712B*).

46. Leave FL 61 (Insured's Group Name) and FL 62 (Insured's Group Number) blank. Because Medicare payers do not use group names or numbers, Astore's insurance information does not list this information.

47. Move the cursor to FL 63 (Treatment Authorization Codes). Refer to Astore's insurance information data, which lists a preauthorization number. Key this number (*01916931*) in FL 63 and press TAB.

48. FL 64 (Document Control Number) is reported on the UB-04 only when filing a replacement or cancellation to a previously processed claim (TOB 0XX7 or 0XX8). Since this is an original claim and not a replacement or a cancellation, press TAB to continue.

49. FL 65 (Employer Name of the Insured) is used to report the insured's employer if applicable. In the case of Gail Astore, since she is not employed, this field is left blank. In general, Medicare requires employer information only when Medicare is secondary to another payer on the claim.

50. The next section of the claim form (FLs 66–75) is used to report the patient's diagnosis and procedure codes. The first field in this section, FL 66 (Diagnosis and Procedure Code Qualifier), is used to report the ICD version that was used for assigning the diagnosis and procedures codes on the claim. Since ICD-9-CM is currently the only version allowable under HIPAA, the qualifier code for ICD-9-CM, code 9, is reported in this field. Key *9* and press TAB to move to FL 67 (Principal Diagnosis Code and POA Indicator).

Tip

When to Use FL 54

FL 54 (Prior Payments—Payer) is used to report any amount the hospital may have received to date from the health plan toward payment of the bill. Completion of this form locator is required for Medicare outpatient claims only when a prior payment has been received. In addition, for an MSP claim, any prior payment amount received from another insurer is reported on the appropriate line in FL 54.

51. The next set of form locators, FLs 67–72, is used to report the patient's diagnosis codes. Refer to the primary and secondary diagnoses listed in Gail Astore's case study information. Diagnosis code 276.1 (the ICD-9-CM code for hyposmolality) is listed as the primary diagnosis code. Therefore, key *2761* in FL 67 (Principal Diagnosis Code and POA Indicator) and press TAB. No periods are required while reporting diagnosis and procedure codes on the UB-04, as these are implied.

52. The cursor moves to the small shaded box to the right of the diagnosis code. The shaded area is used to report the POA (present on admission) indicator. Refer to Gail Astore's diagnosis code data to determine whether the condition of hyposmolality was present on admission. "POA: yes" indicates the condition was present on admission. Therefore, key *Y*, the POA indicator for "Yes," in the shaded area, and press TAB to move to FL 67A.

53. FLs 67 A–Q (Other Diagnosis Codes and POA Indicators) are used to report the any secondary diagnosis codes. Key the required secondary diagnosis code and POA indicator for each secondary diagnosis listed in Astore's case study data. Because certain codes have greater priority than others, key the codes in the order they have been listed, which reflects the order established in the patient's medical record.

54. Leave FL 68 (Unlabeled Field, reserved for national assignment) blank.

55. FL 69 (Admitting Diagnosis) is used on inpatient claims to report the patient's diagnosis at the time of admission. Key the code for Astore's admitting diagnosis, as indicated in her patient data (*78079*). Notice, in Astore's case, this code is different from the principal diagnosis code reported in FL 67. The principal diagnosis code represents the condition established *after study* to be chiefly responsible for causing the hospital admission. Press TAB to move to FL 70.

56. FL 70 (Patient's Reason for Visit) is used to report up to three diagnosis codes indicating the reason for an unscheduled outpatient visit. Since this is an inpatient claim, this field should be kept blank.

57. Completion of FL 71 (PPS Code) and FL 72 (External Cause of Injury) are not required for Medicare billing and are therefore left blank. FL 73 (Unlabeled Field) should also be left blank. This completes the diagnosis code section of the claim.

58. Move the cursor to FL 74 (Principal Procedure Code and Date). FL 74 and FLs 74 a–e (Other Procedure Codes and Dates) represent the procedure code section of the claim. These fields are used to report any surgical or medical procedures, with corresponding dates, that were performed during the billing period. Data is reported in these fields on Medicare inpatient claims only. (Surgical procedures for Medicare outpatient claims are reported with the appropriate surgical-related HCPCS codes in FL 44.) In the case of Gail Astore, no surgical procedures were performed during the hospital stay. Therefore, FLs 74 and 74 a–e are left blank.

59. FL 75 (Unlabeled Field) is also left blank.

60. The next section of the claim (FLs 76–79), contains physician information. Move the cursor to FL 76 (Attending Provider Name and Identifiers). Refer to Astore's patient services data to locate the name and IDs of her attending physician. Key the last name, first name, and NPI in the required fields (*WOOD, JOHN, 1233281192*). The two small boxes to the right of the QUAL box in FL 76 are available to report a secondary identifier for the attending provider when required. When the transition to the NPI

Tip

When to Use FL 71

FL 71 (Prospective Payment System Code) is used to identify the DRG associated with the claim. Completion of this field is not required for Medicare billing. Other payers may request a PPS code as part of their DRG contract with the hospital.

system is complete, secondary identifiers will not be required. For now, a Medicare provider's UPIN number is reported as a secondary identifier. Key the appropriate qualifier code for a UPIN number in the first box (*1G*), followed by the UPIN number itself in the second box (*B18642*).

61. Move the cursor to FL 77 (Operating Provider Name and Identifiers). FL 77 is used to report the last name, first name, NPI, and secondary identifier (if required) for an operating physician. Completion of this field is required on inpatient and outpatient claims when the claim contains a surgical procedure. If the operating physician is the same as the attending provider in FL 76, the same information is repeated in FL 77. Since Gail Astore's claim does not contain a surgical procedure, this field is left blank.

62. FLs 78 and 79 (Other Provider Names and Identifiers) are used to report the names and identifiers for up to two other providers who are involved in the patient's care in connection with the claim. Similar to FLs 76 and 77, an NPI is reported as the primary identifier, and a legacy provider number such as a UPIN number may be used as a secondary identifier. In addition, FLs 78 and 79 require a qualifier code (reported to the left of the NPI field) to indicate the type of provider being reported. For example, qualifier code ZZ is used to report a second operating physician. With regard to Gail Astore's claim, since no other providers were involved in her care, FLs 78 and 79 are left blank.

63. Move the cursor to FL 80 (Remarks). FL 80 is used to report information that is not given anywhere else on the claim but may be required by a third-party payer to process the claim. Often notations are made to explain any noncovered charges, for example. In Astore's claim, it may be helpful to emphasize that her accident occurred at home and that no liability is involved, to eliminate the possibility that another payer was liable. Therefore, in FL 80, make the following notation: *ACCIDENTAL FALL IN HOME, NO LIABILITY.*

64. Move the cursor to the last form locator on the claim, FL 81 (Code-Code Field). FL 81 is used to report overflow codes from other form locators. Although overflow codes are not used on Medicare claims, they are available for other types of claims. FL 81 is also used to report data represented by externally maintained codes sets, such as taxonomy codes. Until the transition to the NPI system is complete, taxonomy codes should be reported on all hospital claims. After that, taxonomy codes will only be reported in certain situations for hospitals having distinct part units. The qualifier code for reporting a taxonomy code, B3, is reported first in FL 81, followed by the taxonomy code itself. Refer to the hospital's billing information to locate the taxonomy code. Report the qualifier code (*B3*) followed by the taxonomy code (*28N00000X*) in the first line of FL 81.

65. This completes the data required for processing the claim. To identify your work, key your initials the last line of FL 80 (Remarks). (Press TAB to move through each line of FL 80.)

66. Now that the claim is complete, you must print it to save a copy of your work. Use the Print option on the File menu to print the first page of the claim. The printout should look like the claim in Figure 16-1 on page 342. If required, make any corrections and print the claim again.

67. Before exiting Adobe Reader, use the Save as Text option on the File menu to save your data entry to a separate text file. Name the text file "Astore Claim." Remember that when you exit Adobe Reader, the data that you have entered in the UB-04 form will be lost automatically.

68. Click the Exit option on the File menu to exit Adobe Reader.

FYI

Secondary Identifier Qualifier Codes for FLs 76–79

Possible qualifier codes for a secondary identifier in FLs 76–79 include:

- 0B: State license number
- 1G: Provider UPIN
- G2: Provider commercial number

Tip

Use FL 80 to Initial Your Work
In the ten case studies that follow in Chapter 17, to identify your work once you have finished a claim, key the Case Study number followed by your initials in FL 80 (Remarks).

Figure 16.1

Sample Completed UB-04 Form

1 HANOVER REGIONAL HOSPITAL 2600 RECORD STREET HANOVER, CT 06783 860-376-2000	2

3a PAT. CNTL # 53820705
b. MED. REC. # 3496815
4 TYPE OF BILL 0111
5 FED. TAX NO. 07-1282340
6 STATEMENT COVERS PERIOD FROM 030410 THROUGH 030910 7

8 PATIENT NAME a	9 PATIENT ADDRESS a 8 RIVER ROAD			
b ASTORE, GAIL	b HARTFORD	c CT	d 06516	e

10 BIRTHDATE	11 SEX	12 DATE	ADMISSION 13 HR.	14 TYPE	15 SRC	16 DHR	17 STAT	CONDITION CODES 18 19 20 21 22 23 24 25 26 27 28	29 ACDT STATE	30
08051936	F	030410	12	1	7	16	06	C5		

31 OCCURRENCE CODE / DATE	32 OCCURRENCE CODE / DATE	33 OCCURRENCE CODE / DATE	34 OCCURRENCE CODE / DATE	35 CODE OCCURRENCE SPAN FROM THROUGH	36 CODE OCCURRENCE SPAN FROM THROUGH	37
a 05 030310	19 060103					
b						

38

	39 CODE VALUE CODES AMOUNT	40 CODE VALUE CODES AMOUNT	41 CODE VALUE CODES AMOUNT
a	45 23 00	80 5 00	
b			
c			
d			

42 REV. CD.	43 DESCRIPTION	44 HCPCS / RATE / HIPPS CODE	45 SERV. DATE	46 SERV. UNITS	47 TOTAL CHARGES	48 NON-COVERED CHARGES	49
1	0121	MED-SURG-GY/SEMI	1080 00		5	5,400 00		1
2	0250	PHARMACY				102 85		2
3	0260	IV THERAPY				101 90		3
4	0272	STERILE SUPPLY				42 39		4
5	0301	CHEMISTRY TESTS				1,858 01		5
6	0305	HEMATOLOGY TESTS				184 82		6
7	0306	BACT & MICRO TESTS				44 18		7
8	0320	DX X-RAY			1	809 25		8
9	0351	CT SCAN/HEAD			1	485 66		9
10	0420	PHYSICAL THERP				177 74		10
11	0424	PHYS THERP/EVAL				154 21		11
12	0450	EMERG ROOM			2	481 50		12
13	0730	EKG/ECG				47 32		13
23	0001	PAGE 1 OF 1	CREATION DATE 031210	TOTALS ➡		9,889 83		23

50 PAYER NAME	51 HEALTH PLAN ID	52 REL INFO	53 ASG BEN	54 PRIOR PAYMENTS	55 EST. AMOUNT DUE	56 NPI 1288561733	
A MEDICARE	00308	Y	Y			57 OTHER PRV ID 070089	A
B							B
C							C

58 INSURED'S NAME	59 P. REL	60 INSURED'S UNIQUE ID	61 GROUP NAME	62 INSURANCE GROUP NO.	
A ASTORE, GAIL	18	102123712B			A
B					B
C					C

63 TREATMENT AUTHORIZATION CODES	64 DOCUMENT CONTROL NUMBER	65 EMPLOYER NAME	
A 01916931			A
B			B
C			C

66 DX 2761	67 2920	A 72889	B 4019	C 30000	D 311	E E8888	F	G	H
9	I	J	K	L	M	N	O	P	Q
									68

69 ADMIT DX 78079	70 PATIENT REASON DX a b c	71 PPS CODE	72 ECI a b c	73

74 PRINCIPAL PROCEDURE CODE / DATE	a OTHER PROCEDURE CODE / DATE	b OTHER PROCEDURE CODE / DATE	75	76 ATTENDING NPI 1233281192 QUAL IG B18642
c OTHER PROCEDURE CODE / DATE	d OTHER PROCEDURE CODE / DATE	e OTHER PROCEDURE CODE / DATE		LAST WOOD FIRST JOHN
				77 OPERATING NPI QUAL
				LAST FIRST

80 REMARKS	81CC a B3 282N00000X	78 OTHER NPI QUAL
ACCIDENTAL FALL IN HOME, NO LIABILITY	b c d	LAST FIRST
		79 OTHER NPI QUAL
		LAST FIRST

UB-04 CMS-1450   APPROVED OMB NO. 0938-0997   **NUBC** National Uniform Billing Committee   THE CERTIFICATIONS ON THE REVERSE APPLY TO THIS BILL AND ARE MADE A PART HEREOF.

Case Studies

B ased on the patient, insurance, and services information supplied in each case study, complete UB-04 claim forms for the following ten cases. The forms may be completed manually or using the simulated UB-04 form, which can be downloaded from the text's Online Learning Center.

To identify your work once you have finished a claim, use FL 80 (Remarks) to key or write the Case Study number followed by your initials.

EXAMPLE (FL 80): CASE STUDY 1, JPM

Simulated UB-04 Form Completion: Read Chapter 16, "Using the Simulated UB-04 Form," before beginning.

Manual Completion: Blank copies of the UB-04 form are provided at the end of the book, following the index.

About the Hospital

Services for each of the cases were provided at:

Name: Hanover Regional Hospital
Address: 2600 Record Street
City/State/ZIP: Hanover, CT 06783
Telephone: 860-376-2000

Federal Tax ID: 07-1282340
NPI: 1288561733
Taxonomy Code: 282N00000X

PATIENT INFORMATION

Patient Name: Merez, Joseph F.

Patient Address: 10 State St.

City/State/Zip: Hartford, CT 06120

Telephone Number: 203-555-1867

Social Security Number: 231-87-9855

Patient Control Number: 76341980

Medical Record Number: 1639870

Date of Birth: 10-11-1960

Occupation: Sales—Full-time employee

Sex: M

Marital Status: Married

Employer: Handelsman Insurance

INSURANCE INFORMATION

Primary Insurance

Insured's Name: Merez, Joseph F.

Patient's Relationship to Insured: self

Insured's ID Number: 46-22

Health Plan: Travelers'

Health Plan ID/Carrier Code: 00890

Group Name/No.: TR-16 / HRI89

Secondary Provider No.: R10

Release of Information on File Y/N: Y

Accepts Assignment Y/N: Y

Preauthorization Number: ---------

Copayment: --------- HMO Y/N: N

PATIENT SERVICES

Date of Service: Admitted 3-15-09, 3:15 P.M. / Discharged 3-15-09, 5:45 P.M.

Date Claim Created: 3-23-09

Notes:

Services	Rev Codes	Dates	Units	Charges
Emergency Room (99283)	0450	3-15-09	1	140.73
Chest X-ray, two views (71020)	0324	3-15-09	1	161.84

Principal Dx: Painful respiration (786.52) Onset of symptoms 3-15-09

Secondary Dx: ---------

Admitting Dx/Reason for Visit: Painful respiration (786.52)

Procedures: ---------   Date of Surgery: ---------

Attending Provider ID: Samuel P. Geller, NPI 4449806712

Secondary Provider ID: 60871T (Commercial No.)

CASE STUDY 2

PATIENT INFORMATION

Patient Name: Wandenberg, Rhonda
Patient Address: 23 Lorry Lane
City/State/Zip: Glastonbury, CT 06883
Telephone Number: 203-555-5545
Social Security Number: 869-46-3629
Patient Control Number: 16530279

Medical Record Number: 5981654
Date of Birth: 5-26-1990
Occupation: ---------
Sex: F
Marital Status: Single
Employer: None

INSURANCE INFORMATION

Primary Insurance

Insured's Name: Wandenberg, Robert G.
Patient's Relationship to Insured: child
Insured's ID Number: TRY-765341028
Health Plan: BCBS
Health Plan ID/Carrier Code: 00650
Group Name/No.: Traditional / C103

Secondary Provider No.: 080
Release of Information on File Y/N: Y
Accepts Assignment Y/N: Y
Preauthorization Number: ---------
Employer: Acme, Inc. (full time)
Copayment: --------- HMO Y/N: N

PATIENT SERVICES

Date of Service: Admitted 3-16-09, 10:30 P.M. / Discharged 3-16-09, 11:45 P.M.
Date Claim Created: 3-23-09
Notes: Patient hit her forearm in the bathtub at about 7 P.M. the night of the visit. Patient student status: full-time nights.

Services	Rev Codes	Dates	Units	Charges
Emergency Room (99283)	0450	3-16-09	1	74.07
Pharmacy	0250	3-16-09	1	15.50
Medical Supplies	0270	3-16-09	1	18.15

Principal Dx: Contusion of forearm (923.10)
Secondary Dx: Hit in bathtub (E917.4)
Admitting Dx/Reason for Visit: Forearm injury (959.3)
Procedures: ---------   **Date of Surgery:** ---------
Attending Provider ID: Roberto Mulkinski, NPI 1455467098
Secondary Provider ID: 43201X (Commercial No.)

CASE STUDY 3

PATIENT INFORMATION

Patient Name: Randall L. Chambless
Patient Address: 21 Ocean Ave.
City/State/Zip: Fairfield, CT 06356
Telephone Number: 203-555-8282
Social Security Number: 432-75-9331
Patient Control Number: 45591124

Medical Record Number: 6548710
Date of Birth: 12-12-1979
Occupation: Accountant
Sex: M
Marital Status: Divorced
Employer: Price and Winterhouse

INSURANCE INFORMATION

Primary Insurance

Insured's Name: Randall L. Chambless
Patient's Relationship to Insured: self
Insured's ID Number: CC12906
Health Plan: ConnCare
Health Plan ID/Carrier Code: 00788
PAT Group Name/No.: PPO-3 / 78-2

Legacy Provider No.: 900015
Release of Information on File Y/N: Y
Accepts Assignment Y/N: Y
Preauthorization Number: RA833
Copayment: $25 HMO Y/N: N

PATIENT SERVICES

Date of Service: Admitted 3-17-09, 6:15 A.M. / Discharged 3-17-09, 1:30 P.M.
Date Claim Created: 3-23-09
Notes:

Services	Rev Codes	Dates	Units	Charges
Treatment Room	0761	3-17-09	3	@ 44.00
Medical Supplies	0270	3-17-09	1	28.30
Pharmacy	0250	3-17-09	1	6.26
OR Services (64721-RT)	0360	3-17-09	1	283.50
Anesthesia	0370	3-17-09	25	@ 2.35

Principal Dx: Carpal Tunnel Syndrome (354.0) made on February 25 of this year
Secondary Dx: Familial hypercholesterolemia (272.0)
Admitting Dx/Reason for Visit: ---------
Procedures: ---------   Date of Surgery: ---------
Attending Provider ID: Roberto Mulkinski, NPI 1455467098
Secondary Provider ID: 43201X (Commercial No.)
Operating Physician ID: Ralph Renito, NPI 1004598765
Secondary Provider ID: 16524F (Commercial No.)

CASE STUDY 4

PATIENT INFORMATION

Patient Name: Juanita Q. Barnes
Patient Address: 118 Center St.
City/State/Zip: Fairfield, CT 06357
Telephone Number: 203-555-6767
Social Security Number: 354-77-9841
Patient Control Number: 12562987

Medical Record Number: 8765000
Date of Birth: 4-16-1935
Occupation: Retired 8-9-02
Sex: F
Marital Status: Widowed
Employer: ---------

INSURANCE INFORMATION

Primary Insurance

Insured's Name: Juanita Q. Barnes
Patient's Relationship to Insured: self
Insured's ID Number: 354779841M
Health Plan: Medicare
Health Plan ID/Carrier Code: 00308
Group Name/No.: ---------
Secondary Provider No.: 070089
Release of Information on File Y/N: Y
Accepts Assignment Y/N: Y
Preauthorization Number: ---------
Copayment: --------- **HMO Y/N:** N

Secondary Insurance

Insured's Name: Juanita Q. Barnes
Patient's Relationship to Insured: self
Insured's ID Number: 5769-P
Health Plan: Health Net
Health Plan ID/Carrier Code: 00700
Group Name/No.: ---------
Secondary Provider No.: JS1007
Release of Information on File Y/N: Y
Accepts Assignment Y/N: Y
Preauthorization Number: ---------
Copayment: --------- **HMO Y/N:** N

PATIENT SERVICES

Date of Service: Admitted to ER 3-15-09, 12:30 P.M. / Discharged 3-15-09, 3:15 P.M.
Date Claim Created: 3-22-09
Notes: Onset of symptoms 3-15-09

CASE STUDY 4

PATIENT SERVICES (cont.)

Services	Rev Codes	Dates	Units	Charges
Lab/Hematology (85024)	0305	3-15-09	1	20.93
Lab/Chemistry (80051)	0301	3-15-09	1	55.04
Lab/Chemistry (82247)	0301	3-15-09	2	@ 13.10
Lab/Chemistry (84450)	0301	3-15-09	1	15.25
Lab/Chemistry (82565)	0301	3-15-09	1	16.33
Lab/Chemistry (82947)	0301	3-15-09	1	12.22
Lab/Chemistry (84520)	0301	3-15-09	1	13.76
Lab/Chemistry (84484)	0301	3-15-09	1	52.05
Lab/Chemistry (82550)	0301	3-15-09	1	25.55
Lab/Chemistry (83690)	0301	3-15-09	1	30.63
Lab/Chemistry (84075)	0301	3-15-09	1	13.76
Lab/Chemistry (84460)	0301	3-15-09	1	17.86
Emergency Room (99283-25)	0450	3-15-09	1	140.73
IV Therapy (Q0081)	0260	3-15-09	3	@ 43.44
Pharmacy	0250	3-15-09	1	13.18
Self-administered Drug, ER	0637	3-15-09	3	@ 2.85 (noncovered)

Principal Dx: Esophageal reflux (530.81)

Secondary Dx: Diabetes mellitus (250.00), Aortocoronary bypass status (V45.81)

Admitting Dx/Reason for Visit: Hyperchlorhydria (536.8)

Procedures: ---------   **Date of Surgery:** ---------

Attending Provider ID: Samuel P. Geller, NPI 4449806712

Secondary Provider ID: 300100 (UPIN)

CASE STUDY 5

PATIENT INFORMATION

Patient Name: Peggy Richards
Patient Address: Sea Breeze Way
City/State/Zip: Fairfield, CT 06357
Telephone Number: 203-555-9988
Social Security Number: 658-33-9425
Patient Control Number: 1652938B

Medical Record Number: 7654209
Date of Birth: 6-1-1940
Occupation: Retired Teacher (6-15-04)
Sex: F
Marital Status: Single
Employer: ---------

INSURANCE INFORMATION

Primary Insurance

Insured's Name: Peggy Richards
Patient's Relationship to Insured: self
Insured's ID Number: 658339425A
Health Plan: Medicare
Health Plan ID/Carrier Code: 00308
Group Name/No.: ---------
Secondary Provider No.: 070089
Release of Information on File Y/N: Y
Accepts Assignment Y/N: Y
Preauthorization Number: ---------
Copayment: --------- **HMO Y/N:** N

Secondary Insurance

Insured's Name: Peggy Richards
Patient's Relationship to Insured: self
Insured's ID Number: WC-18965
Health Plan: Health Net
Health Plan ID/Carrier Code: 00700
Group Name/No.: ---------
Secondary Provider No.: JS1007
Release of Information on File Y/N: Y
Accepts Assignment Y/N: Y
Preauthorization Number: ---------
Copayment: --------- **HMO Y/N:** N

PATIENT SERVICES

Dates of Service: 3-2-09 to 3-16-09
Date Claim Created: 3-20-09
Notes: Pt had Arthroplasty 2-10-09. Physical Therapy plan established 3-2-09.

PATIENT SERVICES (cont.)

Services	Rev Codes	Dates	Units	Charges
Physical Therapy Evaluation (97001)	0424	3-2-09	1	154.98
Physical Therapy Visits:				
Therapeutic exercises (97110)	0421	3-3-09	1	28.05
Manual therapy (97140)	0421	3-4-09	1	29.30
Therapeutic exercises (97110)	0421	3-5-09	1	28.05
Manual therapy (97140)	0421	3-6-09	1	29.30
Therapeutic exercises (97110)	0421	3-9-09	1	28.05
Manual therapy (97140)	0421	3-10-09	1	29.30
Therapeutic exercises (97110)	0421	3-11-09	1	28.05
Manual therapy (97140)	0421	3-12-09	1	29.30
Therapeutic exercises (97110)	0421	3-13-09	1	28.05
Manual therapy (97140)	0421	3-16-09	1	29.30

Principal Dx: Physical Therapy (V57.1)

Secondary Dx: Rotator Cuff syndrome (726.10)

Admitting Dx/Reason for Visit: ---------

Procedures: ---------   **Date of Surgery:** ---------

Attending Provider ID: Alik K. Azodi, NPI 7000598110

Secondary Provider ID: 10340B (UPIN)

PATIENT INFORMATION

Patient Name: Carmen Shoham
Patient Address: 59 Upper County Road
City/State/Zip: Westport, CT 06599
Telephone Number: 203-555-7766
Social Security Number: 276-46-9849
Patient Control Number: RA14264OK

Medical Record Number: 7583518
Date of Birth: 8-19-1938
Occupation: Retired, Dec. 1, 2003
Sex: F
Marital Status: Married
Employer: ---------

INSURANCE INFORMATION

Primary Insurance

Insured's Name: Carmen Shoham
Patient's Relationship to Insured: self
Insured's ID Number: 276469849W
Health Plan: Medicare
Health Plan ID/Carrier Code: 00308
Group Name/No.: ---------
Secondary Provider No.: 070089
Release of Information on File Y/N: Y
Accepts Assignment Y/N: Y
Preauthorization Number: ---------
Copayment: --------- **HMO Y/N:** N

Secondary Insurance

Insured's Name: Carmen Shoham
Patient's Relationship to Insured: self
Insured's ID Number: 756541967
Health Plan: Medicaid
Health Plan ID/Carrier Code: 07655
Group Name/No.: ---------
Secondary Provider No.: CT6543
Release of Information on File Y/N: Y
Accepts Assignment Y/N: Y
Preauthorization Number: ---------
Copayment: --------- **HMO Y/N:** N

PATIENT SERVICES

Date of Service: 4-1-09, 7:00 A.M. / Discharged 4-1-09, 12:30 P.M.
Date Claim Created: 4-6-09
Notes: First of a planned series of outpatient radiation therapy (brachytherapy).

Services	Rev Codes	Dates	Units	Charges
Radiation Therapy (77290)	0333	4-1-09	2	@ 504.00
Radiation Therapy (77334)	0333	4-1-09	2	@ 333.00

Principal Dx: Visit for radiotherapy (V58.0)
Secondary Dx: Malignant neoplasm at the base of the tongue (141.0)
Malignant neoplasm of lymph nodes (196.0)
Admitting Dx/Reason for Visit: ---------
Procedures: ---------   **Date of Surgery:** ---------
Attending Provider ID: Barbara T. Wise-Rivera, NPI 8966680143
Secondary Provider ID: 380010 (UPIN)

PATIENT INFORMATION

Patient Name: John C. Anastasio
Patient Address: 100 Shore Ave.
City/State/Zip: Westport, CT 06587
Telephone Number: 203-555-1100
Social Security Number: 129-89-0634
Patient Control Number: AB88900000

Medical Record Number: 8750372
Date of Birth: 9-11-1919
Occupation: Retired, Jan. 1, 1990
Sex: M
Marital Status: Widowed
Employer: ---------

INSURANCE INFORMATION

Primary Insurance

Insured's Name: John C. Anastasio
Patient's Relationship to Insured: self
Insured's ID Number: 12989063A
Health Plan: Medicare
Health Plan ID/Carrier Code: 00308
Group Name/No.: ---------

Secondary Provider No.: 070089
Release of Information on File Y/N: Y
Accepts Assignment Y/N: Y
Preauthorization Number: ---------
Copayment: --------- HMO Y/N: N

PATIENT SERVICES

Date of Service: 3-16-09, 9:15 P.M. / Discharged 3-21-09, 11:30 A.M.
Date Claim Created: 3-26-09
Notes:

Services	Rev Codes	Units	Charges
Semiprivate Room–2 Bed/Surgical	0121	5	@ 1080.21
Pharmacy	0250	1	87.14
IV Therapy	0260	1	160.00
Lab Charges	0300	21	608.90
ECG	0730	1	178.00
Inhalation Services	0412	1	240.88
Cardiology	0480	1	967.00

Principal Dx: Acute myocardial infarction (410.91) POA: Y
Secondary Dx: Atherosclerosis (414.01) POA: Y
Admitting Dx/Reason for Visit: (410.91)
Procedures: ---------   Date of Surgery: ---------
Attending Provider ID: Louise Fatu, NPI 6015778887
Secondary Provider ID: 58912T (UPIN)

CASE STUDY 8

PATIENT INFORMATION

Patient Name: Marvin Kelly
Patient Address: 46 State St.
City/State/Zip: Hartford, CT 06516
Telephone Number: 203-555-7777
Social Security Number: 364-89-9815
Patient Control Number: XZ6518

Medical Record Number: 1825695
Date of Birth: 3-15-2009
Occupation: ---------
Sex: M
Marital Status: Single
Employer: ---------

INSURANCE INFORMATION

Primary Insurance

Insured's Name: Richard G. Kelly
Patient's Relationship to Insured: child
Insured's ID Number: 002879366
Health Plan: HMO Blue Care
Health Plan ID/Carrier Code: XX142
Group Name/No.: Gartner / AA1

Secondary Provider No.: 4041869
Release of Information on File Y/N: Y
Accepts Assignment Y/N: Y
Preauthorization Number: G21X
Copayment: --------- HMO Y/N: Y
Employer: Gartner, Inc. (full-time)

PATIENT SERVICES

Date of Service: 3-15-09, 5:45 P.M. / Discharged 3-19-09, 3:30 P.M.
Date Claim Created: 3-25-09
Notes: Claim was reviewed and approved by Blue Care UR.

Services	Rev Codes	Units	Charges
Lab–Hematology	0305	1	72.87
Laboratory Pathology–Other	0319	1	35.28
Nursery/Newborn Level I	0171	4	@ 552.00
Medical/Surgical Supplies	0270	1	34.44
Laboratory	0300	1	35.09
Lab–Chemistry	0301	1	517.04

PATIENT SERVICES (cont.)

Principal Dx: Single liveborn, born in hospital (V30.00) **POA:** 1

Secondary Dx: Neonatal jaundice (774.6) **POA:** 1

Diaper rash (691.0) **POA:** 1

Birth injury to scalp (767.1) **POA:** 1

Admitting Dx/Reason for Visit: V30.00

Procedures (ICD-9-CM): Circumcision (64.0) **Date of Surgery:** 3-19-09

Attending Provider ID: Thomas Wong, NPI 9100016533

Secondary Provider ID: 45789R (Commercial No.)

Operating Physician ID: Thomas Wong, NPI 9100016533

Secondary Provider ID: 45789R (Commercial No.)

PATIENT INFORMATION

Patient Name: Mary S. Chung
Patient Address: 56 Gladview Lane
City/State/Zip: Hartford, CT 06514
Telephone Number: 203-555-6655
Social Security Number: 312-22-2420
Patient Control Number: XXB825-99
Medical Record Number: Y172699

Date of Birth: 10-11-1934
Occupation: Husband retired, State of CT, 9-1-03
Sex: F
Marital Status: Married
Employer: ---------

INSURANCE INFORMATION

Primary Insurance

Insured's Name: Mary S. Chung
Patient's Relationship to Insured: self
Insured's ID Number: 312222420B
Health Plan: Medicare
Health Plan ID/Carrier Code: 00308
Group Name/No.: ---------
Secondary Provider No.: 070089
Release of Information on File Y/N: Y
Accepts Assignment Y/N: Y
Preauthorization Number: ---------
Copayment: --------- HMO Y/N: N

Secondary Insurance

Insured's Name: Mary S. Chung
Patient's Relationship to Insured: self
Insured's ID Number: 6653-D
Health Plan: HealthNet
Health Plan ID/Carrier Code: 00700
Group Name/No.: ---------
Secondary Provider No.: JS1007
Release of Information on File Y/N: Y
Accepts Assignment Y/N: Y
Preauthorization Number: ---------
Copayment: --------- HMO Y/N: N

PATIENT SERVICES

Date of Service: 3-15-09, 3:30 P.M. / Discharged 3-20-09, 2:15 P.M.
Date Claim Created: 3-26-09
Notes: Patient discharged to her home under the care of VSN home health service.

CASE STUDY 9

PATIENT SERVICES (cont.)

Services	Rev Codes	Units	Charges
Emergency room	0450	2	481.50
IV therapy	0260	1	101.90
EKG	0730	1	47.32
Lab–Bacteriology	0306	1	44.18
Lab–Chemistry	0301	1	1858.01
Supplies–Sterile	0272	1	42.39
Pharmacy	0250	1	102.85
CT Scan/Head	0351	1	485.66
Radiology-Diagnostic (X ray)	0320	1	809.25
Lab–Hematology	0305	1	184.82
Semiprivate Room–2 Bed/Surgical	0121	5	@ 1080.00
Physical therapy evaluation	0424	1	154.21
Physical therapy	0420	1	177.74

Principal Dx: Hyposmolality (276.1), **POA:** Y

Secondary Dx: Drug withdrawal syndrome (292.0), **POA:** Y

Essential hypertension (401.9), **POA:** Y

Anxiety disorder (300.00), **POA:** Y

Depressive disorder (311), **POA:** Y

Saluretics (E944.3), **POA:** Y

Knee joint replacement (V43.65), **POA:** 1

Admitting Dx/Reason for Visit: Neuromuscular fatigue (780.89)

Procedures: ---------   **Date of Surgery:** ---------

Attending Provider ID: Samuel P. Geller, NPI 4449806712

Secondary Provider ID: 300100 (UPIN)

CASE STUDY 10

PATIENT INFORMATION

Patient Name: Gilbert U. Williams
Patient Address: 201 Magnolia Ave.
City/State/Zip: Fairfield, CT 06357
Telephone Number: 203-555-1111
Social Security Number: 765-45-2817
Patient Control Number: XX871295

Medical Record Number: 7650120
Date of Birth: 9-12-1920
Occupation: Retired, 9-12-85
Sex: M
Marital Status: Married
Employer: ---------

INSURANCE INFORMATION

Primary Insurance
Insured's Name: Gilbert U. Williams
Patient's Relationship to Insured: self
Insured's ID Number: 765452817A
Health Plan: Medicare
Health Plan ID/Carrier Code: 00308
Group Name/No.: ---------

Secondary Provider No.: 070089
Release of Information on File Y/N: Y
Accepts Assignment Y/N: Y
Preauthorization Number: ---------
Copayment: --------- HMO Y/N: N

PATIENT SERVICES

Date of Service: 3-31-09, 9:00 A.M. / Discharged 4-14-09, 7:30 P.M.
Date Claim Created: 4-20-09
Notes:

Services	Rev Codes	Units	Charges
Emergency Room	0450	2	405.41
Radiology-Diagnostic (X ray)	0320	1	433.18
Laboratory	0300	1	4942.66
Nuclear Medicine	0340	1	784.08
CT Scan, Body	0352	4	4075.28
CT Scan, Head	0351	1	1018.82
CT Scan, General	0350	1	421.08
Pharmacy	0250	1	2579.15
Private Room/Surgical	0111	13	@ 720.00
Intensive Care/Surgical	0201	1	@ 1701.00
IV Therapy	0260	1	1545.20

CASE STUDY 10

PATIENT SERVICES (cont.)

Services	Rev Codes	Units	Charges
Medical/Surgical Supplies	0270	1	835.90
Blood Processing and Storage	0392	1	1008.00
Respiratory Services	0410	29	641.56
Cardiology	0480	1	1289.86
EKG	0730	1	96.68
Incremental Nursing Care, General	0230	1	9594.00
Incremental Nursing Care, ICU	0233	1	2027.00
Lab–Chemistry	0301	1	125.00
Peripheral Vascular Lab	0921	1	804.65
Treatment Room	0761	1	54.45

Principal Dx: Pneumonia (486), **POA:** Y

Secondary Dx: Malignant neoplasm of lung (162.8), **POA:** Y

Secondary malignant neoplasm of adrenal gland (198.7), **POA:** Y

Serous pleurisy (511.9), **POA:** Y

Septic shock (785.6), **POA:** N

Chronic obstructive lung disease (496), **POA:** Y

Secondary malignant neoplasm of intrathoracic lymph nodes (196.1), **POA:** Y

Hypertension (401.9), **POA:** Y

Pulmonary congestion (514), **POA:** Y

Admitting Dx/Reason for Visit: Respiratory abnormality (786.00)

Principal Procedure (ICD-9-CM): Arterial puncture (38.98)

Date of Surgery: 3-31-09

Other Procedure (ICD-9-CM): Packed cell transfusion (99.04)

Date of Surgery: 4-3-09

Attending Provider ID: Louise Fatu, NPI 6015778887

Secondary Provider ID: 58912T (UPIN)

Operating Physician ID: Alik K. Azodi, NPI 7000598110

Secondary Provider ID: 10340B (UPIN)

UB-04 Codes

A–1 Type of Bill Codes

Second Digit–Type of Facility

Code	Description
1	Hospital
2	Skilled nursing
3	Home health facility
4	Religious nonmedical health care institution—hospital inpatient
5	Reserved for national assignment
6	Intermediate care
7	Clinic or hospital-based renal dialysis facility
8	Special facility or hospital ASC (ambulatory surgical center)
9	Reserved for national assignment

Third Digit–Bill Classification

Code	Description
1	Inpatient (including Medicare Part A)
2	Inpatient (Medicare Part B only)
3	Outpatient
4	Other (Medicare Part B)
5	Intermediate care–level I
6	Intermediate care–level II
7	Reserved for national assignment
8	Swing bed
9	Reserved for national assignment

Fourth Digit–Frequency of the Bill

Code	Description
0	Nonpayment/zero claim
1	Admit through discharge claim
2	Interim–first claim
3	Interim–continuing claim
4	Interim–last claim
5	Late Charge(s) only claim
6	Reserved for national assignment
7	Replacement of a prior claim
8	Void/cancel of a prior claim
9	Final claim for a home health PPS episode

Occurrence Codes

Code	Description
Accident-Related Codes	
01	Accident/Medical Coverage
02	No-Fault Insurance Involved–Including Auto Accident/Other
03	Accident/Tort Liability
04	Accident/Employment-Related
05	Accident/No Medical or Liability Coverage
06	Crime Victim
07–08	Reserved for National Assignment
Medical Condition Codes	
09	Start of Infertility Treatment Cycle
10	Last Menstrual Period
11	Onset of Symptoms/Illness
12	Date of Onset for a Chronically Dependent Individual (CDI)
13–15	Reserved for National Assignment
Insurance-Related Codes	
16	Date of Last Therapy
17	Date Outpatient Occupational Therapy Plan Established or Last Reviewed
18	Date of Retirement of Patient/Beneficiary
19	Date of Retirement of Spouse
20	Date Guarantee of Payment Began
21	Date UR Notice Received
22	Date Active Care Ended
23	Reserved for Payer Use Only
24	Date Insurance Denied
25	Date Benefits Terminated by Primary Payer
26	Date SNF Bed Became Available
27	Date of Hospice Certification or Recertification

Code	Description
28	Date Comprehensive Outpatient Rehabilitation Plan Established or Last Reviewed
29	Date Outpatient Physical Therapy Plan Established or Last Reviewed
30	Date Outpatient Speech Pathology Plan Established or Last Reviewed
31	Date Beneficiary Notified of Intent to Bill (Accommodations)
32	Date Beneficiary Notified of Intent to Bill (Procedures or Treatments)
33	First Day of the Coordination Period for ESRD Beneficiaries Covered by EGHP
34	Date of Election of Extended Care Facilities
35	Date Treatment Started for Physical Therapy
36	Date of Inpatient Hospital Discharge for Covered Transplant Patient
37	Date of Inpatient Hospital Discharge for Non-covered Transplant Patient
38	Date Treatment Started for Home IV Therapy
39	Date Discharged on a Continuous Course of IV Therapy
Service-Related Codes	
40	Scheduled Date of Admission
41	Date of First Test for Preadmission Testing
42	Date of Discharge
43	Scheduled Date of Cancelled Surgery
44	Date Treatment Started for Occupational Therapy
45	Date Treatment Started for Speech Therapy

Code	Description
46	Date Treatment Started for Cardiac Rehabilitation
47	Date Cost Outlier Status Begins
48–49	Payer Codes
50–69	Reserved for National Assignment
70–99	Reserved for Occurrence Span Codes
A0	Reserved for National Assignment
A1	Birth Date–Insured A
A2	Effective Date–Insured A Policy
A3	Benefits Exhausted—Payer A
A4	Split Bill Date
A5–AZ	Reserved for National Assignment
B0	Reserved for National Assignment

Code	Description
B1	Birth Date–Insured B
B2	Effective Date–Insured B Policy
B3	Benefits Exhausted—Payer B
B4–BZ	Reserved for National Assignment
C0	Reserved for National Assignment
C1	Birth Date–Insured C
C2	Effective Date–Insured C Policy
C3	Benefits Exhausted—Payer C
C4–DQ	Reserved for National Assignment
DR	Reserved for Disaster Related Occurrence Code
DS–LZ	Reserved for National Assignment
M0–ZZ	Reserved for Occurrence Span Codes

Code	Description
General Codes	
01	Most Common Semiprivate Room Rate
02	Hospital Has No Semiprivate Rooms
03	Reserved for National Assignment
04	Professional Component Charges Which Are Combined Billed
05	Professional Component Included in Charges and Also Billed Separately to Carrier
06	Medicare Blood Deductible
07	Reserved for National Assignment
08	Medicare Lifetime Reserve Amount in the First Calendar Year
09	Medicare Coinsurance Amount in the First Calendar Year
10	Medicare Lifetime Reserve Amount in the Second Calendar Year
11	Medicare Coinsurance Amount for Second Calendar Year
12	Working Aged Beneficiary/Spouse with EGHP
13	ESRD Beneficiary in a Medicare Coordination Period with an EGHP
14	No-Fault, Including Auto/Other
15	Workers' Compensation
16	Public Health Service (PHS) or Other Federal Agency
17–20	Reserved for Payer Use Only
21	Catastrophic
22	Surplus
23	Recurring Monthly Income
24	Medicaid Rate Code
25	Offset to the Patient—Payment Amount—Prescription Drugs

Code	Description
26	Offset to the Patient—Payment Amount—Hearing and Ear Services
27	Offset to the Patient—Payment Amount—Vision and Eye Services
28	Offset to the Patient—Payment Amount—Dental Services
29	Offset to the Patient—Payment Amount—Chiropractic Services
30	Preadmission Testing
31	Patient Liability Amount
32	Multiple Patient Ambulance Transport
33	Offset to the Patient—Payment Amount—Podiatric Services
34	Offset to the Patient—Payment Amount—Other Medical Services
35	Offset to the Patient—Payment Amount—Health Insurance Premiums
36	Reserved for National Assignment
37	Pints of Blood Furnished
38	Blood Deductible Pints
39	Pints of Blood Replaced
40	New Coverage Not Implemented by HMO (for inpatient claims only)
41	Black Lung
42	Veterans Affairs
43	Disabled Beneficiary Under Age 65 with LGHP
44	Amount Provider Agreed to Accept from the Primary Insurer When this Amount is Less Than Total Charges, But Greater than the Primary Insurer's Payment

Code	Description
45	Accident Hour
46	Number of Grace Days
47	Any Liability Insurance
48	Hemoglobin Reading
49	Hematocrit Reading
50	Physical Therapy Visits
51	Occupational Therapy Visits
52	Speech Therapy Visits
53	Cardiac Rehabilitation Visits
54	Newborn Birth Weight in Grams
55	Eligibility Threshold for Charity Care
Home Health-Specific and Payer-Specific Codes	
56	Skilled Nurse–Home Visit Hours (HHA Only)
57	Home Health Aid–Home Visit Hours (HHA Only)
58	Arterial Blood Gas (PO_2/PA_2)
59	Oxygen Saturation (O_2SAT/oximetry)
60	HHA Branch MSA
61	Place of Residence Where Service is Furnished (HHA and Hospice)
62–65	Reserved for Payer Use Only
66	Medicaid Spend Down Amount
67	Peritoneal Dialysis
68	EPO–Drug
69	State Charity Care Percent
70–79	Reserved for Payer Use Only
Codes for Covered and Noncovered Days	
80	Covered Days
81	Non-Covered Days
82	Coinsurance Days

Code	Description
83	Lifetime Reserve Days
84–99	Reserved for National Assignment
Alphanumeric Codes	
A0	Special ZIP Code Reporting
A1	Deductible Payer A
A2	Coinsurance Payer A
A3	Estimated Responsibility Payer A
A4	Covered Self-Administrable Drugs— Emergency
A5	Covered Self-Administrable Drugs—Not Self-Administrable in Form and Situation Furnished to Patient
A6	Covered Self-Administrable Drugs— Diagnostic Study and Other
A7	Copayment Payer A
A8	Patient Weight
A9	Patient Height
AA	Regulatory Surcharges, Assessments, Allowances or Health Care Related Taxes Payer A
AB	Other Assessments or Allowances (e.g., Medical Education) Payer A
AC–B0	Reserved for National Assignment
B1	Deductible Payer B
B2	Coinsurance Payer B
B3	Estimated Responsibility Payer B
B4–B6	Reserved for National Assignment
B7	Copayment Payer B
B8–B9	Reserved for National Assignment
BA	Regulatory Surcharges, Assessments, Allowances or Health Care Related Taxes Payer B

Code	Description	Code	Description
BB	Other Assessments or Allowances (e.g., Medical Education) Payer B	D5–DQ	Reserved for National Assignment
		DR	Reserved for Disaster Related Value Code
BC–C0	Reserved for National Assignment	DS–G7	Reserved for National Assignment
C1	Deductible Payer C	G8	Facility Where Inpatient Hospice Service is Delivered
C2	Coinsurance Payer C		
C3	Estimated Responsibility Payer C	G9–OZ	Reserved for National Assignment
C4–C6	Reserved for National Assignment	P0–PZ	Reserved for Public Health Data Reporting
C7	Copayment Payer C		
CA	Regulatory Surcharges, Assessments, Allowances or Health Care Related Taxes Payer C	Q0–Y0	Reserved for National Assignment
		Y1	Part A Demonstration Payment
		Y2	Part B Demonstration Payment
CB	Other Assessments or Allowances (e.g., Medical Education) Payer C	Y3	Part B Coinsurance
		Y4	Conventional Provider Payment Amount for Non-Demonstration Claims
CC–D2	Reserved for National Assignment		
D3	Patient Estimated Responsibility	Y5–ZZ	Reserved for National Assignment
D4	Clinical Trial Number Assigned by NLM/NIH		

A–4 Revenue Codes: Numerical Order

Accommodation Revenue Codes (0001–021X)

Code	Description
0001 Total Charge	
001X Reserved	
002X Health Insurance - Prospective Payment System (HIPPS)	
003X-009X Reserved	
010X All-inclusive Rate	

Subcategory Code	Standard Abbreviation
0 All inclusive room and board plus ancillary	ALL INCL R&B/ANC
1 All-inclusive room and board	ALL INCL R&B

011X R&B—Private (One Bed)

Subcategory Code	Standard Abbreviation
0 General	ROOM-BOARD/PVT
1 Medical/Surgical/Gyn	MED-SURG-GY/PVT
2 Obstetrics (OB)	OB/PVT
3 Pediatric	PEDS/PVT
4 Psychiatric	PSYCH/PVT
5 Hospice	HOSPICE/PVT
6 Detoxification	DETOX/PVT
7 Oncology	ONCOLOGY/PVT
8 Rehabilitation	REHAB/PVT
9 Other	OTHER/PVT

012X R&B—Semi-Private (Two Beds)

Subcategory Code	Standard Abbreviation
0 General	ROOM-BOARD/SEMI
1 Medical/Surgical/Gyn	MED-SURG/GY/SEMI
2 OB	OB/SEMI-PVT
3 Pediatric	PEDS/SEMI-PVT
4 Psychiatric	PSYCH/SEMI-PVT
5 Hospice	HOSPICE/SEMI-PVT
6 Detoxification	DETOX/SEMI-PVY
7 Oncology	ONCOLOGY/SEMI
8 Rehabilitation	REHAB/SEMI-PVT
9 Other	OTHER/SEMI-PVT

013X R&B—Three and Four Beds

Subcategory Code	Standard Abbreviation
0 General	ROOM-BOARD/3&4BED
1 Medical/Surgical/Gyn	MED-SURG-GY/3&4BED
2 OB	OB/3&4BED
3 Pediatric	PEDS/3&4BED
4 Psychiatric	PSYCH/3&4BED
5 Hospice	HOSPICE/3&4BED
6 Detoxification	DETOX/3&4BED
7 Oncology	ONCOLOGY/3&4BED
8 Rehabilitation	REHAB/3&4BED
9 Other	OTHER/3&4BED

014X R&B—Deluxe Private

Subcategory	Standard Abbreviation
0 General	ROOM-BOARD/DLX PVT
1 Medical/Surgical/Gyn	MED-SURG-GY/DLX PVT
2 OB	OB/DLXPVT
3 Pediatric	PEDS/DLXPVT
4 Psychiatric	PSYCH/DLXPVT
5 Hospice	HOSPICE/DLXPVT
6 Detoxification	DETOX/DLXPVT
7 Oncology	ONCOLOGY/DLXPVT

Code	Description
8 Rehabilitation	REHAB/DLXPVT
9 Other	OTHER/DLXPVT

015X R&B—Ward

Subcategory Code	Standard Abbreviation
0 General	ROOM-BOARD/WARD
1 Medical/Surgical/Gyn	MED-SURG-GY/WARD
2 OB	OB/WARD
3 Pediatric	PEDS/WARD
4 Psychiatric	PSYCH/WARD
5 Hospice	HOSPICE/WARD
6 Detoxification	DETOX/WARD
7 Oncology	ONCOLOGY/WARD
8 Rehabilitation	REHAB/WARD
9 Other	OTHER/WARD

016X R&B—Other

Subcategory Code	Standard Abbreviation
0 General	R&B
4 Sterile environment	R&B/STERILE
7 Self care	R&B/SELF
9 Other	R&B/OTHER

017X Nursery

Subcategory Code	Standard Abbreviation
0 General	NURSERY
1 Newborn–Level I	NURSERY/LEVELI
2 Newborn–Level II	NURSERY/LEVELII
3 Newborn–Level III	NURSERY/LEVELIII
4 Newborn–Level IV	NURSERY/LEVELIV
9 Other Nursery	NURSERY-OTHER

018X Leave of Absence (LOA)

Subcategory Code	Standard Abbreviation
0 General	Leave of Absence or LOA

Code	Description
2 Patient convenience	LOA/PT CONV
3 Therapeutic leave	LOA/THERAPEUTIC
5 Nursing home (for hospitalization)	LOA/NURS HOME
9 Other Leave of Absence	LOA/OTHER

019X Subacute Care

Subcategory Code	Standard Abbreviation
0 General	SUBACUTE
1 Subacute care–Level I	SUBACUTE/LEVEL I
2 Subacute care–Level II	SUBACUTE/LEVEL II
3 Subacute care–Level III	SUBACUTE/LEVEL III
4 Subacute care–Level IV	SUBACUTE/LEVEL IV
9 Other subacute care	SUBACUTE/OTHER

020X Intensive Care

Subcategory Code	Standard Abbreviation
0 General	INTENSIVE CARE (ICU)
1 Surgical	ICU/SURGICAL
2 Medical	ICU/MEDICAL
3 Pediatric	ICU/PEDS
4 Psychiatric	ICU/PSYCH
6 Intermediate Intensive Care Unit (ICU)	ICU/INTERMEDIATE
7 Burn care	ICU/BURN CARE
8 Trauma	ICU/TRAUMA
9 Other Intensive Care	ICU/OTHER

021X Coronary Care

Subcategory Code	Standard Abbreviation
0 General	CORONARY CARE (CCU)

Code	Description
1 Myocardial infarction	CCU/MYO INFARC
2 Pulmonary care	CCU/PULMONARY
3 Heart transplant	CCU/TRANSPLANT

Code	Description
4 Intermediate Coronary Care Unit (CCU)	CCU/INTERMEDIATE
9 Other coronary care	CCU/OTHER

Ancillary Revenue Codes (022X–099X)

Code	Description
022X Special Charges	
Subcategory Code	*Standard Abbreviation*
0 General	SPECIAL CHARGE
1 Admission Charges	ADMIT CHARGE
2 Technical support charge	TECH SUPPORT CHG
3 U.R. service charge	UR CHARGE
4 Late discharge, medically necessary	LATE DISCH/ MED NEC
9 Other special charges	OTHER SPEC CHG
023X Incremental Nursing Charge	
Subcategory Code	*Standard Abbreviation*
0 General	NURSING INCREM
1 Nursery	NUR INCR/NURSERY
2 OB	NUR INCR/OB
3 ICU	NUR INCR/ICU
4 CCU	NUR INCR/CCU
5 Hospice	NUR INCR/HOSPICE
9 Other	NUR INCR/OTHER
024X All Inclusive Ancillary	
Subcategory Code	*Standard Abbreviation*
0 General	ALL INCL ANCIL
1 Basic	ALL INCL BASIC
2 Comprehensive	ALL INCL COMP

Code	Description
3 Specialty	ALL INCL SPECIAL
9 Other all inclusive ancillary	ALL INCL ANCIL/ OTHER
025X Pharmacy (see also 063X, an extension of 025X)	
Subcategory Code	*Standard Abbreviation*
0 General	PHARMACY
1 Generic drugs	DRUGS/GENERIC
2 Nongeneric drugs	DRUGS/NONGENERIC
3 Take home drugs	DRUGS/TAKEHOME
4 Drugs incident to other diagnostic services	DRUGS/INCIDENT ODX
5 Drugs incident to radiology	DRUGS/INCIDENT RAD
6 Experimental drugs	DRUGS/EXPERIMT
7 Nonprescription	DRUGS/NONPSCRPT
8 IV solutions	IV SOLUTIONS
9 Other pharmacy	DRUGS/OTHER
026X IV Therapy	
Subcategory Code	*Standard Abbreviation*
0 General	IV THERAPY
1 Infusion pump	IV THER/INFSN PUMP
2 IV therapy/pharmacy services	IV THER/PHARM/ SVC

Code	Description
3 IV therapy/drug/supply/ delivery	IV THER/DRUG/ SUPPLY/DEL
4 IV therapy/supplies	IV THER/SUPPLIES
9 Other IV therapy	IV THERAPY/OTHER

027X Medical/Surgical Supplies and Devices (see also 062X)

Subcategory Code	Standard Abbreviation
0 General	MED-SUR SUPPLIES
1 Nonsterile supply	NON-STER SUPPLY
2 Sterile supply	STERILE SUPPLY
3 Take home supplies	TAKEHOME SUPPLY
4 Prosthetic/orthotic devices	PROSTH/ORTH DEV
5 Pacemaker	PACEMAKER
6 Intraocular lens	INTRA OC LENS
7 Oxygen–Take home	O2/TAKEHOME
8 Other implants	SUPPLY/ IMPLANTS
9 Other supplies/devices	SUPPLY/OTHER

028X Oncology

Subcategory Code	Standard Abbreviation
0 General	ONCOLOGY
9 Other oncology	ONCOLOGY/OTHER

029X DME (Other Than Renal)

Subcategory Code	Standard Abbreviation
0 General	DME
1 Rental	DME-RENTAL
2 Purchase of new DME	DME-NEW
3 Purchase of used DME	DME-USED
4 Supplies/drugs for DME	DME-SUPPLIES/ DRUGS
9 Other equipment	DME-OTHER

030X Laboratory

Subcategory Code	Standard Abbreviation
0 General	LAB
1 Chemistry	CHEMISTRY TESTS
2 Immunology	IMMUNOLOGY TESTS
3 Renal patient (home)	RENAL HOME
4 Nonroutine dialysis	NON-RTNE DIALYSIS
5 Hematology	HEMATOLOGY TESTS
6 Bacteriology & microbiology	BACT & MICRO TESTS
7 Urology	UROLOGY TESTS
9 Other laboratory	OTHER LAB TESTS

031X Laboratory Pathology

Subcategory Code	Standard Abbreviation
0 General	PATHOLOGY LAB
1 Cytology	CYTOLOGY TESTS
2 Histology	HISTOLOGY TESTS
4 Biopsy	BIOPSY TESTS
9 Other Laboratory Pathology	PATH LAB OTHER

032X Radiology—Diagnostic

Subcategory Code	Standard Abbreviation
0 General	DX X-RAY
1 Angiocardiology	DX X-RAY/ANGIO
2 Arthrography	DX X-RAY/ARTHO
3 Arteriography	DX X-RAY/ARTER
4 Chest X-ray	DX X-RAY/CHEST
9 Other Radiology- Diagnostic	DX X-RAY/OTHER

Code	Description
033X Radiology—Therapeutic and/or Chemotherapy Administration	

Subcategory Code	Standard Abbreviation
0 General	RADIOLOGY THERAPY
1 Chemotherapy–Injected	RAD-CHEMO-INJECT
2 Chemotherapy–Oral	RAD-CHEMO-ORAL
3 Radiation Therapy	RAD-RADIATION
5 Chemotherapy–IV	RAD-CHEMO-IV
9 Other Radiology-Therapeutic	RADIOLOGY OTHER

Code	Description
034X Nuclear Medicine	

Subcategory Code	Standard Abbreviation
0 General	NUCLEAR MEDICINE
1 Diagnostic	NUC MED/DX
2 Therapeutic	NUC MED/RX
3 Diagnostic Radiopharmaceuticals	NUC MED/DX RADIOPHARM
4 Therapeutic Radiopharmaceuticals	NUC MED/RX RADIOPHARM
9 Other	NUC MED/OTHER

Code	Description
035X CT Scan	

Subcategory Code	Standard Abbreviation
0 General	CT SCAN
1 Head Scan	CT SCAN/HEAD
2 Body Scan	CT SCAN/BODY
9 Other CT Scans	CT SCAN/OTHER

Code	Description
036X Operating Room Services	

Subcategory Code	Standard Abbreviation
0 General	OR SERVICES
1 Minor surgery	OR/MINOR

Code	Description
2 Organ transplant–Other than kidney	OR/ORGAN TRANS
7 Kidney transplant	OR/KIDNEY TRANS
9 - Other operating room services	OR/OTHER

Code	Description
037X Anesthesia	

Subcategory Code	Standard Abbreviation
0 General	ANESTHESIA
1 Anesthesia incident to Radiology	ANESTH/INCIDENT RAD
2 Anesthesia incident to other diagnostic services	ANESTH/INCIDNT OTHR DX
4 Acupuncture	ANESTH/ACUPUNC
9 Other anesthesia	ANESTH/OTHER

Code	Description
038X Blood and Blood Components	

Subcategory Code	Standard Abbreviation
0 General	BLOOD & BLOOD COMP
1 Packed red cells	BLOOD/PKD RED
2 Whole blood	BLOOD/WHOLE
3 Plasma	BLOOD/PLASMA
4 Platelets	BLOOD/ PLATELETS
5 Leukocytes	BLOOD/ LEUKOCYTES
6 Other blood components	BLOOD/ COMPONENTS
7 Other derivatives (cryoprecipitates)	BLOOD/ DERIVATIVES
9 Other Blood & Blood Components	BLOOD/OTHER

Code	Description
039X Administration, Processing, and Storage for Blood and Blood Components	

Code	Description
Subcategory Code	*Standard Abbreviation*
0 General	BLOOD/ADMIN/STOR
1 Blood administration	BLOOD/ADMIN
2 Processing and storage	BLOOD/STORAGE
9 Other blood handling	BLOOD/ADMIN/STOR/OTHER

040X Other Imaging Services

Code	Description
Subcategory Code	*Standard Abbreviation*
0 General	IMAGING SERVICE
1 Diagnostic mammography	DIAG MAMMOGRAPHY
2 Ultrasound	ULTRASOUND
3 Screening mammography	SCR MAMMOGRAPHY
4 Positron emission tomography	PET SCAN
9 Other imaging services	OTHER IMAGE SVCS

041X Respiratory Services

Code	Description
Subcategory Code	*Standard Abbreviation*
0 General	RESPIRATORY SVC
2 Inhalation services	INHALATION SVC
3 Hyperbaric oxygen therapy	HYPERBARIC 02
9 Other respiratory services	OTHER RESPIR SVCS

042X Physical Therapy

Code	Description
Subcategory Code	*Standard Abbreviation*
0 General	PHYSICAL THERP
1 Visit charge	PHYS THERP/VISIT
2 Hourly charge	PHYS THERP/HOUR

Code	Description
3 Group rate	PHYS THERP/GROUP
4 Evaluation or re-evaluation	PHYS THERP/EVAL
9 Other physical therapy	OTHER PHYS THERP

043X Occupational Therapy

Code	Description
Subcategory Code	*Standard Abbreviation*
0 General	OCCUPATIONAL THER
1 Visit charge	OCCUP THERP/VISIT
2 Hourly charge	OCCUP THERP/HOUR
3 Group Rate	OCCUP THERP/GROUP
4 Evaluation or re-evaluation	OCCUP THERP/EVAL
9 Other occupational OTHER	OCCUP THER/ therapy

044X Speech Therapy-Language Pathology

Code	Description
Subcategory Code	*Standard Abbreviation*
0 General	SPEECH THERAPY
1 Visit charge	SPEECH THERP/VISIT
2 Hourly charge	SPEECH THERP/HOUR
3 Group rate	SPEECH THERP/GROUP
4 Evaluation or re-evaluation	SPEECH THERP/EVAL
9 Other speech-language pathology	OTHER SPEECH THERP

045X Emergency Room

Code	Description
Subcategory Code	*Standard Abbreviation*
0 General	EMERG ROOM
1 EMTALA Emergency medical screening services	ER/EMTALA
2 ER beyond EMTALA screening	ER/BEYOND EMTALA

Code	Description
6 Urgent care	ER/URGENT
9 Other emergency room	OTHER EMERG ROOM

046x Pulmonary Function

Subcategory Code	Standard Abbreviation
0 General	PULMONARY FUNC
9 Other pulmonary function	OTHER PULMONARY FUNC

047X Audiology

Subcategory Code	Standard Abbreviation
0 General	AUDIOLOGY
1 Diagnostic	AUDIOLOGY/DX
2 Treatment	AUDIOLOGY/RX
9 Other audiology	OTHER AUDIOL

048X Cardiology

Subcategory Code	Standard Abbreviation
0 General	CARDIOLOGY
1 Cardiac cath lab	CARDIAC CATH LAB
2 Stress test	STRESS TEST
3 Echocardiology	ECHOCARDIOLOGY
9 Other cardiology	OTHER CARDIOL

049X Ambulatory Surgical Care

Subcategory Code	Standard Abbreviation
0 General	AMBULTRY SURG
9 Other ambulatory surgical care	OTHER AMBL SURG

050X Outpatient Services

Subcategory Code	Standard Abbreviation
0 General	OUTPATIENT SVCS
9 Other outpatient services	OTHER-O/P SERVICES

051X Clinic

Subcategory Code	Standard Abbreviation
0 General	CLINIC
1 Chronic pain center	CHRONIC PAIN CLINIC
2 Dental clinic	DENTAL CLINIC
3 Psychiatric clinic	PSYCHIATRIC CLINIC
4 OB-GYN clinic	OB-GYN CLINIC
5 Pediatric clinic	PEDIATRIC CLINIC
6 Urgent care clinic	URGENT CARE CLINIC
7 Family practice clinic	FAMILY CLINIC
9 Other clinic	OTHER CLINIC

052X Free-Standing Clinic

Subcategory Code	Standard Abbreviation
0 General	FREESTAND CLINIC
1 Rural health—clinic	FS-RURAL/CLINIC
2 Rural health—home	FS-RURAL/HOME
3 Family practice clinic	FS-FAMILY PRACT
6 Urgent care clinic	FR/STD URGENT CLINIC
9 Other freestanding clinic	OTHER FS - CLINIC

053X Osteopathic Services

Subcategory Code	Standard Abbreviation
0 General	OSTEOPATH SVCS
1 Osteopathic therapy	OSTEOPATH RX
9 Other osteopathic services	OTHER OSTEOPATH

054X Ambulance

Subcategory Code	Standard Abbreviation
0 General	AMBULANCE
1 Supplies	AMBUL/SUPPLY

Code	Description
2 Medical transport	AMBUL/MED TRANS
3 Heart mobile	AMBUL/HEART MOB
4 Oxygen	AMBUL/OXYGEN
5 Air ambulance	AIR AMBULANCE
6 Neo-natal ambulance services	AMBUL/NEONAT
7 Pharmacy	AMBUL/PHARMAS
8 EKG transmission	AMBUL/EKG TRANS
9 Other ambulance	AMBUL/OTHER

055X Home Health (HH)—Skilled Nursing

Subcategory Code	Standard Abbreviation
0 General	SKILLED NURSING-HH
1 - Visit charge	SKILLED NURS-VISIT
2 - Hourly charge	SKILLED NURS-HOUR
9 - Other skilled nursing	SKILLED NURS-OTHER

056X Home Health (HH)—Medical Social Services

Subcategory Code	Standard Abbreviation
0 General	MED SOCIAL-HH
1 Visit charge	MED SOC SVCS-VISIT
2 Hourly charge	MED SOC SVCS-HOUR
9 Other med social services	MED SOC SVCS-OTHER

057X Home Health (HH) Aid

Subcategory Code	Standard Abbreviation
0 General	HH AIDE
1 Visit charge	HH AIDE-VISIT
2 Hourly charge	HH AIDE-HOUR
9 Other home health aide	HH AIDE-OTHER

Code	Description
058X Home Health (HH)—Other Visits	

Subcategory Code	Standard Abbreviation
0 General	HH-OTH VIS
1 Visit charge	HH-OTH VIS/VISIT
2 Hourly charge	HH-OTH VIS/HOUR
3 Assessment	HH-OTH VIS/ASSESS
9 Other home health visits	HH-OTH VIS/OTHER

059X Home Health (HH)—Units of Service

Subcategory Code	Standard Abbreviation
0 General	HH-SVCS/UNIT

060X Home Health (HH)—Oxygen

Subcategory Code	Standard Abbreviation
0 General	02/HOME HEALTH
1 Oxygen—Stat/equip/ supply or contents	02/STAT EQUIP/ SUPPL/CONT
2 Oxygen—Stat/equip/ under 1 LPM	02/STAT EQP/ SUPPL<1 LPM
3 Oxygen—Stat/equip/ over 4 LPM	02/STAT EQP/ SUPPL>4 LPM
4 Oxygen—Portable add-on	02/PORTABLE ADD-ON
9 Oxygen—Other	02/OTHER

061X Magnetic Resonance Technology (MRT)

Subcategory Code	Standard Abbreviation
0 General	MRT
1 Brain (including brain stem)	MRI/BRAIN
2 Spinal cord (including spine)	MRI/SPINE
4 MRI—Other	MRI/OTHER
5 MRA—Head and neck	MRA/HEAD & NECK
6 MRA - Lower extremities	MRA/LOWER EXTRM

Code	Description
8 MRA—Other	MRA/OTHER
9 Other MRT	MRT/OTHER

062X Medical/ Surgical Supplies—Extension of 027X

Subcategory Code	Standard Abbreviation
1 Supplies incident to radiology	MED SURG SUPL-INCDT RAD
2 Supplies incident to other diagnostic services	MED SURG SUPL-INCDT ODX
3 Surgical dressings	SURG DRESSINGS
4 FDA investigational devices	FDA INVEST DEVICE

063X Pharmacy—Extension of 025X

Subcategory Code	Standard Abbreviation
1 Single source drug	DRUG/SINGLE
2 Multiple source drug	DRUG/MULTIPLE
3 Restrictive prescription	DRUG/RESTRICT
4 EPO, less than 10,000 units	DRUG/EPO<10,000 UNITS
5 EPO, 10,000 or more units	DRUG/EPO≥10,000 UNITS
6 Drugs requiring detailed coding	DRUGS/DETAIL CODE
7 Self-administrable drugs	DRUGS/SELFADMIN

064X Home IV Therapy Services

Subcategory Code	Standard Abbreviation
0 General	IV THERAPY SVC
1 Nonroutine nursing, central line	NON RT NURSING/ CENTRAL
2 IV site care, central line	IV SITE CARE/ CENTRAL
3 IV start/care, peripheral line	IV STRT&CARE/ PERIPHRL

Code	Description
4 Nonroutine nursing, peripheral line	NONRT NURSING/ PERIPHRL
5 Training patient/ caregiver, central line	TRNG PT/CAREGVR/ CENTRAL
6 Training disabled patient, central line	TRNG DSBLPT/ CENTRAL
7 Training patient/ caregiver, peripheral line	TRNG/PT/CARGVR/ PERIPHRL
8 Training disabled patient, peripheral line	TRNG/DSBLPT/ PERIPHRL
9 Other IV therapy services	OTHER IV THERAPY SVC

065X Hospice Services

Subcategory Code	Standard Abbreviation
0 General	HOSPICE
1 Routine home care	HOSPICE/RTN HOME
2 Continuous home care	HOSPICE/CTNS HOME
5 Inpatient respite care	HOSPICE/IP RESPITE
6 General inpatient care (nonrespite)	HOSPICE/IP NON- RESPITE
7 Physician services	HOSPICE/PHYSICIAN
8 Hospice room & board – nursing facility	HOSPICE/R&B NURSE FAC
9 Other hospice service	HOSPICE/OTHER

066X Respite Care (HHA only)

Subcategory Code	Standard Abbreviation
0 General	RESPITE CARE
1 Hourly charge/nursing	RESPITE/NURSING
2 Hourly charge/home health aide/homemaker/ companion	RESPITE/AIDE/ HMEMKR/COMP
3 Daily respite charge	RESPITE/DAILY
9 Other respite care	RESPITE/OTHER

Code	Description
067X Outpatient Special Residence Charges	
Subcategory Code	*Standard Abbreviation*
0 General	OP SPEC RES
1 Hospital-owned	OP SPEC RES/HOSP OWNED
2 Contracted	OP SPEC RES/ CONTRACTED
9 Other special residence charges	OP SPEC RES/ OTHER
068X Trauma Response	
Subcategory Code	*Standard Abbreviation*
1 Level I Trauma	TRAUMA LEVEL I
2 Level II Trauma	TRAUMA LEVEL II
3 Level III Trauma	TRAUMA LEVEL III
4 Level IV Trauma	TRAUMA LEVEL IV
9 Other Trauma Response	TRAUMA OTHER
069X Not Assigned	
070X Cast Room	
Subcategory Code	*Standard Abbreviation*
0 General	CAST ROOM
071X Recovery Room	
Subcategory Code	*Standard Abbreviation*
0 General	RECOVERY ROOM
072X Labor Room/Delivery	
Subcategory Code	*Standard Abbreviation*
0 General	DELIVERY ROOM/ LABOR
1 Labor	LABOR
2 Delivery room	DELIVERY ROOM
3 Circumcision	CIRCUMCISION

Code	Description
4 Birthing center	BIRTHING CNTR
9 Other labor room/ delivery	OTHER/DELIV- LABOR
073X EKG/ECG (Electrocardiogram)	
Subcategory Code	*Standard Abbreviation*
0 General	EKG/ECG
1 Holter monitor	HOLTER MONT
2 Telemetry	TELEMETRY
9 Other EKG/ECG	OTHER EKG/ ECG
074X EEG (Electroencephalogram)	
Subcategory Code	*Standard Abbreviation*
0 General	EEG
075X Gastro-Intestinal Services	
Subcategory Code	*Standard Abbreviation*
0 General	GASTRO-INTSTL SVCS
076X Specialty Room—Treatment/Observation Room	
Subcategory Code	*Standard Abbreviation*
0 General	SPECIALTY ROOM
1 Treatment room	TREATMENT RM
2 Observation room	OBSERVATION RM
9 Other specialty rooms	OTHER SPECIALTY RMS
077X Preventive Care Services	
Subcategory Code	*Standard Abbreviation*
0 General	PREVENT CARE SVCS
1 Vaccine administration	VACCINE ADMIN
078X Telemedicine	
Subcategory Code	*Standard Abbreviation*
0 General	TELEMEDICINE

Code	Description
079X Extra-Corporeal Shock Wave Therapy	
Subcategory Code	*Standard Abbreviation*
0 General	ESWT
080X Inpatient Renal Dialysis	
Subcategory Code	*Standard Abbreviation*
0 General	RENAL DIALYSIS
1 Inpatient hemodialysis	DIALY/INPATIENT
2 Inpatient peritoneal (Non-CAPD)	DIALY/IP/PER
3 Inpatient continuous ambulatory peritoneal dialysis (CAPD)	DIALY/IP/CAPD
4 Inpatient continuous cycling peritoneal dialysis (CCPD)	DAILY/IP/CCPD
9 Other inpatient dialysis	DIALY/IP/OTHER
081X Acquisition of Body Components	
Subcategory Code	*Standard Abbreviation*
0 General	ORGAN ACQUISIT
1 Living donor	LIVING DONOR
2 Cadaver donor	CADAVER DONOR
3 Unknown donor	UNKNOWN DONOR
4 Unsuccessful organ search donor bank charge	UNSUCCESSFUL SEARCH
9 Other donor	OTHER DONOR
082X Hemodialysis—Outpatient or Home Dialysis	
Subcategory Code	*Standard Abbreviation*
0 General	HEMO/OP OR HOME
1 Hemodialysis/composite or other rate	HEMO/COMPOSITE
2 Home supplies	HEMO/HOME/SUPPL

Code	Description
3 Home equipment	HEMO/HOME/EQUIP
4 Maintenance/100 percent	HEMO/HOME/100%
5 Support services	HEMO/HOME/SUPSERV
9 Other outpatient hemodialysis	HEMO – OTHER OP
083X Peritoneal Dialysis—Outpatient or Home	
Subcategory Code	*Standard Abbreviation*
0 General	PERITONEAL/OP OR HOME
1 Peritoneal/composite or other rate	PERTNL/COMPOSITE
2 Home supplies	PERTNL/HOME/SUPPL
3 Home Equipment	PERTNL/HOME/EQUIP
4 Maintenance/100 percent	PERTNL/HOME/100%
5 Support services	PERTNL/HOME/SUPSERV
9 Other outpatient peritoneal dialysis	PERTNL/HOME/OTHER
084X Continuous Ambulatory Peritoneal Dialysis (CAPD)—Outpatient or Home	
Subcategory Code	*Standard Abbreviation*
0 General	CAPD/OP OR HOME
1 CAPD/composite or other rate	CAPD/COMPOSITE
2 Home supplies	CAPD/HOME/SUPPL
3 Home equipment	CAPD/HOME/EQUIP
4 Maintenance/100 percent	CAPD/HOME/100%
5 Support services	CAPD/HOME/SUPSERV
9 Other outpatient CAPD dialysis	CAPD/HOME/OTHER

Code	Description
085X Continuous Cycling Peritoneal Dialysis (CCPD)—Outpatient or Home	

Subcategory Code	Standard Abbreviation
0 General	CCPD/OP OR HOME
1 CCPD/composite or other rate	CCPD/COMPOSITE
2 Home supplies	CCPD/HOME/SUPPL
3 Home Equipment	CCPD/HOME/EQUIP
4 Maintenance/100 percent	CCPD/HOME/100%
5 Support services	CCPD/HOME/SUPSERV
9 Other outpatient CCPD	CCPD/HOME/OTHER

Code	Description
086X Reserved	
087X Reserved	
088X Miscellaneous Dialysis	

Subcategory Code	Standard Abbreviation
0 General	DIALY/MISC
1 Ultrafiltration	DIALY/ULTRAFILT
2 Home dialysis aid visit	HOME DIALYSIS AID VISIT
9 Other misc. dialysis	DIALY/MISC/OTHER

Code	Description
089X Reserved	
090X Behavioral Health Treatment/Services (also see 091X)	

Subcategory Code	Standard Abbreviation
0 General	BH/TREATMENTS
1 Electroshock treatment	BH/ELECTRO SHOCK
2 Milieu therapy	BH/MILIEU THERAPY
3 Play therapy	BH/PLAY THERAPY
4 Activity therapy	BH/ACTIVITY THERAPY
5 Intensive outpatient services – psychiatric	BH/INTENS OP/ PSYCH

Code	Description
6 Intensive outpatient services – chemical dependency	BH/INTENS OP/ CHEM DEP
7 Community Behavioral Health Program (Day Treatment)	BH/COMMUNITY

Code	Description
091X Behavioral Health Treatments/Services—Ext. of 090X	

Subcategory Code	Standard Abbreviation
1 Rehabilitation	BH/REHAB
2 Partial hospitalization– less intensive	BH/PARTIAL HOSP
3 Partial hospitalization– intensive	BH/PARTIAL INTENSV
4 Individual therapy	BH/INDIV RX
5 Group therapy	BH/GROUP RX
6 Family therapy	BH/FAMILY RX
7 Biofeedback	BH/BIOFEED
8 Testing	BH/TESTING
9 Other behavioral health treatments	BH/OTHER

Code	Description
092X Other Diagnostic Services	

Subcategory Code	Standard Abbreviation
0 General	OTHER DX SVCS
1 Peripheral vascular lab	PERI VASCUL LAB
2 Electromyelogram	EMG
3 Pap smear	PAP SMEAR
4 Allergy test	ALLERGY TEST
5 Pregnancy test	PREG TEST
9 Other diagnostic service	OTHER DX SVCS

Code	Description
093X Medical Rehabilitation Day Program	
Subcategory Code	*Standard Abbreviation*
1 Half day	HALF DAY
2 Full day	FULL DAY
094X Other Therapeutic Services (See also 095X)	
Subcategory Code	*Standard Abbreviation*
0 General	OTHER RX SVCS
1 Recreational therapy	RECREATION RX
2 Education/training	EDUC/TRAINING
3 Cardiac rehabilitation	CARDIAC REHAB
4 Drug rehabilitation	DRUG REHAB
5 Alcohol rehabilitation	ALCOHOL REHAB
6 Complex medical equipment-routine	COMPLX MED EQUIP-ROUT
7 Complex medical equipment-ancillary	COMPLX MED EQUIP-ANC
8 Pulmonary rehabilitation	PULMONARY REHAB
9 Other therapeutic services	ADDITIONAL RX SVCS
095X Other Therapeutic Services—Extension of 094X	
Subcategory Code	*Standard Abbreviation*
1 Athletic training	ATHLETIC TRAINING
2 Kinesiotherapy	KINESIOTHERAPY
096X Professional Fees (See also 097X and 098X)	
Subcategory Code	*Standard Abbreviation*
0 General	PRO FEE
1 Psychiatric	PRO FEE/PSYCH
2 Ophthalmology	PRO FEE/EYE
3 Anesthesiologist (MD)	PRO FEE/ANEST MD
4 Anesthetist (CRNA)	PRO FEE/ANEST CRNA
9 Other professional fees	PRO FEE/OTHER

Code	Description
097X Professional Fees—Extension of 096X	
Subcategory Code	*Standard Abbreviation*
1 Laboratory	PRO FEE/LAB
2 Radiology–diagnostic	PRO FEE/RAD/DX
3 Radiology–therapeutic	PRO FEE/RAD/RX
4 Radiology–nuclear medicine	PRO FEE/NUC MED
5 Operating room	PRO FEE/OR
6 Respiratory therapy	PRO FEE/RESPIR
7 Physical therapy	PRO FEE/PHYSI
8 Occupational therapy	PRO FEE/OCCUPA
9 Speech pathology	PRO FEE/SPEECH
098X Professional Fees—Extension of 096X and 097X	
Subcategory Code	*Standard Abbreviation*
1 Emergency room services	PRO FEE/ER
2 Outpatient services	PRO FEE/OUTPT
3 Clinic	PRO FEE/CLINIC
4 Medical social services	PRO FEE/SOC SVC
5 EKG	PRO FEE/EKG
6 EEG	PRO FEE/EEG
7 Hospital visit	PRO FEE/HOS VIS
8 Consultation	PRO FEE/CONSULT
9 Private duty nurse	PRO FEE/PVT NURSE
099X Patient Convenience Items	
Subcategory Code	*Standard Abbreviation*
0 General	PT CONVENIENCE
1 Cafeteria/guest tray	CAFETERIA
2 Private linen service	LINEN
3 Telephone/telecom	TELEPHONE

Code	Description
4 TV/radio	TV/RADIO
5 Nonpatient room rentals	NONPT ROOM RENT
6 Late discharge charge	LATE DISCHARGE
7 Admission kits	ADM KITS
8 Beauty shop/barber	BARBER/BEAUTY
9 Other convenience items	PT CONV/OTHER

100X Behavioral Health Accommodations

Subcategory Code	Standard Abbreviation
0 General	BH R&B
1 Residential Treatment – Psychiatric	BH R&B RES/PSYCH
2 Residential Treatment – Chemical Dependency	BH R&B RES/CHEM
3 Supervised Living	BH R&B SUP LIVING
4 Halfway House	BH R&B HALFWAY HOUSE
5 Group Home	BH R&B GROUP HOME

101X to 209X Reserved

210X Alternative Therapy Services

Subcategory Code	Standard Abbreviation
0 General	ALTTHERAPY
1 Acupuncture	ACUPUNCTURE
2 Acupressure	ACUPRESSURE
3 Massage	MASSAGE
4 Reflexology	REFLEXOLOGY
5 Biofeedback	BIOFEEDBACK
6 Hypnosis	HYPNOSIS
9 Other alternative therapy services	OTHER ALTTHERAPY

211X to 309X Reserved

310X Adult Care

Subcategory Code	Standard Abbreviation
1 Adult Day Care, Medical & Social Hourly	ADULT MED/SOC HR
2 Adult Day Care, Social – Hourly	ADULT SOC HR
3 Adult Day Care, Medical & Social-Daily	ADULT MED/SOC DAY
4 Adult Day Care, Social-Daily	ADULT SOC DAY
5 Adult Foster Care, Daily	ADULT FOSTER DAY
9 Other Adult Care	OTHER ADULT

311X to 999X Reserved

Description	Revenue Code	Description	Revenue Code
Acupressure	2102	Anesthesia	0370
Activity Therapy, Behavioral Health	0904	Anesthesia incident to other diagnostic services	0372
Acupuncture (Alternative Therapy)	2101	Anesthesia incident to RAD	0371
Acupuncture (Anesthesia)	0374	Angiocardiology	0321
Admission Charge	0221	Arteriography	0323
Admission Kit	0997	Arthrography	0322
Adult Day Care, Med/Soc - Hourly	3101	Athletic Training - Therapeutic	0951
		Audiology	0470
Adult Day Care, Soc – Hourly	3102	Audiology - Diagnostic	0471
Adult Day Care, Med/Soc – Daily	3103	Audiology - Treatment	0472
		Bacteriology and Microbiology	0306
Adult Day Care, Soc – Daily	3104	Barber Shop	0998
Alcohol Rehabilitation	0945	Beauty Shop	0998
All Inclusive Ancillary	0240	Behavioral Health Treatment/ Services	0900
All Inclusive IP Rate plus ancillaries	0100	Biofeedback (Alternative Therapy)	2105
All Inclusive IP Room and Board, no ancillaries	0101	Biofeedback (Behavioral Health Treatments)	0917
Allergy Test	0924	Biopsy	0314
Alternative Therapy Services	2100	Birthing Center	0724
Ambulance	0540	Blood	0380
Ambulance - Air	0545	Blood Administration	0391
Ambulance - Heartmobile	0543	Blood - Leukocytes	0385
Ambulance - Medical Transport	0542	Blood - Other Components	0386
Ambulance - Neo-natal services	0546	Blood - Other Derivatives (Cryoprecipitates)	0387
Ambulance - Oxygen	0544	Blood - Packed Red Cells	0381
Ambulance - Pharmacy	0547	Blood - Plasma	0383
Ambulance - Supplies	0541	Blood - Platelets	0384
Ambulance – EKG transmission	0548	Blood Processing and Storage	0392
Ambulatory Surgical Care	0490	Blood - Whole	0382
Ancillary Charge - All-inclusive	0240		

Revenue Codes: Alphabetical Order (Selected)

Description	Revenue Code	Description	Revenue Code
Burn Care - ICU	0207	CCU - Heart Transplant	0213
Cafeteria Tray	0991	CCU - Intermediate Care	0214
CAPD - Continuous Ambulatory Peritoneal Dialysis, OP or Home	0840	CCU - Myocardial Infarction	0211
		CCU - Pulmonary Care	0212
CAPD/Composite or Other Rate – OP or Home	0841	Chemistry	0301
		Chemotherapy - Injected	0331
CAPD Home Equipment – OP or Home	0843	Chemotherapy - IV	0335
		Chemotherapy - Oral	0332
CAPD Home Supplies – OP or Home	0842	Chest X-Ray	0324
CAPD Maintenance/100 percent – OP or Home	0844	Chronic Pain Center	0511
		Circumcision	0723
CAPD Support Services – OP or Home	0845	Clinic - Chronic Pain Center	0511
		Clinic - Dental	0512
Cardiac Catheterization Lab	0481	Clinic - Family Practice	0517
Cardiac Rehabilitation	0943	Clinic - Family Practice Free Standing	0523
Cardiology	0480		
Cast Room	0700	Clinic - Free Standing	0520
CCPD - Continuous Cycling Peritoneal Dialysis, IP	0804	Clinic - General	0510
		Clinic - OB-GYN	0514
CCPD - Continuous Cycling Peritoneal Dialysis, OP or Home	0850	Clinic - Pediatric	0515
		Clinic - Psychiatric	0513
CCPD/Composite or Other Rate, OP or Home	0851	Clinic - Rural Health Free Standing	0521
CCPD Home Equipment, OP or Home	0853	Clinic - Urgent Care	0516
CCPD Home Supplies, OP or Home	0852	Clinic - Urgent Care Free Standing	0526
CCPD Maintenance/100 percent, OP or Home	0854	Community Behavioral Health Program	0907
CCPD Support Services, OP or Home	0855	Complex Medical Equipment - Ancillary	0947
CCU - Coronary Care Unit	0210	Complex Medical Equipment - Routine	0946

Description	Revenue Code	Description	Revenue Code
Continuous Ambulatory Peritoneal Dialysis (CAPD), IP	0803	Drugs - Erythropoietin (EPO), 10,000 + units	0635
Continuous Ambulatory Peritoneal Dialysis (CAPD), OP or Home	0840	Drugs - Experimental	0256
		Drugs - IV Solutions	0258
Continuous Cycling Peritoneal Dialysis (CCPD), IP	0804	Drugs Incident to Other Diagnostic Services	0254
Continuous Cycling Peritoneal Dialysis (CCPD), OP or Home	0850	Drugs Incident to Radiology	0255
		Drugs – Non-Prescription	0257
Coronary Care	0210	Drugs – Requiring Detailed Coding	0636
CT Scan	0350	Drugs – Restrictive Prescription	0633
CT Scan - Body	0352	Drugs – Self-administrable	0637
CT Scan - Head	0351	Drugs – Take Home	0253
Cytology	0311	Durable Medical Equipment (See also: DME)	0290
Delivery Room	0722		
Dental Clinic	0512	ECG	0730
Devices - Medical	0270	Echocardiology	0483
Devices - Surgical	0270	Education/Training (Therapeutic)	0942
Diagnostic Services - Other	0920	EEG	0740
Dialysis – Home aid visit	0882	EKG	0730
Dialysis - Miscellaneous	0880	Electrocardiogram	0730
Dialysis – Ultrafiltration	0881	Electroencephalogram	0740
DME - Durable Medical Equipment	0290	Electromyelogram	0922
		Electroshock Treatment	0901
DME - Purchase of New DME	0292	Emergency Room	0450
DME - Purchase of Used DME	0293	Emergency Room - Urgent Care	0456
DME - Rental	0291	EMTALA Emergency Medical Screening services	0451
DME - Supplies/Drugs for DME - Home Health Agency only	0294		
		EPO - Erythropoietin	0634 or 0635
Drug Rehabilitation	0944	ER beyond EMTALA Screening	0452
Drugs - Erythropoietin (EPO), <10,000 units	0634		
		Experimental Drugs	0256

Revenue Codes: Alphabetical Order (Selected)

Description	Revenue Code
Extra-Corporeal Shock Wave Therapy	0790
Family Practice Clinic	0517
Family Practice Freestanding Clinic	0523
Family Therapy, Behavioral Health	0916
FDA Investigational Devices	0624
Freestanding Clinic	0520
Gastro-Intestinal Services	0750
Generic Drugs	0251
Group Therapy, Behavioral Health	0915
Guest Tray	0991
Health Insurance Prospective Payment System (HIPPS)	002X
Heart Transplant CCU	0213
Heart Mobile - Ambulance	0543
Hematology	0305
Hemodialysis, IP	0801
Hemodialysis, OP or Home	0820
Hemodialysis/Composite or Other Rate	0821
Hemodialysis - Home Equipment	0823
Hemodialysis - Home Supplies	0822
Hemodialysis - Maintenance/ 100 percent	0824
Hemodialysis - Support Services	0825
Histology	0312
Holter Monitor	0731
Home Health Aide - Home Health Agency only	0570
Home Health Aide, Visit	0571
Home Health Aide, Hourly	0572

Description	Revenue Code
Home Health - Other Visits	0580
Home Health – Other, Visit	0581
Home Health – Other, Hourly	0582
Home Health, Other, Assessment	0583
Home Health - Units of Service	0590
Home IV Therapy Services	0640
Hospice	0650
Hyperbaric Oxygen Therapy	0413
Hypnosis	2106
ICU - Burn Care	0207
ICU - Intensive Care Unit	0200
ICU - Intermediate ICU	0206
ICU - Medical	0202
ICU - Pediatric	0203
ICU - Psychiatric	0204
ICU - Surgical	0201
ICU - Trauma	0208
Imaging Services, Other	0400
Immunology	0302
Incremental Nursing Charge	0230
Incremental Nursing Charge, Nursery	0231
Incremental Nursing Charge, OB	0232
Incremental Nursing Charge, ICU	0233
Incremental Nursing Charge, CCU	0234
Incremental Nursing Charge, Hospice	0235
Individual Therapy, Behavioral Health	0914
Infusion Pump	0261
Inhalation Services	0412

Description	Revenue Code
Inpatient Renal Dialysis	0800
Intensive Care Unit	0200
Intensive Care Unit – Surgical	0201
Intermediate Coronary Care Unit (CCU)	0214
Intermediate Intensive Care Unit (ICU)	0206
Intraocular Lens	0276
IV Solutions - Drugs	0258
IV Therapy	0260
IV Therapy - Pharmacy Svcs	0262
IV Therapy - Supplies	0264
IV Therapy – Drug/Supply/ Delivery	0263
Kinesiotherapy - Therapeutic	0952
Kidney Transplant	0367
Lab - Non-Routine Dialysis	0304
Lab - Renal Patient (Home)	0303
Labor Room - General	0721
Labor Room/Delivery	0720
Laboratory	0300
Laboratory – Chemistry	0301
Laboratory – Hematology	0305
Laboratory – Bacteriology & Microbiology	0306
Laboratory Pathology	0310
Laboratory Pathology – Other	0319
Language Pathology	0440
Language Pathology, Evaluation or Re-evaluation	0444
Late Discharge Charge - Non-Medical	0996

Description	Revenue Code
Late Discharge, Medically Necessary	0224
Leave of Absence (See also: LOA)	0180
Leukocytes	0385
Linen Service - Private	0992
LOA - Leave of Absence	0180
LOA - Nursing home (for hospitalization)	0185
LOA - Patient Convenience	0182
LOA - Therapeutic Leave	0183
Magnetic Resonance Technology - MRT	0610
Mammography, Diagnostic	0401
Mammography, Screening	0403
Massage	2103
Medical Care – ICU	0202
Medical Rehabilitation Day Program - Half Day	0931
Medical Rehabilitation Day Program - Full Day	0932
Medical Social Services - Home Health Agency only	0560
Medical/Surgical Supplies and Devices	0270
Medical Transport - Ambulance	0542
Microbiology	0306
Milieu Therapy – Behavioral Health	0902
Minor Surgery	0361
MRA - Head and Neck	0615
MRA - Lower Extremities	0616
MRA – Other	0618

Revenue Codes: Alphabetical Order (Selected)

Description	Revenue Code
MRI - Brain (Including Brain Stem)	0611
MRI - Spinal Cord (Including Spine)	0612
MRI – Other	0614
Multiple Source Drug	0632
Myocardial Infarction - CCU	0211
Non-Generic Drugs	0252
Non-Prescription Drugs	0257
Nuclear Medicine	0340
Nuclear Medicine - Diagnostic	0341
Nuclear Medicine - Therapeutic	0342
Nursery	0170
Nursery - Newborn - Level I	0171
Nursery - Newborn - Level II	0172
Nursery - Newborn - Level III	0173
Nursery - Newborn - Level IV	0174
Nursing Increments - Charge Rate	0230
OB-GYN Clinic	0514
Observation Room	0762
Occupational Therapy	0430
Occupational Therapy Evaluation or re-evaluation	0434
Occupational Therapy Group Rate	0433
Occupational Therapy Hourly charge	0432
Occupational Therapy Visit charge	0431
Oncology	0280
Operating Room Services	0360
Organ Acquisition	0810
Organ Donor - Cadaver	0812

Description	Revenue Code
Organ Donor - Living	0811
Organ Donor - Unknown	0813
Organ Transplant - Other than Kidney	0362
Osteopathic Services	0530
Osteopathic Therapy	0531
Outpatient Services	0500
Outpatient Services – Intensive Psych.	0905
Outpatient Services – Intensive Chemical Dependency	0906
Outpatient Special Residence Charges	0670
Oxygen - Home Health Agency only	0600
Oxygen Take Home	0277
Pacemaker	0275
Packed Red Blood Cells	0381
Pap Smear	0923
Partial Hospitalization, Psych - Intensive	0913
Partial Hospitalization, Psych - Less Intensive.	0912
Patient Convenience Items	0990
Patient Convenience Items - Admission Kits	0997
Patient Convenience Items - Beauty Shop/Barber	0998
Patient Convenience Items - Cafeteria/Guest Tray	0991
Patient Convenience Items - Non-Patient Room Rentals	0995

Description	Revenue Code
Patient Convenience Items - Private Linen Service	0992
Patient Convenience Items - Telephone/Telecom	0993
Patient Convenience Items - TV/Radio	0994
Pediatric Care – ICU	0203
Pediatric Clinic	0515
Peripheral Vascular Lab	0921
Peritoneal Dialysis (non-CAPD), IP	0802
Peritoneal Dialysis, OP or Home	0830
Peritoneal Dialysis/Composite or other rate	0831
Peritoneal Dialysis - Home Equipment	0833
Peritoneal Dialysis - Home Supplies	0832
Peritoneal Dialysis - Maintenance/100 percent	0834
Peritoneal Dialysis - Support Services	0835
PET Scan - Positron Emission Tomography	0404
Pharmacy	0250
Physical Therapy	0420
Physical Therapy - Visit	0421
Physical Therapy - Evaluation or Re-evaluation	0424
Plasma	0383
Platelets	0384
Play Therapy, Behavioral Health	0903
Positron Emission Tomography	0404
Pregnancy Test	0925

Description	Revenue Code
Preventive Care Services	0770
Private-duty Nurse	0989
Professional Fees	0960
Professional Fees - Anesthesiologist (MD)	0963
Professional Fees - Anesthetist (CRNA))	0964
Professional Fees - Clinic	0983
Professional Fees - Consultation	0988
Professional Fees - EEG	0986
Professional Fees - EKG	0985
Professional Fees - Emergency Room	0981
Professional Fees - Hospital Visit	0987
Professional Fees - Laboratory	0971
Professional Fees - Medical Social Services	0984
Professional Fees - Occupational Therapy	0978
Professional Fees - Ophthalmology	0962
Professional Fees - Outpatient Services	0982
Professional Fees - Physical Therapy	0977
Professional Fees - Private-duty Nurse	0989
Professional Fees - Psychiatric	0961
Professional Fees - Radiology - Diagnostic	0972
Professional Fees - Radiology - Nuclear Medicine	0974
Professional Fees - Radiology - Therapeutic	0973

Revenue Codes: Alphabetical Order (Selected)

Description	Revenue Code	Description	Revenue Code
Professional Fees - Respiratory Therapy	0976	Room & Board - Private 1 bed - Hospice	0115
Professional Fees - Speech Pathology	0979	Room & Board - Private 1 bed - Medical/Surgical/Gyn	0111
Prosthetic/Orthotic Devices	0274	Room & Board - Private 1 Bed - OB	0112
Psychiatric Care - ICU	0204	Room & Board - Private 1 Bed - Oncology	0117
Psychiatric Clinic	0513	Room & Board - Private 1 Bed - Pediatric	0113
Pulmonary Care - CCU	0212	Room & Board - Private 1 Bed - Psychiatric	0114
Pulmonary Function	0460	Room & Board - Private 1 Bed – Rehabilitation	0118
Pulmonary Rehabilitation	0948	Room & Board – Deluxe Private	0140
Radiation Therapy	0333	Room & Board – Deluxe Private – Detoxification	0146
Radiology - Diagnostic	0320	Room & Board – Deluxe Private - Hospice	0145
Radiology – Therapeutic and/or Chemotherapy	0330	Room & Board – Deluxe Private - Medical/Surgical/Gyn	0141
Radiopharmaceuticals, Diagnostic	0343	Room & Board – Deluxe Private - OB	0142
Radiopharmaceuticals, Therapeutic	0344	Room & Board – Deluxe Private - Oncology	0147
Recovery Room	0710	Room & Board – Deluxe Private - Pediatric	0143
Recreational Therapy	0941	Room & Board – Deluxe Private - Psychiatric	0144
Reflexology	2104	Room & Board – Deluxe Private – Rehabilitation	0148
Rehabilitation, Behavioral Health	0911	Room & Board – Self care	0167
Renal Dialysis - Inpatient	0800	Room & Board - Semi-Private 2 Bed - (Medical or General)	0120
Respiratory Services	0410		
Respite Care - Home Health Agency only	0660		
Room & Board - All inclusive IP Rate plus ancillaries	0100		
Room & Board - All inclusive IP Rate, no ancillaries	0101		
Room & Board - Private 1 Bed (Medical or General)	0110		
Room & Board - Private 1 Bed – Detoxification	0116		

Description	Revenue Code
Room & Board - Semi-Private 2 Bed – Detoxification	0126
Room & Board - Semi-Private 2 Bed – Hospice	0125
Room & Board - Semi-Private 2 Bed - Medical/Surgical/Gyn	0121
Room & Board - Semi-Private 2 Bed - OB	0122
Room & Board - Semi-Private 2 Bed - Oncology	0127
Room & Board - Semi-Private 2 Bed – Pediatric	0123
Room & Board - Semi-Private 2 Bed – Psychiatric	0124
Room & Board - Semi-Private 2 Bed – Rehabilitation	0128
Room & Board – Sterile environment	0164
Room & Board - 3 & 4 Beds - General	0130
Room & Board - 3 & 4 Beds - Detoxification	0136
Room & Board - 3 & 4 Beds - Hospice	0135
Room & Board - 3 & 4 Beds - Medical/Surgical/Gyn	0131
Room & Board - 3 & 4 Beds - OB	0132
Room & Board - 3 & 4 Beds - Oncology	0137
Room & Board - 3 & 4 Beds - Pediatric	0133
Room & Board - 3 & 4 Beds - Psychiatric	0134

Description	Revenue Code
Room & Board - 3 & 4 Beds - Rehabilitation	0138
Room & Board - Ward - 5 or More Beds (Medical or General)	0150
Room & Board - Ward - Detoxification	0156
Room & Board - Ward - Hospice	0155
Room & Board - Ward - Medical/Surgical/Gyn	0151
Room & Board Ward - OB	0152
Room & Board - Ward - Oncology	0157
Room & Board - Ward - Pediatric	0153
Room & Board - Ward - Psychiatric	0154
Room & Board - Ward - Rehabilitation	0158
Rural Health Freestanding Clinic	0521
Rural Health Home Freestanding Clinic	0522
Self-administrable Drugs	0637
Skilled Nursing – Home Health	0550
Skilled Nursing – Home Health, Visit	0551
Skilled Nursing – Home Health, Hourly	0552
Single Source Drug	0631
Special Charges	0220
Specialty Room – Treatment/ Observation	0760
Speech - Language Pathology	0440
Speech - Language Pathology Evaluation or re-evaluation	0444

Revenue Codes: Alphabetical Order (Selected)

Description	Revenue Code	Description	Revenue Code
Speech Therapy	0440	Take-home Supplies	0273
Speech Therapy Evaluation or re-evaluation	0444	Telemedicine	0780
		Telemetry	0732
Speech Therapy Group Rate	0443	Telephone Service	0993
Speech Therapy Hourly Charge	0442	Testing, Behavioral Health	0918
Speech Therapy Visit Charge	0441	Therapeutic Services - Other	0940
Sterile environment, Room & Board	0164	Total Charges	0001
Stress Test	0482	Training - Caregiver of Home IV Therapy Services, peripheral line	0647
Subacute Care	0190	Training - Patient of Home IV Therapy Services, peripheral line	0647
Subacute Care - Level I	0191		
Subacute Care - Level II	0192	Trauma Care - ICU	0208
Subacute Care - Level III	0193	Trauma Response – Level I	0681
Subacute Care - Level IV	0194	Treatment Room	0761
Supplies - Incident to Other Diagnostic Services	0622	TV Service	0994
		Ultrasound	0402
Supplies - Incident to Radiology	0621	Units of Service (Home Health)	0590
Supplies – Medical	0270	Urgent Care - In Emergency Room	0456
Supplies - Non-Sterile	0271		
Supplies - Sterile	0272	Urgent Care Clinic	0516
Supplies - Surgical	0270	Urgent Care Freestanding Clinic	0526
Supplies – Surgical dressings	0623		
Supplies - Take-Home	0273	Urology	0307
Surgical Care - ICU	0201	Vaccine Administration	0771
Take-home Drugs	0253	Whole Blood	0382

Abbreviations

AAPC   American Academy of Professional Coders

AAMT   American Association for Medical Transcription

ABN   Advance Beneficiary Notice of Noncoverage

AHIMA   American Health Information Management Association

AMA   American Medical Association

ANSI   American National Standards Institute

APC   ambulatory patient classification

AR   accounts receivable

ASC   ambulatory surgical center

ASU   ambulatory surgical unit

BCBS   Blue Cross and Blue Shield

CAH   critical access hospital

CC   comorbidities and complications

CCI   Correct Coding Initiative (Medicare)

CCYY   year, indicates entry of four digits for the century (CC) and year (YY)

CDM   charge description master

CE   covered entity

CHAMPVA   Civilian Health and Medical Program of the Department of Veterans Affairs

CLIA   Clinical Laboratory Improvement Amendment

CMI   case mix index

CMS   Centers for Medicare and Medicaid Services

CMS-1450   UB-04; hospital claim form

CMS-1500   physician claim form

COB   coordination of benefits

COBRA   Consolidated Omnibus Budget Reconciliation Act of 1985

CORF   comprehensive outpatient rehabilitation facility

CPT-4   Current Procedural Terminology, Fourth Edition

CRCS   Civil Service Retirement System

CWF   Common Working File (Medicare)

DCN   Document Control Number

DEERS   Defense Enrollment Eligibility Reporting System (TRICARE)

DME   durable medical equipment

DMERC   Durable Medical Equipment Regional Carrier

DNFB   discharged/not final bill

DOS   date of service

DRG   diagnosis-related group

Dx   diagnosis

E/M code   Evaluation and Management code

EDI   electronic data interchange

EGHP   employer-group health plan

EHR   electronic health record

EIN   Employer Identification Number

EMC   electronic media claim

EMTALA   Emergency Medical Treatment and Labor Act of 1986

EOB   explanation of benefits

EOC   episode of care

EPSDT   Early and Periodic Screening, Diagnosis, and Treatment

ER   emergency room

ERA   electronic remittance advice

ERISA Employee Retirement Income Security Act of 1974

ESRD end-stage renal disease

FECA Federal Employee Compensation Act

FEHBP Federal Employees Health Benefits Program

FERS Federal Employees Retirement System

FI fiscal intermediary

FICA Federal Insurance Contribution Act

FL form locator

FMAP Federal Medicaid Assistance Percentage

FMR focused medical review

GHP group health plan

HCIN health insurance claim number

HCPCS Health Care Common Procedure Coding System

HHA home health agency

HHS Health and Human Services Department

HIM health information management

HINN Hospital-Issued Notice of Noncoverage

HIPAA Health Insurance Portability and Accountability Act of 1996

HIPPS Health Insurance Prospective Payment System

HMO health maintenance organization

ICD-9-CM International Classification of Diseases, Ninth Revision, Clinical Modification

ICF intermediate care facility

ICN Internal Control Number

ID, I.D. identification

IP inpatient

IPPS (acute care hospital) Inpatient Prospective Payment System

IV intravenous

JCAHO Joint Commission (formerly Joint Commission on Accreditation of Healthcare Organizations)

LCD local coverage determination (Medicare)

LGHP large group health plan

LOA leave of absence days

LOS length of stay

LRD Lifetime Reserve Days

MAC Medicare Administrative Contractor

MCC major complication or comorbidity

MCE Medicare Code Editor

MCM Medicare Carriers Manual

MCO managed care organization

MDC major diagnostic category

MFS Medicare fee schedule

MS-DRG Medicare-Severity DRG

MSN Medicare summary notice

MSP Medicare Secondary Payer

MTF military treatment facility

NCCI National Correct Coding Initiative

NCD national coverage determination (Medicare)

NCHS National Center for Health Statistics

NCQA National Committee for Quality Assurance

NPI National Provider Identifier

NPP Notice of Privacy Practices

NUBC National Uniform Billing Committee

NUCC National Uniform Claim Committee

OCE Outpatient Code Editor

OCR Office of Civil Rights

OIG Office of the Inspector General

OMP Original Medicare Plan

OP outpatient

OPPS Outpatient Prospective Payment System

OR operating room

OSHA Occupational Safety and Health Administration

OWCP Office of Workers' Compensation Programs

PCM primary care manager (TRICARE)

PCP primary care physician

Abbreviations

PHI protected health information

PHS Public Health Service

PIN provider identifier number

PM program memorandum

POA present on admission

POS (1) place of service; (2) point of service

PPO preferred provider organization

PPS prospective payment system

QUAL qualifier

QIO Quality Improvement Organization

RA remittance advice

RW relative weight

SAD self-administered drug

SI status indicator

SNF skilled nursing facility

TCS (HIPAA Electronic) Transaction and Code Sets

TOB type of bill

TOS time of service

TPO treatment, payment, and operations

TRICARE formerly CHAMPUS (Civilian Health and Medical Program of the Uniformed Services)

UB-04 hospital claim form; CMS-1450

UHDDS Uniform Hospital Discharge Data Set

UPIN unique physician identifier number

UR utilization review

URAC Utilization Review Accreditation Commission (also American Accreditation Healthcare Commission)

VA Veterans Affairs

Glossary

abuse   Improper billing practices, such as billing for a noncovered service or misusing codes on a claim.

access   The ability to obtain needed health care services.

accommodation revenue code   A revenue code that reports a particular bed/accommodation/board charge of a facility on a UB-04 claim.

accounts receivable (AR)   Amount of money owed to a facility by patients and payers.

accredited   Health care organization or facility that has met quality standards set by private national groups.

acute care facility   A health care facility that provides continuous professional medical care to patients with acute conditions or illnesses.

adjustment   An amount (positive or negative) entered in a billing program to change an account balance.

Administrative Simplification   A part of HIPAA that requires the health care industry to use certain standards for the electronic exchange of health care data to protect confidentiality of patient's records. It is in Title II.

admission   The registration process in which patients enter the facility for care.

admission date   The date a patient was admitted for inpatient care, outpatient service, or start of care.

admitting diagnosis (ADX)   The disease or condition that is the reason for the patient's admission for care.

Advance Beneficiary Notice of Noncoverage (ABN)   A notice that a facility should give a Medicare beneficiary to sign if Medicare will probably not pay for the services that the patient will receive; used to establish the patient's responsibility for payment.

aging   The classification of accounts receivable by the amount of time they are past due.

all-inclusive rate   A fixed amount charged on a daily basis during a patient's hospitalization or a total rate charged for an entire stay.

ambulatory payment classification (APC)   A Medicare payment classification for outpatient services.

ambulatory surgical center (ASC)   A health care facility providing surgical services only on an outpatient basis.

ancillary charge   Fee for services other than room and board provided during a patient's hospitalization, such as anesthesia, pharmacy, supplies, and therapies.

ancillary service revenue code   A revenue code used on a UB-04 claim to report services, other than routine room and board charges, that are incidental to the hospital stay.

American Academy of Professional Coders (AAPC)   National association that fosters the establishment and maintenance of professional, ethical, and educational standards for all parties concerned with procedural coding.

American Association for Medical Transcription (AAMT)   National association fostering the profession of medical transcription.

American Health Information Management Association (AHIMA)   A National association of health information management professionals; promotes valid, accessible, yet confidential health information and advocates quality health care.

American Medical Association (AMA)   Member organization for physicians; goals are to promote the art and science of medicine, improve public health, and promote ethical, educational, and clinical standards for the medical profession.

American National Standards Institute (ANSI)   Organization that sets standards for electronic date interchange on a national level.

appeal   A request sent to a payer for reconsideration of a claim denial or partial payment.

assignment of benefits   Authorization by a policyholder that allows a payer to pay benefits directly to a health care provider. Under Medicare, when the payment is made directly to a provider who is accepting assignment, the assignment is also an agreement to accept Medicare's payment as payment in full and not to bill the patient for any amount that exceeds the DRG or allowance amount, except for a deductible and/or coinsurance amount or for noncovered services.

attending physician   The clinician primarily responsible for the care of the patient from the hospital admission through discharge or transfer.

base rate   Under the Medicare Inpatient Prospective Payment System, a number which is calculated based on a hospital's costs, wage index, and location, and is used in determining what a hospital will be paid for a particular DRG.

basic medical care plan   An insurance plan that provides limited hospital, surgical, and medical benefits.

benchmark   To compare something against a standard, such as an activity looked at in an audit that is compared against a HIPAA standard.

beneficiary   A person eligible to receive benefits under a health plan.

benefit period   The method used by Medicare to measure a beneficiary's use of hospital and skilled nursing facility services; see also *spell of illness.*

capitation   A fixed amount per person, per time period paid by a purchaser, such as a health plan, to a health care provider to supply covered health services to beneficiaries during the period.

carrier   (1) An insurance company; (2) a private company that has a contract with Medicare to process Medicare Part B bills.

carrier code   The code assigned to an insurance carrier for UB-04 claim processing.

case mix   The mix of patients treated in a facility based on a patient classification system such as DRGs.

case mix index (CMI)   A measure of the clinical severity or resource requirements of the patients in a particular hospital or treated by a particular clinician during a specific time period.

cash deductible   The amount of a patient's payment that is applied to a patient's deductible for a particular health plan.

CCI column 1/column 2 code pair edits   Medicare code edit under which CPT codes in column 2 will not be paid if reported for the same patient on the same day of service by the same provider as the column 1 code.

CCI mutually exclusive edits   CCI edits for codes for services that could not have reasonably been done during a single patient encounter, so both will not be paid by Medicare. Only the lower-paid code is reimbursed.

CC and MCC lists   Medicare lists containing the ICD-9-CM codes for the secondary diagnoses that are considered significant acute diseases, acute exacerbations of significant chronic diseases, or other chronic conditions that have an effect on the use of hospital resources and can therefore be assigned as CCs or MCCs under the MS-DRG system.

Centers for Medicare and Medicaid Services (CMS)   Federal agency within the Department of Health and Human Services that runs Medicare, Medicaid, Clinical Laboratories, and other governmental health programs. Formerly known as the Health Care Financing Administration (HCFA).

charge description master (CDM)   A hospital's list of the codes and charges for its services.

charge explode   A billing system feature that stores all charges for particular services; when a service is provided, the system automatically bills all of its component charges.

charge slip   A form that lists the typical major services a facility department provides.

Civilian Health and Medical Program of the Veterans Administration (CHAMPVA)   The Civilian Health and Medical Program of the Veterans Administration (now known as the Department of Veterans Affairs) that shares health care costs for families of veterans with 100 percent service-connected disability and the surviving spouses and children of veterans who die from service-connected disabilities.

claim denial   A payer's determination that a claim will not be paid; a denial can be appealed.

claim rejection   A payer's determination that a claim is not ready for processing; the claim is returned to the sender for revision.

clean claim   A claim that meets all of a payer's specifications and edits.

clearinghouse A company that offers providers, for a fee, the service of receiving electronic/paper claims, checking and preparing them for processing, and transmitting them in proper data format to the correct carriers.

clinic An outpatient facility that provides scheduled medical services for patients.

CMS-1450 The Medicare-required Part A (hospital) claim form; also known as the UB-04 and formerly called the HCFA-1450.

CMS-1500 The Medicare-required Part B (physician) claim form; also known as the Universal Health Insurance Claim form and formerly called the HCFA-1500.

code set Alphabetic and/or numeric representations for data. Medical code sets are systems of medical terms that are required for HIPAA transactions. Administrative (nonmedical) code sets, such as taxonomy codes and ZIP codes, are also used in HIPAA transactions.

coinsurance The portion of charges that an insured person must pay for health care services after payment of the deductible amount; usually stated as a percentage.

coinsurance days Under Medicare Part A, for the 61st through 90th day of hospitalization in a benefit period, a daily amount (equal to 25% of the inpatient hospital deductible) for which the beneficiary is responsible.

comorbidity Admitted patient's coexisting condition that affects the length of the hospital stay or the course of treatment.

complete procedure Under the CPT procedural coding system, most surgical codes represent groups of procedures that include all routine elements, such as the operation, local anesthesia, and routine follow-up care. Facilities report these codes to charge for their service associated with the procedure.

compliance Actions that satisfy official guidelines and requirements.

compliance plan A medical practice's written plan for the following: the appointment of a compliance officer and committee; a code of conduct for physicians' business arrangements and employees' compliance; training plans; properly prepared and updated coding tools such as job reference aids, encounter forms, and documentation templates; rules for prompt identification and refunding of overpayments; and ongoing monitoring and auditing of claim preparation.

compliance program guidance Guidance issued by the Office of the Inspector General (OIG) for a specific covered entity with descriptions of what that entity should include in their compliance plan in order to uncover and correct compliance problems connected with HIPAA violations, fraud, and abuse.

complication Condition an admitted patient develops after surgery or treatment that affects the length of hospital stay or the course of further treatment.

comprehensive outpatient rehabilitation facility (CORF) A facility that provides physician-supervised rehabilitation services, such as physical, occupational, and speech therapies, to patients who do not require an overnight stay.

condition code A two-digit numeric or alphanumeric code used to report a special condition or unique circumstance about a claim.

conditional payment A payment from Medicare requested in advance of a primary payer's payment when Medicare is the secondary payer and the provider believes the primary payer will not pay promptly (within 100 days) due to liability issues.

consumer-driven health plan (CDHP) Type of medical insurance that combines a high-deductible health plan with a medical savings plan which covers some out-of-pocket expenses.

continuing claim A claim that is submitted after an initial or subsequent bill has been sent for the same confinement or course of treatment; it is anticipated that subsequent bills will be submitted.

conventions Typographic techniques or standard practices that provide visual guidelines for understanding printed material.

coordination of benefits (COB) A clause in an insurance policy that explains how the policy will pay if more than one insurance policy applies to the claim.

copayment (copay) An amount that an insured person must pay for each health care service encounter.

Correct Coding Initiative (CCI) Medicare's national coding policy, under which mutually exclusive services and comprehensive/component edits are set up as the basis for computerized claim review.

cost-based reimbursement The method Medicare initially used to pay health care facilities for services furnished to beneficiaries. Payment was based on providers' costs as reported annually.

cost outlier Payment made by Medicare in addition to a regular DRG payment when a patient in a particular DRG has an exceptionally high cost compared to other similar patients.

covered days The number of days of inpatient care that are covered by primary insurance benefits.

covered entity A health plan, a health care clearinghouse, or a health care provider who transmits any health information in electronic form in connection with a HIPAA transaction.

covered services The patient services that are covered by primary insurance benefits.

critical access hospital (CAH) A freestanding hospital emergency department.

crosswalk A comparison or map of the codes for the same or similar classifications under two coding systems; it serves as a guide for selecting the closest match.

Current Procedural Terminology,* Fourth Edition *(CPT) Publication of the American Medical Association containing a standardized classification system for reporting medical procedures and services.

deductible An amount that an insured person must pay, usually on an annual basis, for health care services before a payer's insurance payment begins.

de-identified health information Medical data from which individual identifiers have been removed; also known as a redacted or blinded record.

delimiter A character or symbol used in printed material to visually separate one group of words or values from another.

demographics Information about a patient, such as name, address, Social Security number, employment, and insurance carrier data.

detail-level code The fourth digit of a revenue code defines the detail description of the code; the general classification is indicated by a zero (such as 0430, the general classification for Occupational Therapy) and the detail-level codes—the numbers 1 through 9—represent different details for that particular revenue code (such as 0443 to report a group rate for Occupational Therapy).

development The process of determining the primary payer for an insurance claim; often used with the Medicare Secondary Payer program to describe the series of questions asked of patients to find out whether they are beneficiaries of insurance other than Medicare.

diagnosis A physician's opinion of the nature of a patient's illness or injury.

diagnosis code The number assigned to a diagnosis in the *International Classification of Diseases.*

diagnosis-related groups (DRGs) A system of analyzing conditions and treatments for similar groups of patients used to establish Medicare fees for hospital inpatient services; patients are classified by their principal diagnosis, surgical procedure, age, and other factors.

discharge Release of a patient from a facility, including those who have died and those who are transferred to another facility.

discharge date Date a patient is released from a facility.

DNFB (discharged/not final bill) list A hospital list containing the accounts of patients who have been discharged but whose claims have not yet been transmitted to payers, used by hospitals to measure the timeliness of their billing process.

DRG weight Under the Medicare Inpatient Prospective Payment System, a national relative amount assigned to each DRG that represents the average resources required to care for cases in that particular DRG relative to the average resources used to treat cases in all DRGs.

durable medical equipment (DME) Medicare term for reusable physical supplies such as wheelchairs and hospital beds.

Durable Medical Equipment Regional Carriers (DMERCs) Medicare contractors that process claims for durable medical equipment, prosthetics, orthotics, and supplies.

E code An alphanumeric code in the ICD that identifies an external cause of injury or poisoning.

edits Computer programs that third-party payers use to find coding problems and inconsistencies on insurance claims.

837I HIPAA-mandated electronic transaction for hospital claims.

837P HIPAA-mandated electronic transaction for professional claims.

elective admission Hospital admission of a patient whose health is not at risk; often scheduled in advance.

electronic data interchange (EDI) The system-to-system exchange of data in a standardized format.

electronic health record (EHR) system A running collection of health information that provides immediate electronic access by authorized users.

electronic media claim (EMC) A computerized insurance claim form transmitted electronically from a provider to a payer's computer system.

emergency A situation in which a delay in the treatment of the patient would lead to a significant increase in the threat to life or body part.

emergency department Hospital department providing health care for patients who would have a significant increase in the threat to life or body part if treatment were delayed.

employer group health plan (EGHP) A health plan offered by an employer of more than 20 people that provides medical benefits to employees, former employees, and their families.

encounter form A listing of the services, procedures, and revenue departments for collecting charges for a patient's visit; also called a charge ticket or superbill.

end-stage renal disease (ESRD) Permanent kidney failure that requires a regular course of dialysis or kidney transplantation to maintain life.

excluded (noncovered) services Medical care that is not covered by a health plan; in Medicare, most preventive care and services that are not medically necessary are excluded.

explanation of benefits (EOB) A document from a payer to a patient or a provider that shows how the amount of a benefit was determined.

external audit A formal examination in which an agency, such as the OIG, selects certain records for review.

Federal Employees' Compensation Act (FECA) A federal law that provides workers' compensation insurance for civilian employees of the federal government.

Federal Employees Health Benefits Program (FEHBP) The health insurance program that covers employees of the federal government.

Federal Employees Retirement System (FERS) Disability program for employees of the federal government.

Federal Insurance Contribution Act (FICA) The federal law that authorizes payroll deductions for the Social Security Disability Program.

Federal Medicaid Assistance Percentage (FMAP) Basis for federal government Medicaid allocations to individual states.

Federal Register A publication of the Office of the Federal Register (OFR), which is responsible for publishing federal laws, presidential documents, administrative regulations and notices, and descriptions of federal organizations, programs, and activities.

fee schedule List of charges for services performed.

fiscal intermediary (FI) A government contractor that processes claims for Medicare Part A claims.

focused medical review (FMR) The CMS process of closely examining Medicare claims considered to be associated with the greatest probability of inappropriate payments.

form locator (FL) A numeric indicator that directs the reader to a specific box or space on a data collection form; there are 81 form locators on the UB-04 claim form.

fraud Under Medicare, fraud is an intentional misrepresentation that is known to be false and could result in unauthorized benefit, such as claiming costs for non-covered items and intentionally double billing for the same services.

guarantee of payment provision Policy that Medicare will pay for hospital inpatient services—even if the patient's benefits were exhausted before the admission—if the hospital acted in good faith in admitting the patient.

guarantor The person who is responsible for the payment of a patient's bill for medical services.

guardian An adult responsible for care and custody of a minor.

Health Care Common Procedure Coding System (HCPCS) Procedure codes for Medicare claims, made up of CPT-4 codes (Level I) and national codes (Level II).

health insurance claim number (HICN) A number issued by the Social Security Administration to individuals or beneficiaries who are entitled to Medicare benefits. The HIC number, as recorded on the beneficiary's Medicare card, is the source of beneficiary information that is required for processing Medicare claims.

Health Insurance Portability and Accountability Act (HIPAA) of 1996 Federal government act that set forth guidelines for standardizing the electronic data interchange of administrative and financial transactions, exposing fraud and abuse in government programs, and protecting the security and privacy of health information.

Health Insurance Prospective Payment System (HIPPS) Procedural coding system used in association with the skilled nursing facilities (SNF) and home health prospective payment systems.

Health Insurance Prospective Payment System (HIPPS) rate code A five-digit alphanumeric payment code used under the Prospective Payment Systems associated with skilled nursing facilities, home health providers, and inpatient rehabilitation facilities.

health maintenance organization (HMO) A managed health care system in which providers agree to offer health care to the organization's members for fixed periodic payments from the plan; usually members must receive medical services only from the plan's providers.

health plan Under HIPAA, an individual or group plan that either provides or pays for the cost of medical care; includes group health plans, health insurance issuers, HMOs, Medicare Part A or B, Medicaid, TRICARE, and other government and nongovernment plans.

HIPAA claim Generic term for the HIPAA X12N 837 institutional or professional health care claim transaction.

HIPAA Electronic Health Care Transactions and Code Sets (TCS) HIPAA standards governing the electronic exchange of health information using standard formats and standard code sets.

HIPAA Privacy Rule Law that regulates the use and disclosure of patients' protected health information (PHI).

HIPAA Security Rule Security standards that require appropriate administrative, physical, and technical safeguards to protect the privacy of protected health information against unintended disclosure through breach of security.

home health agency (HHA) Health care provider, licensed under state or local law, that provides skilled nursing and other therapeutic services, such as visiting nurse associations and hospital-based home care programs.

hospice Care for the terminally ill that emphasizes emotional support and coping with pain and death.

hospital-acquired condition A secondary condition developed during a hospital stay; for certain of these conditions, CMS will not assign a higher paying DRG for treatment unless it is documented as present on admission.

Hospital-Issued Notice of Noncoverage (HINN) A hospital notice to a beneficiary that is provided to inform the patient that the inpatient care the beneficiary is receiving or about to receive is not covered.

ICD-9-CM *Official Guidelines for Coding and Reporting* Written by NCHS (National Center for Health Statistics) and CMS and approved by the cooperating parties, it provides rules for selecting and sequencing diagnosis codes in both the inpatient and the outpatient environments.

indemnity plan An insurance company's agreement to reimburse a policyholder for covered losses if required payments have been made.

inpatient A person admitted to a health care facility for services that require an overnight stay.

inpatient-only procedures Surgical procedures which, due to their invasive nature and the need for a twenty-four-hour recovery time, Medicare has designated will only be paid for if performed on an inpatient basis.

Inpatient Prospective Payment System (IPPS) Medicare payment system for hospital services; based on diagnosis-related groups (DRGs).

interim bill A bill that does not cover a complete hospital or SNF stay; used after a minimum stay of 30 days when it is expected that additional claims will be submitted for the same confinement.

intermediate care facility (ICF) A health care facility providing care to patients who do not require professional medical or skilled nursing services.

internal audit Self-audit conducted by a staff member or consultant as a routine check of compliance with reporting regulations.

***International Classification of Diseases*, Ninth Revision, *Clinical Modification* (ICD-9-CM)** A publication that classifies diseases and injuries according to a system developed by the World Health Organization and modified for use in the United States.

Joint Commission Organization that reviews accreditation of hospitals and other organizations/programs; previously know as the Joint Commission on Accreditation of Healthcare Organizations (JCAHO).

large group health plan (LGHP) A group health plan that covers employees of either an employer or employee organization that has more than 100 employees.

leave of absence (LOA) days Days on which a patient is temporarily released from the hospital.

lifetime reserve days (LRD) The 60 days of reduced-cost hospitalization coverage that Medicare benefits allow a patient for use after a benefit period is used up; for each lifetime reserve day, Medicare pays all covered costs except for a daily coinsurance.

lifetime reserve days coinsurance rate An amount set annually that is always equal to 25 percent of the Medicare Part A annual inpatient deductible.

lifetime reserve days rate An amount set annually that is always equal to 50 percent of the Medicare Part A annual inpatient deductible.

local coverage determination (LCD) Notice sent to providers with detailed and updated information about the coding and medical necessity of a specific Medicare service.

local medical review policy (LMRP) See *local coverage determination*.

major CC (MCC) Secondary diagnosis classified by the Inpatient Prospective Payment System as severe when assigning the DRG.

major diagnostic category (MDC) Under the Inpatient Prospective Payment System, a classification of principal diagnoses based on groups of patients who are similar clinically and who require similar hospital resources.

major medical benefit plan An insurance plan that provides comprehensive hospital, surgical, and medical benefits.

managed care organization (MCO) Organization offering some type of managed health care plan.

manifestation Characteristic sign or symptom of a disease.

Medicaid A federal/state assistance program that pays for health care services for people who cannot afford them.

medical necessity Payment criterion of payers that requires medical treatments to be appropriate and provided in accordance with generally accepted standards of medical practice.

medical/health record number A number assigned by a facility to a patient's medical record.

Medicare administrative contractors (MACs) New entities assigned by CMS to replace the numerous FIs and carriers that currently administer the Medicare Part A and Part B programs; fifteen of them will process and pay Medicare Part A and Part B claims within specified multistate jurisdictions.

Medicare Advantage Medicare plans other than the Original Medicare Plan.

Medicare blood deductible Under Medicare, a patient must either replace or pay for the first 3 pints of blood used each calendar year.

Medicare Code Editor (MCE) A computer program used by Medicare to find billing problems and inconsistencies on inpatient claims, and to verify compliance with Medicare coverage rules.

Medicare Common Working File (CWF) CMS databases containing the histories of Medicare beneficiaries used by FIs and carriers to check eligibility, use of benefits, and other insurance coverage.

Medicare Conditional Payment request See *conditional payment*.

Medicare distinct part unit A distinct unit or a unique level of care in a hospital, such as a psychiatric or rehabilitation unit, that operates under its own payment system and therefore requires a separate claim to the payer.

Medicare Part A The part of the Medicare program that pays for hospitalization, care in a skilled nursing facility, home health care, and hospice care.

Medicare Part B The part of the Medicare program that pays for physician services, outpatient hospital services, durable medical equipment, and other services and supplies.

Medicare Secondary Payer (MSP) Under MSP, Medicare does not pay for services if payment has been

Glossary

made or can reasonably be expected to be made by another payer. For example, Medicare is secondary to workers compensation, automobile, medical no-fault, and liability insurance. Medicare is also secondary to GHPs and certain group health plans covering aged and disabled beneficiaries. MSP cases are identified by CMS through the development process, which includes beneficiary questionnaires, provider identification of third-party coverage during the admissions process, data transfers with other state and federal agencies, and Common Working File edits.

Medicare-Severity DRGs (MS-DRGs)   Medicare Inpatient Prospective Payment System revision that takes into account whether certain conditions were present on admission.

Medicare Summary Notice (MSN)   The explanation of Part A and Part B benefits supplied by Medicare to beneficiaries in the Original Medicare Plan.

Medigap   Medicare supplemental insurance sold by private companies to Original Medicare Plan beneficiaries to fill the "gaps" of coverage.

minimum necessary standard   Principle that individually identifiable health information should be disclosed only to the extent needed to support the purpose of the disclosure.

modifier   A two-digit number in the CPT-4 coding system used to report special circumstances involved with a procedure or service.

MS Grouper   A software program used by Medicare and hospitals to assign DRGs and determine payments for inpatient claims.

MSP value code   One of nine value codes and its corresponding amount that indicates the amount paid on behalf of the beneficiary that is the portion of payment from the primary payer; Medicare is being billed as secondary for the Medicare-covered services on the claim.

national coverage determination (NCD)   Medicare policy stating whether and under what circumstances a service is covered by the Medicare program.

National Provider Identifier (NPI)   Under HIPAA, unique 10-digit identifier assigned to each provider by the National Provider System; replaces both the UPIN and Medicare PIN.

National Provider Identifier (NPI) Registry   The query-only portion of the NPPES (National Plan and

Provider Enumeration System) database which is maintained as part of the CMS website and which contains a complete list of NPIs and other provider data that can be made available to the public.

non-CCs   Under the MS-DRG system, a category of secondary conditions with the lowest of three levels of severity, representing chronic conditions that do not require additional hospital resources.

noncovered days   Days of inpatient care that are not covered by a patient's primary insurance.

observation services   Physician-ordered care provided to a patient admitted to evaluate a condition or determine a course of treatment.

occurrence codes   Two-digit numeric or alphanumeric codes that define a significant event in connection with a claim which has an effect on its processing and payment; an associated date must also be reported.

occurrence span codes   Two-digit numeric or alphanumeric codes that identify significant events which occur over a span of time and which affect the processing and payment of the claim; associated "from" and "through" dates must also be reported.

Office of the Inspector General (OIG)   Federal agency that investigates and prosecutes fraud against government health care programs such as Medicare.

Original Medicare Plan (OMP)   A pay-per-visit health plan with two parts, Medicare Part A and Part B, requiring the beneficiary to pay a premium (Part B), a deductible, and coinsurance.

outlier   A hospital case that incurs unusually high costs for its DRG classification and therefore may qualify for an outlier payment.

outlier payment   A supplemental payment made to a hospital, in addition to the base payment for the DRG, if its costs for treating a particular case exceed the usual Medicare payment for that case by a set threshold.

outpatient   A person who receives health care in a medical setting without an overnight admission; the length of stay is generally less than 23 hours.

Outpatient Code Editor (OCE)   The computer program used by Medicare to review claims for hospital-based outpatient services.

Outpatient Prospective Payment System (OPPS) The Medicare payment system for outpatients, which sets payment amounts in advance for services and procedures based on ambulatory payment classifications (APCs).

paper claim Insurance claim submitted to a payer as a printed or typed form; it an be an optical character recognition (OCR) claim that is designed to be read by a scanner or a claim that is converted to electronic format by the payer.

patient control number A unique alphanumeric identifier assigned by the provider to each patient and generally displayed on payment checks and vouchers.

patient discharge status A patient's discharge status as of the "through" date of the billing period; the options are routine discharge, discharged to another facility, still a patient, or expired.

patient's reason for visit For unscheduled outpatient encounters, such as an emergency department visit, the condition the patient states is responsible for the hospital visit.

pay-for-performance programs Quality initiative programs that align financial incentives with the delivery of high-quality care.

payer General term for an insurance carrier or government program that provides benefits for patients of a facility.

per diem A payment method that reimburses a set rate for each inpatient day according to the case category.

point of origin for admission or visit On the UB-04 form, a field (FL 15) for reporting the patient's point of origin for the emergency, elective, or other type of inpatient admission, as well as the point of origin for outpatient services, previously referred to as the source of admission.

precertification Prior authorization from a payer that must be received before elective hospital-based or outpatient surgeries are covered; also *preauthorization* or *authorization*.

preferred provider organization (PPO) A managed care network of health care providers who agree to perform services for plan members at discounted fees; usually, plan members can receive services from non-network providers for a higher cost.

premium The periodic amount of money paid to an insurance company for an insurance plan.

present on admission (POA) Indicator required by Medicare that identifies whether a coded condition was present at the time of hospital admission.

present on admission (POA) exempt list List of conditions that do not require a POA (present on admission) indicator.

primary care physician (PCP) In a health maintenance organization (HMO), the physician assigned to direct all aspects of a patient's care, including routine services, referrals to specialists within the system, and supervision of hospital admissions; also known as *gatekeeper*.

primary diagnosis Diagnosis that represents the patient's major illness or condition for an encounter.

primary insurance The insurance carrier that pays benefits first when a patient is covered by more than one medical plan.

principal diagnosis The condition that after study is established as chiefly responsible for a patient's admission to a hospital.

principal procedure The main service performed for the condition listed as the principal diagnosis for a hospital inpatient.

procedure code A code that identifies medical or diagnostic services.

professional services The work of physicians—such as surgeons, anesthesiologists, and patients' private doctors—that is billed to patients by the physician rather than by the facility.

prospective payment A method of payment that sets a predetermined rate for each category of patient illness or for services provided for a standard type of case.

Prospective Payment System (PPS) The Medicare payment system for inpatients, which sets payment amounts in advance for services based on diagnosis-related groups (DRGs).

protected health information (PHI) Individually identifiable health information that is transmitted or maintained by electronic media.

provider Person or entity that supplies medical or health services and bills for or is paid for the services in the normal course of business. A provider may be a professional member of the health care team, such as a physician, or a facility, such as a hospital or skilled nursing home.

provider number A number assigned to a provider of health care services by a payer entered in FL57 on the UB-04 claim form; Medicare uses a six-digit provider number whose last four digits indicate the type of facility with which the provider is connected. When the NPI system is fully in place, it will replace the provider numbering system and provider numbers will no longer be required on the UB-04.

qualifier codes Two-digit code for a type of provider identification number other than the National Provider Identifier (NPI).

Quality Improvement Organization (QIO) An organization hired by CMS to determine the medical necessity, appropriateness, and quality of patients' treatments; formerly *Peer Review Organization (PRO)*.

quality measures A specified set of measures based on scientific evidence that are used to gauge how well an entity provides care to its patients.

referring physician The physician who orders a patient's services.

remittance advice (RA) The document sent by a payer to a provider that itemizes the patients, claims, and explanations for payment decisions included in the attached payment.

revenue code A code that reports a particular accommodation or ancillary charge on a UB-04 claim.

revenue code series The component subcategories of a four-digit revenue code that are described using the convention of an X in the last position (instead of a number from 0 to 9); for example, revenue code 013X stands for the revenue code series "Room & Board — Three and Four Beds."

routine charge The total of the costs of all supplies that are customarily used to provide the service; items included in the routine charge should not be billed separately.

secondary identifiers Provider identifiers that may be required by various plans in addition to the NPI, such as a plan identification number.

secondary insurance The insurance plan that pays benefits after the primary payer when a patient is covered by more than one medical insurance plan.

self-referral A patient who requests outpatient services without a physician referral.

72-hour rule Hospital coding rule for Medicare beneficiaries that allows outpatient services performed within 72 hours of an inpatient admission to be reported on the claim as part of the inpatient stay so long as the services are related to the inpatient stay; also known as the *three-day window rule*.

skilled nursing facility (SNF) A health care facility that provides skilled nursing care and related services for patients who need nursing care or rehabilitation services.

source of admission The source for a patient's admission, such as a referral, a transfer from another facility, or a newborn (such as a normal delivery).

spell of illness A period of hospitalization as defined by a health plan. Medicare beneficiaries' spell of illness—a benefit period—begins with a hospital admission and ends when the patient has not received inpatient care for 60 consecutive days.

statement covers period The "from" and "through" dates that represent the beginning and ending dates of service for the period covered by the bill.

status indicator (SI) Letters assigned to each CPT/HCPCS code identifying the payment rules established by CMS for that code.

subcategory code See *detail-level code*.

supplemental insurance An insurance plan, such as Medigap, that provides benefits for services which are not normally covered by a primary plan.

swing bed hospital A hospital with a Medicare-approved swing bed agreement under which an acute-care bed can be used to provide long-term care services similar to a skilled nursing facility.

taxonomy code Administrative code set under HIPAA used to report a physician's specialty or an institutional provider's type of facility when it affects payment.

technical component (TC) The technician's work and the equipment and supplies used in performing a procedure; billable by the facility rather than the physician.

three-day window rule See *72-hour rule*.

time of service The patient's encounter with the provider; payments may be due and collected at the time of service, such as copayments, rather than billed after the service was provided.

transitional pass-through payment Temporary additional reimbursement under APCs for new drugs or other treatments not included in the payment rate.

treatment, payment, and health care operations (TPO) Under HIPAA, the rule that patients' protected health information may be shared without authorization for the purposes of treatment, payment, and operations.

TRICARE The Civilian Health and Medical Program of the Uniformed Services that serves spouses and children of active-duty service members, military retirees and their families, some former spouses, and survivors of deceased military members; formerly CHAMPUS.

triggered reviews An audit or review triggered by certain events or certain repeated actions indicating noncompliance.

type of bill (TOB) A four-digit code; the first digit is a leading zero, the second digit identifies the type of facility where services were rendered, the third digit classifies the type of care being billed, and the fourth digit, a "frequency" code, indicates the sequence of the bill within a given episode of care.

UB-04 The uniform bill introduced in 2004 by the National Uniform Billing Committee (NUBC) for submitting Medicare Part A inpatient and outpatient claims to Medicare fiscal intermediaries; used by most other payers as well because it meets the billing requirements of many types of provider facilities. The UB-04 officially replaced its predecessor, the UB-92, on March 1, 2007.

uncollectible account A patient's balance that the billing department has determined cannot be collected from the debtor and is written off.

Uniform Hospital Discharge Data Set (UHDDS) Classification system for inpatient health data.

unlisted procedure code A service that is not listed in CPT-4; requires a special report when used.

UPIN (unique physician identification number) In the past, a number assigned by CMS to identify physicians and suppliers who provided medical services or supplies to Medicare beneficiaries. Each physician had a unique six-character, alphanumeric identification number designed to track payment and utilization information for individual physicians. The UPIN has gradually been replaced by the NPI under HIPAA.

urgent An admission category that indicates the patient is suffering from a physical or mental disorder that requires immediate attention and should be admitted as soon as a suitable bed is available, within 24 to 48 hours; prolonged delay will threaten the patient's life or well-being.

utilization review (UR) A formal review to determine the appropriateness and usage of hospital-based health care services delivered to a member of a plan; may be conducted on a prospective, concurrent, or retrospective basis.

V code An alphanumeric code in the ICD-9-CM that identifies factors that influence health status and encounters that are not due to illness or injury.

value code A code reported along with an amount—a dollar figure or other unit of measure—to provide financial information on the UB-04 claim form such as the charge for a semiprivate room.

Volume 1 (Tabular List) ICD-9-CM Tabular List of Disease and Injuries.

Volume 2 (Alphabetic Index) ICD-9-CM Alphabetic Index to Disease and Injuries.

Volume 3 (Procedures) ICD-9-CM Alphabetic Index and Tabular List of Procedures.

working aged person In Medicare, the term for a patient or his/her spouse who is over age 65 and who is eligible for group health insurance through employment or the employment of his/her spouse; Medicare is the secondary payer.

workers' compensation A state or federal plan that covers medical care and other benefits for employees who suffer accidental injury or become ill as a result of employment.

write off (*noun* write-off) To deduct an amount from a patient's account because of a contractual agreement to accept a payer's allowed charge or other reason.

Index

Note: **Bold** page numbers indicate material in tables or figures.

1			2		3a PAT. CNTL #		4 TYPE OF BILL
					b. MED. REC. #		
					5 FED. TAX NO.	6 STATEMENT COVERS PERIOD FROM THROUGH	7

8 PATIENT NAME	a		9 PATIENT ADDRESS	a			
b			b		c	d	e

10 BIRTHDATE	11 SEX	12 DATE	ADMISSION 13 HR	14 TYPE	15 SRC	16 DHR	17 STAT	18	19	20	21	CONDITION CODES 22	23	24	25	26	27	28	29 ACDT STATE	30

31 OCCURRENCE CODE DATE	32 OCCURRENCE CODE DATE	33 OCCURRENCE CODE DATE	34 OCCURRENCE CODE DATE	35 OCCURRENCE SPAN CODE FROM THROUGH	36 OCCURRENCE SPAN CODE FROM THROUGH	37
a						a
b						b

38		39 CODE VALUE CODES AMOUNT	40 CODE VALUE CODES AMOUNT	41 CODE VALUE CODES AMOUNT
	a			
	b			
	c			
	d			

42 REV. CD.	43 DESCRIPTION	44 HCPCS / RATE / HIPPS CODE	45 SERV. DATE	46 SERV. UNITS	47 TOTAL CHARGES	48 NON-COVERED CHARGES	49
1							1
2							2
3							3
4							4
5							5
6							6
7							7
8							8
9							9
10							10
11							11
12							12
13							13
14							14
15							15
16							16
17							17
18							18
19							19
20							20
21							21
22							22
23	PAGE ____ OF ____	CREATION DATE	TOTALS ➤				23

50 PAYER NAME	51 HEALTH PLAN ID	52 REL INFO	53 ASG BEN	54 PRIOR PAYMENTS	55 EST. AMOUNT DUE	56 NPI	
A						57 OTHER PRV ID	A
B							B
C							C

58 INSURED'S NAME	59 P.REL	60 INSURED'S UNIQUE ID	61 GROUP NAME	62 INSURANCE GROUP NO.	
A					A
B					B
C					C

63 TREATMENT AUTHORIZATION CODES	64 DOCUMENT CONTROL NUMBER	65 EMPLOYER NAME	
A			A
B			B
C			C

66 DX	67	A	B	C	D	E	F	G	H	68
		I	J	K	L	M	N	O	P	Q

69 ADMIT DX	70 PATIENT REASON DX a b c	71 PPS CODE	72 ECI a b c	73

74 PRINCIPAL PROCEDURE CODE DATE	a. OTHER PROCEDURE CODE DATE	b. OTHER PROCEDURE CODE DATE	75	76 ATTENDING NPI		QUAL	
c. OTHER PROCEDURE CODE DATE	d. OTHER PROCEDURE CODE DATE	e. OTHER PROCEDURE CODE DATE		LAST FIRST			
				77 OPERATING NPI		QUAL	
				LAST FIRST			

80 REMARKS	81CC a		78 OTHER NPI		QUAL	
	b		LAST FIRST			
	c		79 OTHER NPI		QUAL	
	d		LAST FIRST			

UB-04 CMS-1450   APPROVED OMB NO. 0938-0997   **NUBC**™ National Uniform Billing Committee   THE CERTIFICATIONS ON THE REVERSE APPLY TO THIS BILL AND ARE MADE A PART HEREOF.

Submission of this claim constitutes certification that the billing information as shown on the face hereof is true, accurate and complete. That the submitter did not knowingly or recklessly disregard or misrepresent or conceal material facts. The following certifications or verifications apply where pertinent to this Bill:

1. If third party benefits are indicated, the appropriate assignments by the insured /beneficiary and signature of the patient or parent or a legal guardian covering authorization to release information are on file. Determinations as to the release of medical and financial information should be guided by the patient or the patient's legal representative.

2. If patient occupied a private room or required private nursing for medical necessity, any required certifications are on file.

3. Physician's certifications and re-certifications, if required by contract or Federal regulations, are on file.

4. For Religious Non-Medical facilities, verifications and if necessary recertifications of the patient's need for services are on file.

5. Signature of patient or his representative on certifications, authorization to release information, and payment request, as required by Federal Law and Regulations (42 USC 1935f, 42 CFR 424.36, 10 USC 1071 through 1086, 32 CFR 199) and any other applicable contract regulations, is on file.

6. The provider of care submitter acknowledges that the bill is in conformance with the Civil Rights Act of 1964 as amended. Records adequately describing services will be maintained and necessary information will be furnished to such governmental agencies as required by applicable law.

7. For Medicare Purposes: If the patient has indicated that other health insurance or a state medical assistance agency will pay part of his/her medical expenses and he/she wants information about his/her claim released to them upon request, necessary authorization is on file. The patient's signature on the provider's request to bill Medicare medical and non-medical information, including employment status, and whether the person has employer group health insurance which is responsible to pay for the services for which this Medicare claim is made.

8. For Medicaid purposes: The submitter understands that because payment and satisfaction of this claim will be from Federal and State funds, any false statements, documents, or concealment of a material fact are subject to prosecution under applicable Federal or State Laws.

9. For TRICARE Purposes:

   (a) The information on the face of this claim is true, accurate and complete to the best of the submitter's knowledge and belief, and services were medically necessary and appropriate for the health of the patient;

   (b) The patient has represented that by a reported residential address outside a military medical treatment facility catchment area he or she does not live within the catchment area of a U.S. military medical treatment facility, or if the patient resides within a catchment area of such a facility, a copy of Non-Availability Statement (DD Form 1251) is on file, or the physician has certified to a medical emergency in any instance where a copy of a Non-Availability Statement is not on file;

   (c) The patient or the patient's parent or guardian has responded directly to the provider's request to identify all health insurance coverage, and that all such coverage is identified on the face of the claim except that coverage which is exclusively supplemental payments to TRICARE-determined benefits;

   (d) The amount billed to TRICARE has been billed after all such coverage have been billed and paid excluding Medicaid, and the amount billed to TRICARE is that remaining claimed against TRICARE benefits;

   (e) The beneficiary's cost share has not been waived by consent or failure to exercise generally accepted billing and collection efforts; and,

   (f) Any hospital-based physician under contract, the cost of whose services are allocated in the charges included in this bill, is not an employee or member of the Uniformed Services. For purposes of this certification, an employee of the Uniformed Services is an employee, appointed in civil service (refer to 5 USC 2105), including part-time or intermittent employees, but excluding contract surgeons or other personal service contracts. Similarly, member of the Uniformed Services does not apply to reserve members of the Uniformed Services not on active duty.

   (g) Based on 42 United States Code 1395cc(a)(1)(j) all providers participating in Medicare must also participate in TRICARE for inpatient hospital services provided pursuant to admissions to hospitals occurring on or after January 1, 1987; and

   (h) If TRICARE benefits are to be paid in a participating status, the submitter of this claim agrees to submit this claim to the appropriate TRICARE claims processor. The provider of care submitter also agrees to accept the TRICARE determined reasonable charge as the total charge for the medical services or supplies listed on the claim form. The provider of care will accept the TRICARE-determined reasonable charge even if it is less than the billed amount, and also agrees to accept the amount paid by TRICARE combined with the cost-share amount and deductible amount, if any, paid by or on behalf of the patient as full payment for the listed medical services or supplies. The provider of care submitter will not attempt to collect from the patient (or his or her parent or guardian) amounts over the TRICARE determined reasonable charge. TRICARE will make any benefits payable directly to the provider of care, if the provider of care is a participating provider.

SEE http://www.nubc.org/ FOR MORE INFORMATION ON UB-04 DATA ELEMENT AND PRINTING SPECIFICATIONS

1		2		3a PAT. CNTL #			4 TYPE OF BILL
				b. MED. REC. #			
				5 FED. TAX NO.	6 STATEMENT COVERS PERIOD FROM THROUGH		7

8 PATIENT NAME	a		9 PATIENT ADDRESS	a			
b			b		c	d	e

| 10 BIRTHDATE | 11 SEX | 12 DATE | ADMISSION 13 HR 14 TYPE 15 SRC | 16 DHR | 17 STAT | 18 19 20 21 CONDITION CODES 22 23 24 25 26 27 28 | 29 ACDT STATE | 30 |

31 OCCURRENCE CODE DATE	32 OCCURRENCE CODE DATE	33 OCCURRENCE CODE DATE	34 OCCURRENCE CODE DATE	35 OCCURRENCE SPAN CODE FROM THROUGH	36 OCCURRENCE SPAN CODE FROM THROUGH	37
a						a
b						b

38			39 CODE VALUE CODES AMOUNT	40 CODE VALUE CODES AMOUNT	41 CODE VALUE CODES AMOUNT
		a			
		b			
		c			
		d			

42 REV. CD.	43 DESCRIPTION	44 HCPCS / RATE / HIPPS CODE	45 SERV. DATE	46 SERV. UNITS	47 TOTAL CHARGES	48 NON-COVERED CHARGES	49	
1								1
2								2
3								3
4								4
5								5
6								6
7								7
8								8
9								9
10								10
11								11
12								12
13								13
14								14
15								15
16								16
17								17
18								18
19								19
20								20
21								21
22								22
23	PAGE ____ OF ____	CREATION DATE		TOTALS ➡				23

50 PAYER NAME	51 HEALTH PLAN ID	52 REL INFO	53 ASG BEN.	54 PRIOR PAYMENTS	55 EST. AMOUNT DUE	56 NPI		
A						57 OTHER PRV ID		A
B								B
C								C

58 INSURED'S NAME	59 P.REL	60 INSURED'S UNIQUE ID	61 GROUP NAME	62 INSURANCE GROUP NO.	
A					A
B					B
C					C

63 TREATMENT AUTHORIZATION CODES	64 DOCUMENT CONTROL NUMBER	65 EMPLOYER NAME	
A			A
B			B
C			C

66 DX	67 A B C D E F G H I J K L M N O P Q				68

69 ADMIT DX	70 PATIENT REASON DX a b c	71 PPS CODE	72 ECI a b c	73

74 PRINCIPAL PROCEDURE CODE DATE	a. OTHER PROCEDURE CODE DATE	b. OTHER PROCEDURE CODE DATE	75	76 ATTENDING NPI		QUAL
c. OTHER PROCEDURE CODE DATE	d. OTHER PROCEDURE CODE DATE	e. OTHER PROCEDURE CODE DATE		LAST	FIRST	
				77 OPERATING NPI		QUAL
				LAST	FIRST	

80 REMARKS	81CC a	78 OTHER NPI		QUAL
	b	LAST	FIRST	
	c	79 OTHER NPI		QUAL
	d	LAST	FIRST	

UB-04 CMS-1450   APPROVED OMB NO. 0938-0997   **NUBC**™ National Uniform Billing Committee   THE CERTIFICATIONS ON THE REVERSE APPLY TO THIS BILL AND ARE MADE A PART HEREOF.

Submission of this claim constitutes certification that the billing information as shown on the face hereof is true, accurate and complete. That the submitter did not knowingly or recklessly disregard or misrepresent or conceal material facts. The following certifications or verifications apply where pertinent to this Bill:

1. If third party benefits are indicated, the appropriate assignments by the insured /beneficiary and signature of the patient or parent or a legal guardian covering authorization to release information are on file. Determinations as to the release of medical and financial information should be guided by the patient or the patient's legal representative.

2. If patient occupied a private room or required private nursing for medical necessity, any required certifications are on file.

3. Physician's certifications and re-certifications, if required by contract or Federal regulations, are on file.

4. For Religious Non-Medical facilities, verifications and if necessary recertifications of the patient's need for services are on file.

5. Signature of patient or his representative on certifications, authorization to release information, and payment request, as required by Federal Law and Regulations (42 USC 1935f, 42 CFR 424.36, 10 USC 1071 through 1086, 32 CFR 199) and any other applicable contract regulations, is on file.

6. The provider of care submitter acknowledges that the bill is in conformance with the Civil Rights Act of 1964 as amended. Records adequately describing services will be maintained and necessary information will be furnished to such governmental agencies as required by applicable law.

7. For Medicare Purposes: If the patient has indicated that other health insurance or a state medical assistance agency will pay part of his/her medical expenses and he/she wants information about his/her claim released to them upon request, necessary authorization is on file. The patient's signature on the provider's request to bill Medicare medical and non-medical information, including employment status, and whether the person has employer group health insurance which is responsible to pay for the services for which this Medicare claim is made.

8. For Medicaid purposes: The submitter understands that because payment and satisfaction of this claim will be from Federal and State funds, any false statements, documents, or concealment of a material fact are subject to prosecution under applicable Federal or State Laws.

9. For TRICARE Purposes:

(a) The information on the face of this claim is true, accurate and complete to the best of the submitter's knowledge and belief, and services were medically necessary and appropriate for the health of the patient;

(b) The patient has represented that by a reported residential address outside a military medical treatment facility catchment area he or she does not live within the catchment area of a U.S. military medical treatment facility, or if the patient resides within a catchment area of such a facility, a copy of Non-Availability Statement (DD Form 1251) is on file, or the physician has certified to a medical emergency in any instance where a copy of a Non-Availability Statement is not on file;

(c) The patient or the patient's parent or guardian has responded directly to the provider's request to identify all health insurance coverage, and that all such coverage is identified on the face of the claim except that coverage which is exclusively supplemental payments to TRICARE-determined benefits;

(d) The amount billed to TRICARE has been billed after all such coverage have been billed and paid excluding Medicaid, and the amount billed to TRICARE is that remaining claimed against TRICARE benefits;

(e) The beneficiary's cost share has not been waived by consent or failure to exercise generally accepted billing and collection efforts; and,

(f) Any hospital-based physician under contract, the cost of whose services are allocated in the charges included in this bill, is not an employee or member of the Uniformed Services. For purposes of this certification, an employee of the Uniformed Services is an employee, appointed in civil service (refer to 5 USC 2105), including part-time or intermittent employees, but excluding contract surgeons or other personal service contracts. Similarly, member of the Uniformed Services does not apply to reserve members of the Uniformed Services not on active duty.

(g) Based on 42 United States Code 1395cc(a)(1)(j) all providers participating in Medicare must also participate in TRICARE for inpatient hospital services provided pursuant to admissions to hospitals occurring on or after January 1, 1987; and

(h) If TRICARE benefits are to be paid in a participating status, the submitter of this claim agrees to submit this claim to the appropriate TRICARE claims processor. The provider of care submitter also agrees to accept the TRICARE determined reasonable charge as the total charge for the medical services or supplies listed on the claim form. The provider of care will accept the TRICARE-determined reasonable charge even if it is less than the billed amount, and also agrees to accept the amount paid by TRICARE combined with the cost-share amount and deductible amount, if any, paid by or on behalf of the patient as full payment for the listed medical services or supplies. The provider of care submitter will not attempt to collect from the patient (or his or her parent or guardian) amounts over the TRICARE determined reasonable charge. TRICARE will make any benefits payable directly to the provider of care, if the provider of care is a participating provider.

SEE http://www.nubc.org/ FOR MORE INFORMATION ON UB-04 DATA ELEMENT AND PRINTING SPECIFICATIONS

UB-04 Claim Form fields:

1

2

3a PAT. CNTL. #

b. MED. REC. #

4 TYPE OF BILL

5 FED. TAX NO.

6 STATEMENT COVERS PERIOD FROM THROUGH

7

8 PATIENT NAME a | b

9 PATIENT ADDRESS a | b | c | d | e

10 BIRTHDATE | 11 SEX | 12 DATE ADMISSION 13 HR | 14 TYPE | 15 SRC | 16 DHR | 17 STAT | 18 19 20 21 CONDITION CODES 22 23 24 25 26 27 28 | 29 ACDT STATE | 30

31 OCCURRENCE CODE DATE | 32 OCCURRENCE CODE DATE | 33 OCCURRENCE CODE DATE | 34 OCCURRENCE CODE DATE | 35 OCCURRENCE SPAN CODE FROM THROUGH | 36 OCCURRENCE SPAN CODE FROM THROUGH | 37

a | b

38

39 CODE VALUE CODES AMOUNT | 40 CODE VALUE CODES AMOUNT | 41 CODE VALUE CODES AMOUNT

a | b | c | d

42 REV. CD. | 43 DESCRIPTION | 44 HCPCS / RATE / HIPPS CODE | 45 SERV. DATE | 46 SERV. UNITS | 47 TOTAL CHARGES | 48 NON-COVERED CHARGES | 49

1 – 23

PAGE ___ OF ___ | CREATION DATE | TOTALS

50 PAYER NAME | 51 HEALTH PLAN ID | 52 REL INFO | 53 ASG BEN. | 54 PRIOR PAYMENTS | 55 EST. AMOUNT DUE | 56 NPI

57 OTHER PRV ID

A | B | C

58 INSURED'S NAME | 59 P. REL | 60 INSURED'S UNIQUE ID | 61 GROUP NAME | 62 INSURANCE GROUP NO.

A | B | C

63 TREATMENT AUTHORIZATION CODES | 64 DOCUMENT CONTROL NUMBER | 65 EMPLOYER NAME

A | B | C

66 DX | 67 A B C D E F G H I J K L M N O P Q | 68

69 ADMIT DX | 70 PATIENT REASON DX a b c | 71 PPS CODE | 72 ECI a b c | 73

74 PRINCIPAL PROCEDURE CODE DATE | a. OTHER PROCEDURE CODE DATE | b. OTHER PROCEDURE CODE DATE | 75 | 76 ATTENDING NPI QUAL | LAST FIRST

c. OTHER PROCEDURE CODE DATE | d. OTHER PROCEDURE CODE DATE | e. OTHER PROCEDURE CODE DATE | 77 OPERATING NPI QUAL | LAST FIRST

80 REMARKS | 81CC a b c d | 78 OTHER NPI QUAL | LAST FIRST | 79 OTHER NPI QUAL | LAST FIRST

UB-04 CMS-1450 | APPROVED OMB NO. 0938-0997 | NUBC™ National Uniform Billing Committee | THE CERTIFICATIONS ON THE REVERSE APPLY TO THIS BILL AND ARE MADE A PART HEREOF.

Submission of this claim constitutes certification that the billing information as shown on the face hereof is true, accurate and complete. That the submitter did not knowingly or recklessly disregard or misrepresent or conceal material facts. The following certifications or verifications apply where pertinent to this Bill:

1. If third party benefits are indicated, the appropriate assignments by the insured /beneficiary and signature of the patient or parent or a legal guardian covering authorization to release information are on file. Determinations as to the release of medical and financial information should be guided by the patient or the patient's legal representative.

2. If patient occupied a private room or required private nursing for medical necessity, any required certifications are on file.

3. Physician's certifications and re-certifications, if required by contract or Federal regulations, are on file.

4. For Religious Non-Medical facilities, verifications and if necessary recertifications of the patient's need for services are on file.

5. Signature of patient or his representative on certifications, authorization to release information, and payment request, as required by Federal Law and Regulations (42 USC 1935f, 42 CFR 424.36, 10 USC 1071 through 1086, 32 CFR 199) and any other applicable contract regulations, is on file.

6. The provider of care submitter acknowledges that the bill is in conformance with the Civil Rights Act of 1964 as amended. Records adequately describing services will be maintained and necessary information will be furnished to such governmental agencies as required by applicable law.

7. For Medicare Purposes: If the patient has indicated that other health insurance or a state medical assistance agency will pay part of his/her medical expenses and he/she wants information about his/her claim released to them upon request, necessary authorization is on file. The patient's signature on the provider's request to bill Medicare medical and non-medical information, including employment status, and whether the person has employer group health insurance which is responsible to pay for the services for which this Medicare claim is made.

8. For Medicaid purposes: The submitter understands that because payment and satisfaction of this claim will be from Federal and State funds, any false statements, documents, or concealment of a material fact are subject to prosecution under applicable Federal or State Laws.

9. For TRICARE Purposes:

   (a) The information on the face of this claim is true, accurate and complete to the best of the submitter's knowledge and belief, and services were medically necessary and appropriate for the health of the patient;

   (b) The patient has represented that by a reported residential address outside a military medical treatment facility catchment area he or she does not live within the catchment area of a U.S. military medical treatment facility, or if the patient resides within a catchment area of such a facility, a copy of Non-Availability Statement (DD Form 1251) is on file, or the physician has certified to a medical emergency in any instance where a copy of a Non-Availability Statement is not on file;

   (c) The patient or the patient's parent or guardian has responded directly to the provider's request to identify all health insurance coverage, and that all such coverage is identified on the face of the claim except that coverage which is exclusively supplemental payments to TRICARE-determined benefits;

   (d) The amount billed to TRICARE has been billed after all such coverage have been billed and paid excluding Medicaid, and the amount billed to TRICARE is that remaining claimed against TRICARE benefits;

   (e) The beneficiary's cost share has not been waived by consent or failure to exercise generally accepted billing and collection efforts; and,

   (f) Any hospital-based physician under contract, the cost of whose services are allocated in the charges included in this bill, is not an employee or member of the Uniformed Services. For purposes of this certification, an employee of the Uniformed Services is an employee, appointed in civil service (refer to 5 USC 2105), including part-time or intermittent employees, but excluding contract surgeons or other personal service contracts. Similarly, member of the Uniformed Services does not apply to reserve members of the Uniformed Services not on active duty.

   (g) Based on 42 United States Code 1395cc(a)(1)(j) all providers participating in Medicare must also participate in TRICARE for inpatient hospital services provided pursuant to admissions to hospitals occurring on or after January 1, 1987; and

   (h) If TRICARE benefits are to be paid in a participating status, the submitter of this claim agrees to submit this claim to the appropriate TRICARE claims processor. The provider of care submitter also agrees to accept the TRICARE determined reasonable charge as the total charge for the medical services or supplies listed on the claim form. The provider of care will accept the TRICARE-determined reasonable charge even if it is less than the billed amount, and also agrees to accept the amount paid by TRICARE combined with the cost-share amount and deductible amount, if any, paid by or on behalf of the patient as full payment for the listed medical services or supplies. The provider of care submitter will not attempt to collect from the patient (or his or her parent or guardian) amounts over the TRICARE determined reasonable charge. TRICARE will make any benefits payable directly to the provider of care, if the provider of care is a participating provider.

SEE http://www.nubc.org/ FOR MORE INFORMATION ON UB-04 DATA ELEMENT AND PRINTING SPECIFICATIONS

1	
2	
3a PAT. CNTL #	
b. MED. REC. #	
4 TYPE OF BILL	
5 FED. TAX NO.	
6 STATEMENT COVERS PERIOD FROM THROUGH	
7	

8 PATIENT NAME a

b

9 PATIENT ADDRESS a

b   c   d   e

| 10 BIRTHDATE | 11 SEX | 12 DATE | ADMISSION 13 HR | 14 TYPE | 15 SRC | 16 DHR | 17 STAT | 18 19 20 21 CONDITION CODES 22 23 24 25 26 27 28 | 29 ACDT STATE | 30 |

| 31 OCCURRENCE CODE DATE | 32 OCCURRENCE CODE DATE | 33 OCCURRENCE CODE DATE | 34 OCCURRENCE CODE DATE | 35 OCCURRENCE SPAN CODE FROM THROUGH | 36 OCCURRENCE SPAN CODE FROM THROUGH | 37 |

a
b

38

39 CODE VALUE CODES AMOUNT	40 CODE VALUE CODES AMOUNT	41 CODE VALUE CODES AMOUNT
a		
b		
c		
d		

42 REV. CD.	43 DESCRIPTION	44 HCPCS / RATE / HIPPS CODE	45 SERV. DATE	46 SERV. UNITS	47 TOTAL CHARGES	48 NON-COVERED CHARGES	49
1							1
2							2
3							3
4							4
5							5
6							6
7							7
8							8
9							9
10							10
11							11
12							12
13							13
14							14
15							15
16							16
17							17
18							18
19							19
20							20
21							21
22							22
23	PAGE ____ OF ____	CREATION DATE		TOTALS ➡			23

50 PAYER NAME	51 HEALTH PLAN ID	52 REL INFO	53 ASG. BEN.	54 PRIOR PAYMENTS	55 EST. AMOUNT DUE	56 NPI
A						
B						57 OTHER PRV ID
C						

58 INSURED'S NAME	59 P.REL	60 INSURED'S UNIQUE ID	61 GROUP NAME	62 INSURANCE GROUP NO.
A				
B				
C				

63 TREATMENT AUTHORIZATION CODES	64 DOCUMENT CONTROL NUMBER	65 EMPLOYER NAME
A		
B		
C		

| 66 DX | 67 A B C D E F G H | 68 |
| | I J K L M N O P Q | |

| 69 ADMIT DX | 70 PATIENT REASON DX a b c | 71 PPS CODE | 72 ECI a b c | 73 |

74 PRINCIPAL PROCEDURE CODE DATE	a. OTHER PROCEDURE CODE DATE	b. OTHER PROCEDURE CODE DATE	75	76 ATTENDING NPI	QUAL
c. OTHER PROCEDURE CODE DATE	d. OTHER PROCEDURE CODE DATE	e. OTHER PROCEDURE CODE DATE		LAST FIRST	
				77 OPERATING NPI	QUAL
				LAST FIRST	

80 REMARKS	81CC a	78 OTHER NPI	QUAL
	b	LAST FIRST	
	c	79 OTHER NPI	QUAL
	d	LAST FIRST	

UB-04 CMS-1450   APPROVED OMB NO. 0938-0997   **NUBC** National Uniform Billing Committee   THE CERTIFICATIONS ON THE REVERSE APPLY TO THIS BILL AND ARE MADE A PART HEREOF.

Submission of this claim constitutes certification that the billing information as shown on the face hereof is true, accurate and complete. That the submitter did not knowingly or recklessly disregard or misrepresent or conceal material facts. The following certifications or verifications apply where pertinent to this Bill:

1. If third party benefits are indicated, the appropriate assignments by the insured /beneficiary and signature of the patient or parent or a legal guardian covering authorization to release information are on file. Determinations as to the release of medical and financial information should be guided by the patient or the patient's legal representative.

2. If patient occupied a private room or required private nursing for medical necessity, any required certifications are on file.

3. Physician's certifications and re-certifications, if required by contract or Federal regulations, are on file.

4. For Religious Non-Medical facilities, verifications and if necessary recertifications of the patient's need for services are on file.

5. Signature of patient or his representative on certifications, authorization to release information, and payment request, as required by Federal Law and Regulations (42 USC 1935f, 42 CFR 424.36, 10 USC 1071 through 1086, 32 CFR 199) and any other applicable contract regulations, is on file.

6. The provider of care submitter acknowledges that the bill is in conformance with the Civil Rights Act of 1964 as amended. Records adequately describing services will be maintained and necessary information will be furnished to such governmental agencies as required by applicable law.

7. For Medicare Purposes: If the patient has indicated that other health insurance or a state medical assistance agency will pay part of his/her medical expenses and he/she wants information about his/her claim released to them upon request, necessary authorization is on file. The patient's signature on the provider's request to bill Medicare medical and non-medical information, including employment status, and whether the person has employer group health insurance which is responsible to pay for the services for which this Medicare claim is made.

8. For Medicaid purposes: The submitter understands that because payment and satisfaction of this claim will be from Federal and State funds, any false statements, documents, or concealment of a material fact are subject to prosecution under applicable Federal or State Laws.

9. For TRICARE Purposes:

   (a) The information on the face of this claim is true, accurate and complete to the best of the submitter's knowledge and belief, and services were medically necessary and appropriate for the health of the patient;

   (b) The patient has represented that by a reported residential address outside a military medical treatment facility catchment area he or she does not live within the catchment area of a U.S. military medical treatment facility, or if the patient resides within a catchment area of such a facility, a copy of Non-Availability Statement (DD Form 1251) is on file, or the physician has certified to a medical emergency in any instance where a copy of a Non-Availability Statement is not on file;

   (c) The patient or the patient's parent or guardian has responded directly to the provider's request to identify all health insurance coverage, and that all such coverage is identified on the face of the claim except that coverage which is exclusively supplemental payments to TRICARE-determined benefits;

   (d) The amount billed to TRICARE has been billed after all such coverage have been billed and paid excluding Medicaid, and the amount billed to TRICARE is that remaining claimed against TRICARE benefits;

   (e) The beneficiary's cost share has not been waived by consent or failure to exercise generally accepted billing and collection efforts; and,

   (f) Any hospital-based physician under contract, the cost of whose services are allocated in the charges included in this bill, is not an employee or member of the Uniformed Services. For purposes of this certification, an employee of the Uniformed Services is an employee, appointed in civil service (refer to 5 USC 2105), including part-time or intermittent employees, but excluding contract surgeons or other personal service contracts. Similarly, member of the Uniformed Services does not apply to reserve members of the Uniformed Services not on active duty.

   (g) Based on 42 United States Code 1395cc(a)(1)(j) all providers participating in Medicare must also participate in TRICARE for inpatient hospital services provided pursuant to admissions to hospitals occurring on or after January 1, 1987; and

   (h) If TRICARE benefits are to be paid in a participating status, the submitter of this claim agrees to submit this claim to the appropriate TRICARE claims processor. The provider of care submitter also agrees to accept the TRICARE determined reasonable charge as the total charge for the medical services or supplies listed on the claim form. The provider of care will accept the TRICARE-determined reasonable charge even if it is less than the billed amount, and also agrees to accept the amount paid by TRICARE combined with the cost-share amount and deductible amount, if any, paid by or on behalf of the patient as full payment for the listed medical services or supplies. The provider of care submitter will not attempt to collect from the patient (or his or her parent or guardian) amounts over the TRICARE determined reasonable charge. TRICARE will make any benefits payable directly to the provider of care, if the provider of care is a participating provider.

SEE http://www.nubc.org/ FOR MORE INFORMATION ON UB-04 DATA ELEMENT AND PRINTING SPECIFICATIONS

1		2			3a PAT. CNTL #			4 TYPE OF BILL
					b. MED. REC. #			
					5 FED. TAX NO.	6 STATEMENT COVERS PERIOD FROM THROUGH	7	

8 PATIENT NAME	a		9 PATIENT ADDRESS	a				
b			b			c	d	e

| 10 BIRTHDATE | 11 SEX | 12 DATE | ADMISSION 13 HR | 14 TYPE | 15 SRC | 16 DHR | 17 STAT | 18 | 19 | 20 | 21 | CONDITION CODES 22 | 23 | 24 | 25 | 26 | 27 | 28 | 29 ACDT STATE | 30 |

31 OCCURRENCE CODE DATE	32 OCCURRENCE CODE DATE	33 OCCURRENCE CODE DATE	34 OCCURRENCE CODE DATE	35 OCCURRENCE SPAN CODE FROM THROUGH	36 OCCURRENCE SPAN CODE FROM THROUGH	37
a						a
b						b

38		39 VALUE CODES CODE AMOUNT	40 VALUE CODES CODE AMOUNT	41 VALUE CODES CODE AMOUNT
	a			
	b			
	c			
	d			

42 REV. CD.	43 DESCRIPTION	44 HCPCS / RATE / HIPPS CODE	45 SERV. DATE	46 SERV. UNITS	47 TOTAL CHARGES	48 NON-COVERED CHARGES	49
1							1
2							2
3							3
4							4
5							5
6							6
7							7
8							8
9							9
10							10
11							11
12							12
13							13
14							14
15							15
16							16
17							17
18							18
19							19
20							20
21							21
22							22
23	PAGE ___ OF ___	CREATION DATE		TOTALS ➡			23

50 PAYER NAME	51 HEALTH PLAN ID	52 REL INFO	53 ASG BEN.	54 PRIOR PAYMENTS	55 EST. AMOUNT DUE	56 NPI	
A						57 OTHER	A
B						OTHER	B
C						PRV ID	C

58 INSURED'S NAME	59 P.REL	60 INSURED'S UNIQUE ID	61 GROUP NAME	62 INSURANCE GROUP NO.	
A					A
B					B
C					C

63 TREATMENT AUTHORIZATION CODES	64 DOCUMENT CONTROL NUMBER	65 EMPLOYER NAME	
A			A
B			B
C			C

66 DX	67	A	B	C	D	E	F	G	H	68
	I	J	K	L	M	N	O	P	Q	

69 ADMIT DX	70 PATIENT REASON DX a b c	71 PPS CODE	72 ECI a b c	73

74 PRINCIPAL PROCEDURE CODE DATE	a. OTHER PROCEDURE CODE DATE	b. OTHER PROCEDURE CODE DATE	75	76 ATTENDING NPI QUAL
				LAST FIRST
c. OTHER PROCEDURE CODE DATE	d. OTHER PROCEDURE CODE DATE	e. OTHER PROCEDURE CODE DATE		77 OPERATING NPI QUAL
				LAST FIRST

80 REMARKS	81CC a		78 OTHER NPI QUAL
	b		LAST FIRST
	c		79 OTHER NPI QUAL
	d		LAST FIRST

UB-04 CMS-1450   APPROVED OMB NO. 0938-0997   **NUBC** National Uniform Billing Committee   THE CERTIFICATIONS ON THE REVERSE APPLY TO THIS BILL AND ARE MADE A PART HEREOF.

Submission of this claim constitutes certification that the billing information as shown on the face hereof is true, accurate and complete. That the submitter did not knowingly or recklessly disregard or misrepresent or conceal material facts. The following certifications or verifications apply where pertinent to this Bill:

1. If third party benefits are indicated, the appropriate assignments by the insured /beneficiary and signature of the patient or parent or a legal guardian covering authorization to release information are on file. Determinations as to the release of medical and financial information should be guided by the patient or the patient's legal representative.

2. If patient occupied a private room or required private nursing for medical necessity, any required certifications are on file.

3. Physician's certifications and re-certifications, if required by contract or Federal regulations, are on file.

4. For Religious Non-Medical facilities, verifications and if necessary recertifications of the patient's need for services are on file.

5. Signature of patient or his representative on certifications, authorization to release information, and payment request, as required by Federal Law and Regulations (42 USC 1935f, 42 CFR 424.36, 10 USC 1071 through 1086, 32 CFR 199) and any other applicable contract regulations, is on file.

6. The provider of care submitter acknowledges that the bill is in conformance with the Civil Rights Act of 1964 as amended. Records adequately describing services will be maintained and necessary information will be furnished to such governmental agencies as required by applicable law.

7. For Medicare Purposes: If the patient has indicated that other health insurance or a state medical assistance agency will pay part of his/her medical expenses and he/she wants information about his/her claim released to them upon request, necessary authorization is on file. The patient's signature on the provider's request to bill Medicare medical and non-medical information, including employment status, and whether the person has employer group health insurance which is responsible to pay for the services for which this Medicare claim is made.

8. For Medicaid purposes: The submitter understands that because payment and satisfaction of this claim will be from Federal and State funds, any false statements, documents, or concealment of a material fact are subject to prosecution under applicable Federal or State Laws.

9. For TRICARE Purposes:

   (a) The information on the face of this claim is true, accurate and complete to the best of the submitter's knowledge and belief, and services were medically necessary and appropriate for the health of the patient;

   (b) The patient has represented that by a reported residential address outside a military medical treatment facility catchment area he or she does not live within the catchment area of a U.S. military medical treatment facility, or if the patient resides within a catchment area of such a facility, a copy of Non-Availability Statement (DD Form 1251) is on file, or the physician has certified to a medical emergency in any instance where a copy of a Non-Availability Statement is not on file;

   (c) The patient or the patient's parent or guardian has responded directly to the provider's request to identify all health insurance coverage, and that all such coverage is identified on the face of the claim except that coverage which is exclusively supplemental payments to TRICARE-determined benefits;

   (d) The amount billed to TRICARE has been billed after all such coverage have been billed and paid excluding Medicaid, and the amount billed to TRICARE is that remaining claimed against TRICARE benefits;

   (e) The beneficiary's cost share has not been waived by consent or failure to exercise generally accepted billing and collection efforts; and,

   (f) Any hospital-based physician under contract, the cost of whose services are allocated in the charges included in this bill, is not an employee or member of the Uniformed Services. For purposes of this certification, an employee of the Uniformed Services is an employee, appointed in civil service (refer to 5 USC 2105), including part-time or intermittent employees, but excluding contract surgeons or other personal service contracts. Similarly, member of the Uniformed Services does not apply to reserve members of the Uniformed Services not on active duty.

   (g) Based on 42 United States Code 1395cc(a)(1)(j) all providers participating in Medicare must also participate in TRICARE for inpatient hospital services provided pursuant to admissions to hospitals occurring on or after January 1, 1987; and

   (h) If TRICARE benefits are to be paid in a participating status, the submitter of this claim agrees to submit this claim to the appropriate TRICARE claims processor. The provider of care submitter also agrees to accept the TRICARE determined reasonable charge as the total charge for the medical services or supplies listed on the claim form. The provider of care will accept the TRICARE-determined reasonable charge even if it is less than the billed amount, and also agrees to accept the amount paid by TRICARE combined with the cost-share amount and deductible amount, if any, paid by or on behalf of the patient as full payment for the listed medical services or supplies. The provider of care submitter will not attempt to collect from the patient (or his or her parent or guardian) amounts over the TRICARE determined reasonable charge. TRICARE will make any benefits payable directly to the provider of care, if the provider of care is a participating provider.

SEE http://www.nubc.org/ FOR MORE INFORMATION ON UB-04 DATA ELEMENT AND PRINTING SPECIFICATIONS